Advanced Critical Care in

MEDICAL, SURGICAL AND NEONATAL NURSING

Advanced Critical Care in

MEDICAL, SURGICAL AND NEONATAL NURSING

(As per INC Syllabus)

SN Nanjunde Gowda MSc (N) DPN PhD
Professor and Principal
Anil Baghi College of Nursing
Ferozepur, Punjab, India
Formerly, Principal
Padmashree Institute of Nursing
Ikon Nursing College
Dayananda Sagar College of Nursing
Bengaluru, Karnataka, India

Jyothi Nanjunde Gowda MSc (N) DPN
Vice-Principal
Anil Baghi College of Nursing
Ferozepur, Punjab, India
Formerly, Deputy Principal
and Nursing Officer
Nizwa Hospital, Ministry of Health
Sultanate of Oman

Foreword
Nagarajaiah

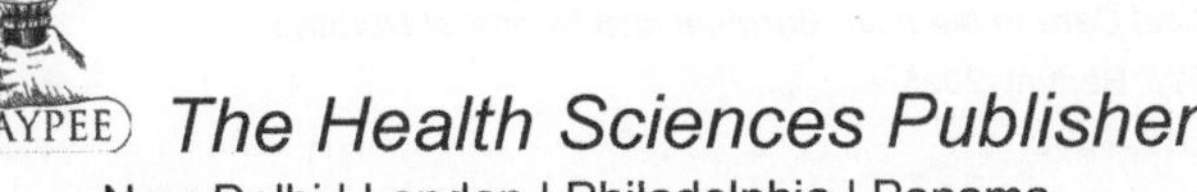

The Health Sciences Publisher
New Delhi | London | Philadelphia | Panama

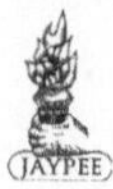

Jaypee Brothers Medical Publishers (P) Ltd

Headquarters

Jaypee Brothers Medical Publishers (P) Ltd
4838/24, Ansari Road, Daryaganj
New Delhi 110 002, India
Phone: +91-11-43574357
Fax: +91-11-43574314
Email: jaypee@jaypeebrothers.com

Overseas Offices

J.P. Medical Ltd
83 Victoria Street, London
SW1H 0HW (UK)
Phone: +44 20 3170 8910
Fax: +44(0) 20 3008 6180
Email: info@jpmedpub.com

Jaypee-Highlights Medical Publishers Inc
City of Knowledge, Bld. 235, 2nd Floor
Clayton, Panama City, Panama
Phone: +1 507-301-0496
Fax: +1 507-301-0499
Email: cservice@jphmedical.com

JP Medical Inc
325 Chestnut Street
Ste 412, Philadelphia, PA 19106, USA
Phone: +1 267-519-9789
Email: support@jpmedus.com

Jaypee Brothers Medical Publishers (P) Ltd
17/1-B Babar Road, Block-B, Shaymali
Mohammadpur, Dhaka-1207
Bangladesh
Phone: +08801912003485
Email: jaypeedhaka@gmail.com

Jaypee Brothers Medical Publishers (P) Ltd
Bhotahity, Kathmandu, Nepal
Phone: +977-9741283608
Email: kathmandu@jaypeebrothers.com

Website: www.jaypeebrothers.com
Website: www.jaypeedigital.com

Inquiries for bulk sales may be solicited at: jaypee@jaypeebrothers.com

Advanced Critical Care in Medical, Surgical and Neonatal Nursing

First Edition: 2017, Reprint: **2025**

ISBN 978-93-86150-46-2

Printed in India

Foreword

It is important for the nurse to recognize the great development in child care in the country. Such an understanding is essential not only for the nurse as a professional caregiver but also for a parent and community member, which helps in recognition and appreciation of children as unique individuals with special needs and qualities. The term holism is applicable to our perception of children. It is important to consider the child as composed of physical, intellectual, emotional and spiritual natures, and to relate the child as a whole or biopsychosocial individual. As a result of this thought, child care has been shifted from treatment of diseases to prevention of diseases and promotion of health. Nurses are no longer solely involved in the episodic care of children during an acute illness. They are increasingly responsible for providing comprehensive and distributive care that attempts to meet the needs of children and their families.

The presentation of this book, *Advanced Critical Care in Medical, Surgical and Neonatal Nursing*, is with practical procedures for Post Basic BSc Nursing, which includes modern concept of child health care, healthy child, nursing care of neonate, nursing management of common childhood diseases, and also the practicum is formulated. The content of this book will be a great resource for both nurse educators and students, in an effective manner to teach and learn better by utilizing information.

I recommend this book to be used for Post Basic BSc Nursing as well as nurse educators; should be a reference book for every student and teacher.

I congratulate the author who has brought together the most important ideas from the old and new nursing principles under one roof of advanced critical care.

Nagarajaiah
Formerly, Associate Professor
National Institute of Mental Health
and Neurosciences (NIMHANS)
Bengaluru, Karnataka, India

Preface

It gives us great pleasure and satisfaction to introduce the first edition of *Advanced Critical Care in Medical, Surgical and Neonatal Nursing* to Post Basic BSc Nursing students and teachers, and nursing community. In offering this title, we remain grateful to readers, specially nursing teachers, who supported our books such as *Foundations of Nursing, Fundamentals of Nursing for General Nursing and Midwifery, Intravenous Therapy for Nurses, Perioperative Nursing Manual, Clinical Practice Dairy, Cumulative Record of Clinical Learning Experience for Post Basic BSc Nursing* and *A to Z Guideline Manual in Nursing Performance Evaluation Tool (for Practitioners and Students)*.

One of the ways to improve quality of care could be use of new technology to manage complex health issues of children. Health promotion depends on development of new health policy and the responsibility of healthcare providers, especially nurses who involve in educating the community on lifestyle, prevention of disease and health promotion, particularly the child health.

This first edition deals with modern concept of child health care, healthy child, nursing care of neonate, nursing management of common childhood diseases and surgical aspects, including the practicum formulated. This book has been written as a basic textbook for Post Basic BSc Nursing students. We hope that the content of this textbook will help students and educators in providing guidance; as a result, future nurses achieve the goal of the profession.

Our sincere thought—if the nursing teachers, students and other healthcare personnel apply scientific principles, which are described in this book, our hard work will be recognized. We sincerely welcome constructive criticism from readers that will help us to enrich our knowledge to contribute more to the profession.

SN Nanjunde Gowda
Jyothi Nanjunde Gowda

Preface

[illegible]

[illegible]

[illegible]

[illegible]

[illegible]

Acknowledgments

The development of this book resulted from the combined effort of many talented professionals. As authors, we acknowledge their dedication, skill and professionalism. We are very proud to be associated with such fine individuals.

We are deeply indebted to Dr YG Patil and Dr Shylaja Patil, Senior Specialist, Sultanate of Oman, whose help, stimulating suggestions and encouragement helped us all the time in producing this book.

Our special thanks to the professional members who offered suggestions and supported for completion of this book.

Our warm appreciation and thanks goes to Shri Jitendar P Vij (Group Chairman), Mr Ankit Vij (Group President) and Mr Tarun Duneja (Director-Publishing) of M/s Jaypee Brothers Medical Publishers (P) Ltd, New Delhi, India, for sharing our vision for this book and giving us the chance to turn vision into reality.

I, Dr Nanjunde Gowda, express deepest gratitude toward my loving wife, daughter and son-in-law, who has been my support throughout the process.

Above all, we are thankful to Almighty God for bestowing His bountiful grace for the successful completion of this book.

Syllabus as per Indian Nursing Council (INC)

Selected Topic from BSc(N) Syllabus

Units	Topics
VI	*Nursing management of patient (adult including elderly) with genitourinary problems* • Review of anatomy and physiology of genitourinary system • Nursing assessment—history and physical assessment • Nursing management of: – Nephritic – Nephritic syndrome – Renal calculus – Tumors – Acute renal failure – Chronic renal failure – End stage renal disease – Dialysis and renal transplant
Selected Topic from MSc(N) Nephrourology Syllabus	
X	*Dialysis* • Dialysis history, types, principles • Hemodialysis, vascular access sites, temporary and permanent • Peritoneal dialysis • Dialysis procedure—steps, equipment, maintenance • Role of nurse—predialysis, intra- and post-dialysis • Complication • Counseling • Patient educations • Record and report
Selected Topic from BSc(N) Medical Surgical Nursing	
V	*Management of patient with blood and cardiovascular problems* • Coronary artery disease • Ischemic heart disease • Coronary atherosclerosis • Angina pectoris • Myocardial infarction • Congenital and acquired • Rheumatic heart disease • Cardiac emergencies
IX	*Nursing management of patient in critical care unit* • Nursing assessment—history and physical assessment • Principles of critical care nursing

Contd...

Contd...

IX	• Protocols, equipment and supplies • Special equipment, ventilators, cardiac monitors, defibrillators • Drugs used in critical care unit
Selected Topic from BSc(N) Child Health Nursing	
III	*Nursing care of neonate* • Nursing care of a normal newborn/Essential newborn care • Neonatal resuscitation • Nursing management of low-birth-weight baby • Nursing management of common neonatal disorder • Organization of neonatal unit • Identification of nursing management of common congenital malformation
IV	• Integrated management of neonatal childhood illness
V	*Nursing management in common childhood disease* • Respiratory disorders and infection • Cardiovascular problem, congenital defect and rheumatic fever
Selected Topic from PB BSc(N) Child Health Nursing	
Units	*Nursing care of neonate* • Nursing care of a normal newborn/Essential newborn care • Neonatal resuscitation • Nursing management of low-birth-weight baby • Kangaroo mother care • Nursing management of common neonatal disorders • Organization of neonatal unit
Selected Topic from GNM Medical Surgical Nursing—Practical	
Units ICU	• Connect and monitor ECG and pulse oximetry • Assist in endotracheal intubation and suctioning; provide care for a patient on ventilator • Handling emergency drug/Trolley/Crash cart • Assisting in insertion of central line and monitoring central venous pressure
Cardiology ward/ICCU/ Cardiothoracic and velcro	• Perform cardiac vascular assessment recording ECG and identify basic changes in ECG • Monitoring of patient on cardiac monitor • Preparing and assisting frequently performed diagnostic, therapeutic, noninvasive and invasive procedures • Administer cardiac drug • Advance/Basic cardiac life support (ACLS/BCLS) • Monitoring and caring for patient with chest drainage • Assist in defibrillation • Monitoring patient in ICU • Maintain flow sheet • Perform endotracheal suction • Demonstrate use of ventilator

Contd...

Contd...

	• Physical examination • Collect specimen and interpret ABG analysis • Assist with arterial puncture • Maintain CVP Line • Bag-mask ventilation • Administration of drug

Contents

Section 1: Management of Shock/Unconsciousness

1. Introduction **3**

Advanced Critical Care Nursing 3
Organization of Critical Care Area 4
Prehospital Care in Critically Ill Patient 6
Admission Criteria in Critical Care Area 10

2. Management of Client with Shock **12**

Classification of Shock 12
Stages of Shock 14
Risk Factors 14
Clinical Manifestations 14
Diagnostic Assessment 15
Management 15

3. Therapeutic Management of Cardiovascular System **20**

Nursing Assessment of Cardiac System 20
Coronary Artery Disease 24
Angina Pectoris 25
Acute Myocardial Infarction (Acute Coronary Syndrome) 27
Management of Patients with Cardiac Monitor 31
Cardiac Arrhythmias 37
Defibrillation 41
Nursing Care of the Patient with Central
Venous Pressure 45
Hemodynamic Monitoring 54

4. Nursing Management of Unconscious Patient **60**

Consciousness 60
Unconsciousness 60

5. Preparation of Drug Infusion **69**

Preparation 69
Emergency/Crash Trolley and Drug Tray 69
Drug Infusion Guidelines 70
Replacement of Potassium 79

6. Therapeutic Management of Respiratory System **80**

Acute Respiratory Distress Syndrome 80
Pulmonary Embolism 81
Pleurisy 84
Pleural Effusion 84
Emphysema 85
Oxygen Administration 85

Nursing Assessment of Respiratory System 93
Diagnostic Tests 96
Arterial Blood Gas Analysis 97
Pulmonary Function Test 100
Chest Drainage 101
Deep Vein Thrombosis and Thromboembolism Prophylaxis 104
Pneumothorax 105
Hemothorax 107
Tracheostomy 108
Endotracheal Intubation 109

7. Managing Diabetic Emergencies **118**
Hypoglycemia 118
Diabetic Ketoacidosis (in Adult) 119
Non-ketotic Hyperosmolar Hyperglycemic Coma 121
Lactic Acidosis 121
Chronic Complications of Diabetes Mellitus 122
Management of Patient with Burns 126

8. Mechanical Ventilation **132**
Terminology 132
Mechanical Ventilator 132
Method of Mechanical Ventilation 132
Indications 133
Criteria/Preparations for Using Ventilator 133
Classification 134
Modes of Ventilation 135
Setting of Mechanical Ventilation/Monitoring and Nursing Management 136
Weaning from Mechanical Ventilator 137
Ventilator Checklist 138
Nutritional Support of Patient on Ventilator 139
Cleaning and Asepsis of Ventilator 140
Change of Breathing Circuit of Ventilators 140
Change of Condenser Humidifier of Ventilator 140
Nursing Intervention for Patient on Mechanical Ventilation 141

9. Immediate Postoperative Care in Recovery Room or Postanesthesia Care Unit **143**
Competency for PACU Nurses 143
Admission to Postanesthesia Care Unit 143
Postoperative Report and General Nursing Care for all Patients in Recovery Room 144
Postoperative Nursing 147
Discharge Criteria from Critical Care Area 154
Infection Control Procedure in Intensive Care Unit 155
Visitor Policy in Critical Care Area 156
Change of Patients' Position in Bed 157

Section 2: Critical Care in Nephrology/Urology

10. Genitourinary Disorders and Nursing Management **161**

Structure of the Kidney 161
Main Functions of the Kidneys 162
Renal System: Essential Concepts 162
Assessment and Diagnostic Measures 164
Urinary Tract Infection 168
Nephrotic Syndrome 172
Acute Poststreptococcal Glomerulonephritis 173
Wilms' Tumor 174

11. Urological Disorders and Nursing Management **176**

Urinary Tract Infection 176
Nephrotic Syndrome 180
Acute Poststreptococcal Glomerulonephritis 183
Cryptorchidism (Undescended Testicle) 185
Hypospadias 187
Renal Calculus 188
Renal Failure 190

12. Dialysis **195**

Principles of Dialysis 195
Indication for Dialysis 196
Vascular Access 196
Predialysis Assessment of Hemodialysis Patient 197
Priming of Hemodialysis Bloodlines and Dialyzer 199
Hemodialysis 202
Connecting a Patient with Arteriovenous Fistula to Hemodialysis Machine 204
Disconnecting a Patient with Arteriovenous Fistula from Hemodialysis Machine 208
Postdialysis Assessment of Hemodialysis Patient 213
Continuous Ambulatory Peritoneal Dialysis with Temporary Access to Hemodialysis Machine 215
Disconnecting a Patient with Temporary Access from Hemodialysis Machine 217
Preoperative and Postoperative Care of Arteriovenous Fistula 224
Management of Hypotension During Hemodialysis 227
Prevention and Management of Air Embolism 227
Hemodialysis Hazards 230
Disinfection, Cleaning, Decalcification and Maintenance of Hemodialysis Machine 235
Blood Transfusion During Hemodialysis 237
Hemodialysis Shunt Graft and Fistula Care 240

13. Peritoneal Dialysis **243**
Continuous Ambulatory Peritoneal Dialysis 243
Plasmapheresis 260
Preoperative Preparation of Patient for Insertion of Tenckhoff Catheter 263
Postoperative Care of Patient with Tenckhoff Catheter 264
Continuous Venous Hemofiltration with Hemodialysis 266

14. Stress and Adaptation **268**
Concept of Stress 268
Manifestation of Stress 269
Nursing Management of Stress 271

15. Defense Against Injury **275**
Physical Barriers and the Immune System 275

16. Fluid, Electrolyte and Acid-Base Balance **278**
Body Fluid Distribution 278
Fluid Imbalance: Dehydration 282
Electrolyte Imbalance 285
Nursing Process: Fluid and Electrolyte Imbalance 290

17. Management of Patients in Pain **295**
Components of Pain 295
Types of Pain 295
Clinical Manifestation of Pain 296
Factors that Influence Responses to Pain 297
Guidelines for Assessment of the Patient in Pain 297
Nursing Diagnosis 298

Section 3: Critical Care for Neonates and Children

18. Neonatal Critical Care **305**
Terminologies 303
Organization of Neonatal Unit 303
Health Education 304
Breastfeeding 304
Provision of Infection Control 305
Aim and Objectives 305
Admission to Neonatal Care Unit 305
Child Morbidity and Mortality 306
Changing Trends in Hospital Care: Preventive, Promotive and Curative Aspects of Child Health 308
Child Health Assessment 310
Reflexes in the Neonate 315

19. High-risk Neonate **316**
Hyaline Membrane Disease 316
Transient Tachypnea of the Newborn 316
Meconium Aspiration Syndrome 317

Sepsis 317
Hyperbilirubinemia 318
Isoimmune Hemolytic Disease of the Neonate 319
Sexually Transmitted Disease 320
Hydrocephaly 321
Phenylketonuria 321
Torch Syndrome 322
Prematurity 323
Postmaturity 324

20. Nursing Care of Newborn **325**
Preparing for Birth 325
Admission Routine 325
Observations 325
Care 326

21. Examination of the Newborn by the Pediatrician **331**
History 331
Formal Examination 331
Observation 333

22. Common Parental Questions/Concerns and its Answers **334**
Fontanel 334
Breasts 334
Bumps and Bruises 334
Birthmarks and Spots 334
Jaundice 334
Cradle Cap 335
Eczema 335
Bonding and Breastfeeding 335
Bathing a Baby 338

23. Neonatal Resuscitation **340**
Immediate Newborn Conditions or Problems 340
Management 340
Resuscitation 341
Technique of Artificial Ventilation 345
Emergency Drugs 347

24. Nursing Care in Different Conditions **349**
Care of the Newborn Infant from HIV- or HBsAg-positive Mother 349
Hypoglycemia in Newborn 351
Convulsion in the Newborn 352
Jaundice in the Newborn 354
Nursing Management of a Low-birth-weight Baby 356
Care of Baby in Incubator 358
Respiratory System 359
Assist in Exchange Transfusion 373

Guide to Some of the Conditions, Which may be Recognized 377
Relief of Choking in Infants 380

25. Genetic Influences in Child Health **383**
Genetics 383
Genes and Chromosomes 383
Karyotype 383
Cell Division and Reproduction 384
Behavioral Genetics 384
Genetic Abnormalities 385
Prenatal Diagnosis 387
Postnatal Diagnosis 387
Therapeutic Management of Genetic Disease 387

26. Principles of Preoperative Care of Infants and Children **390**
Preoperative Nursing Management 390
Differences between Children and Adults 393

27. Congenital Heart Disease **395**
Acyanotic Heart Defects 395
Congestive Heart Failure 400
Rheumatic Fever 403

28. Child with Special Needs **406**
Overview 406
Trends in Health Care 406
Mental Retardation 407
Parents of a Child with Special Needs 410
Behavioral Disorders in Children 414
Socialization of Children 414
Destructive Behaviors Disorders 415
Anxiety Disorders 417
Bed Wetting 418
Anorexia Nervosa 419
Physically Challenged Children 420
Fractures (Orthopedics Disorders) 421
Cancer in Children (Essential Concepts) 424
Leukemia 430
Psychosocial Care 432
Lymphomas 433

29. Pediatric Emergencies **439**
Congenital Heart Disease 439
Pediatric Asthma 439
Croup 440
Intestinal Obstruction 441
Poisoning 442
Burns 444

Appendices ***451***

Appendix I: Emergency Drugs Required During Resuscitation 451
Appendix II: Advantages of Breastfeeding vs Formula 453
Appendix III: Composition of Breast Milk 454
Appendix IV: Process of Breastfeeding 456
Appendix V: Common Problems Encountered During Breastfeeding and its Solutions 458
Appendix VI: Breastfeeding Policy 460
Appendix VII: Important Milestones 461
Appendix VIII: Problems of Immediate Newborn 467
Appendix IX: Signs and Symptoms in Abnormal Newborn 468
Appendix X: Developmental Examination 469

Index ***471***

Section 1

Management of Shock/Unconsciousness

Chapter 1 Introduction

ADVANCED CRITICAL CARE NURSING

Critically ill care and nursing has evolved over the last couple of decades into full pledge specialty. Critical care nursing requires not only knowledge and understanding of the human physiology, but also special procedure skills and wisdom to handle technology, knowledge and medical advances judiciously. The practice of critical care nursing is essentially team work and training, involves the health restoration functions for the individual patients and handling of the families and clients response to their illness in their hours of utmost need.

Critical Care Team

The critical care team includes a diverse group of highly trained professionals, who provide care in a specialized area known intensive care unit (ICU). This team works toward the best outcome possible for seriously ill patients. All members of the team may be asked to teach patients and their families various strategies to improve health, healing, coping and well-being, specific to their area of expertise. Members of the team include:

- Physician
- Surgeon
- Specialist from internal medicine
- Pediatrician
- Anesthetist.

Critical Care Nurses

Critical care nurses provide a high level of skilled nursing for total patient care and often facilitate communication among all of the people involved in the care of patient. Their expertise and continuous presence allows early recognition of subtle, but significant changes in patient conditions, thereby preventing worsening conditions and minimizing complications that arise from critical illness or injury. Because of their close contact with the family and patient, critical care nurses often serve as the patient's advocate and become integral to the decision-making process of the patient, family and critical care team. Additionally, some critical care nurses are recognized as a critical care registered nurse (CCRN) (with special training). They have received more specialized education, training and testing and are certified by the authorized authority.

Intensivists

Intensivists may be assigned to the ICU on a full-time basis and work with other critical care team members to provide their patients with ongoing and consistent care. It may also coordinate the administrative environment of the ICU by setting policies, developing protocols and facilitating communication among primary care physicians, specialists, patients and their families.

Dietitian

Dietitian is a vital part of the medical team that consults with physicians, nurses, therapists and family members in the ICU. The registered dietitian works to improve the nutritional health and promotes recovery of the critically ill or injured patient.

Social Worker

A social worker is a licensed professional that works with the ICU interdisciplinary team to provide a link between treatment plans for the critically ill or injured patient and family members. Special knowledge that is acquired through formal—professional and social work education, welfare policies and services, and social welfare systems and community resources guide the practice of social work.

Respiratory Therapist

Respiratory therapists work with the critical care team to monitor and assists with airway management of the critically ill patient. This may include oxygen therapy, mechanical ventilation management (breathing machine), aerosol medication therapy, cardiorespiratory monitoring, patient and caregiver education.

Physical Therapist or Occupational Therapist

The physical therapist provides services that restore function, improve mobility, relieve pain and prevent or limit permanent physical disabilities. The occupational therapist is trained to make a complete evaluation of the impact of disease on the activities of critically ill patient.

ORGANIZATION OF CRITICAL CARE AREA

There are varieties of environment factors that affect patient on ICU or critical care area. They all interact with each other and can have significant effects on the health, well-being and outcome of critically ill patient. A lot of time, effort and money are invested in the technologies advances of critical care unit and also involvement of dedicated sympathetic multidisciplinary team.

Intensive care unit was developed as a consequence of the poliomyelitis epidemics of the 1950s, when extensive use of ventilation was required, since then the technology available to support the critically ill patient, has become more sophisticated and complex. Critical care unit consist of the following area:

- Patient care area
- Clinical support area consists of patient room and adjacent area
- Unit support area, refer to areas of the unit where administrative, material management and staff function occurs
- Family support area refer to area designed to support families and visitors
- Design for an optimal functioning unit will consider the requirements of daily workflow.

Requirement of Critical Care Area

1. Unit design begins with an in-depth analysis of patient care and support functions. An inventory of equipment and supply, both current and future, will help to determine space requirement. The design should reduce travel distance to staff, placing frequently needed space, equipment or material as close as possible to site of use.
2. Care giver must be able to observe patient from many point within the unit.
3. Many experts proposed units or patient room ranging from minimum of 6 beds to maximum of 8–12 beds, patient care area, single or multibed room and clear floor area, door and windows.
4. Pleasant surrounding for patient, ward should include secure storage of patient and family clothing.
5. The efficient unit is small enough for care providers to be fully aware of all activities on the unit.
6. Electrical outlet need to be accessible from each side of the patient bed and arranged to provide enough room for multiple simultaneous procedures.
7. The oxygen system must also be easy to access during intubation or extubation procedure.
8. Each patient room may be equipped with television and educational entertainment system should be available.
9. Medical gas vacuum.
10. Supplies, in room storage and handling of patient care supplies must minimize on hand inventory and waste, while economizing efforts of bedside staff.
11. Infection control is an important consideration and storage for clean and soiled items must prevent cross-contamination by visitors and staff.
12. Specify the area location availability and usage for hand hygiene, toilets facilities and fluid disposal.
13. For sharp object, container should be provided.

14. Emergency eyewash area will be used to address the issues.
15. Nursing work station, clearly organized workplace for unit staff and patient care to improve communication. This area should include dedicated computer, telephone, paper, forms fax machine and digital technology within easy reach of staff.
16. Preparing and dispensing patient medication: -
    - Medication delivery system may be automated
    - Medication should be easily accessible in life-threatening situation
    - Medication room should provide adequate space for medication storage.
17. Storage location for electrical devices should provide adequate electrical outlet for charging.
18. Hazardous waste, storage space for hazardous materials such as red bags and prompt removal of these materials should be planned.
19. Emergency equipment and supplies and should be a sufficient space for storing emergency equipment, e.g. crash trolley life-support equipment.
20. Within concurrence of the consultant microbiologist, infection control nurse and infection control team. Infection control precaution procedure should be agreed and enforced regarding:
    - Antibiotic policy
    - Clothing of staff and visitors
    - Aseptic precaution for invasive procedure
    - Use of disposable
    - Filtering of patient respired air
    - Changes of patient catheter, humidifier, ventilator and equipment
    - Cleaning of the unit
    - Isolation precaution.
21. The limitation in communication, eating and movement all add to the stress experienced by the critical care patient.
22. Patient has to rely on nurses to perform personnel hygiene, feeding and changing position in the bed, drug and equipment; patient should not feel they are not able to maintain privacy.

PREHOSPITAL CARE IN CRITICALLY ILL PATIENT

Ill Patient

Recognition that time is critical factor in determining whether an individual can survive trauma is old one. Baron Larry developed a system to expeditiously remove the wounded in Napoleon's armies from the war field more than 200 years ago. The concept used today in prehospital care is exactly the same as Larry's.

In 1962, physician Deck Farrington JD (father of modern emergency medicine services) and Sam Banks instituted the first trauma course for ambulance. The course was started with Chicago Committee on trauma in Chicago Fire Academy with it. Farrington initiated the concept, now known as prehospital care and a true ambulance service.

Aim

The aims of prehospital care in critically ill patients include:

- Rapid assessment
- Appropriate airway management
- Field control of hemorrhage
- Stabilization of fractures and initiation of volume replacement enroute to hospital standard that the field time should be no longer than 10 minutes
- Ambulance and the personal trained to provide initial resuscitation and triage are the elements of prehospital care.

Adams Cowley's statement is, you think people die from heart attacks or accidents, but they really do not directly. Those things produce shock, which is sluggish or non-existent circulation and that is what kills you. If you stay in shock for very long, you are dead. Maybe you will die in 10 minutes or maybe you will die next week, but you are dead, so if you are in shock, we have to work fast. You have at most 60 minutes. If I can get to you and stop your bleeding and restore your blood pressure, within an hour of your accident then I can probably save you. I call that the golden hour.

Phases of Prehospital Care

- Development updating and approval of treatment protocols
- Initial training and education of relevant personal
- Purchasing, repairing and equipping of vehicles
- Staffing of units, resupply of units.

Immediate Phase

- Emergency medical service (EMS) access system
- Observation of situation by emergency medical technician (EMT)
- Assessment of patients and starting of treatment and physician at the hospital is notified of the situation, the number of patients their condition and the treatment that has been initiated.

Retrospective Phase

The retrospective component involves the development of continuing education program to bring new information to attention of the system's EMT. Continuing education in trauma care should include prehospital trauma life support of basic trauma life.

Features of Prehospital Care

- Extrication of causality and protection of cervical spine
- Airway control
- Control of hemorrhage
- Venous access and intravenous (IV) fluids.

Treatment of Prehospital Care

- Cardiac arrest
- Cardiac tamponade
- Tension pneumothorax
- Evisceration of viscera
- Splinting of fracture.

Administration of Drugs

- Analgesics
- Antibiotics
- Tetanus prophylaxis.

All the features enumerated above firms, which is termed as advanced life support (ALS), when airway is supported by endotracheal intubation, circulation is supported by venous access and IV fluid administration.

Prehospital Care Protocols

Extrication Casualties and Protection of Spine

Extrication problems are acute in railway accident, house collapse and air disaster, although it does not pose much problem in road traffic accident. Cervical spine should be protected with rigid collar and patient is extricated and loaded on the stretcher in a single piece.

Airway

With airway begins the ABC of resuscitation, i.e. airway, breathing, circulation. Airway must be cleared of blood, mucus, vomit, foreign body or dentures. Tongue is pulled out and jaw braced forward and oropharyngeal airway placed in situ. In unconscious patient, endotracheal tube may be inserted to obtain positive airway control. In desperate condition, a 16 gauze needle pushed in cricothyroid space and connected to oxygen at the rate of 10–12 L/min.

Breathing

Once the airway is cleared, the patient's respiratory effort is observed. Any sucking chest wound is closed by applying adhesive dressing and closing on three sides with adhesive plaster. In suspicion of tension pneumothorax

16 gauze needle with a finger stall at the other end with a small hole is pushed into second intercostal space. Patient with chest trauma if not contraindicated due to other injuries should travel propped up.

Circulation

Most trauma patients have bleeding either external or internal. Pressure dressing is adequate for external bleeding, in case external bleeding not assessed by pressure dressing, pneumatic tourniquet should be used which can released intermittently.

Administration of Intravenous Fluid

In case of cardiac arrest:

- Immediate establishment of airway, KVO is keep vein open
- Ventilation with 100% oxygen
- If feasible with an endotracheal tube
- Initiation of external cardiac massage.

Cardiac tamponade is difficult to diagnose in field settings pericardiocentesis not feasible. Intravenous fluid loading and inotropic agents can tie over.

Immobilization

- Splinting of fractured limbs
- Patients must be strapped well on stretcher without pillow in supine position, if spinal injury is suspected.

Eviscerated of Viscera

Eviscerated of viscera not only give a ghostly look but also increase the shock, bleeding and subsequent infection. Clean sterile towel is enough to cover these and bandage loosely strapped and no attempt made to push intensive to avoid strangulation and twisting.

Prehospital Transport

The aim of transport is to decrease the time lag between the accident and definitive care. Prehospital transport systems are:

- Ground ambulance
- ALS ambulance
- Air ambulance.

Status of Prehospital Care in India

Prehospital care is still in its infancy in India as compared to Europe and western countries. A large number of rural road accidents occur due to nonavailability of immediate care and delay in transport for definitive care to hospitals.

Centralized Accident and Trauma Services (CATS) was started in Delhi on 15th March, 1991 with 27 ambulances. This is connected with wireless services at various points and manned with two paramedics and equipped with basic first aid and cardiopulmonary resuscitation (CPR) measures. But a very few people know the access number of CATS (1099). In Karnataka, State Highway accident service was started, service provided by Government of Karnataka. So, there is need for an area-based planning to provide early care and there is immediate need for training program in the area of first aid services and integrated trauma care.

ADMISSION CRITERIA IN CRITICAL CARE AREA

Diagnosis Model

1. **Cardiac system:** Acute myocardial infarction with complications:
   - Cardiogenic shock
   - Complex arrhythmias requiring close monitoring and intervention
   - Acute congestive heart failure with respiratory failure and/or requiring hemodynamic support
   - Hypertensive emergencies
   - Unstable angina, particularly with dysrhythmias, hemodynamic instability or persistent chest pain
   - Sudden cardiac arrest
   - Cardiac tamponade
   - Dissecting aortic aneurysms
   - Complete heart block.
2. **Pulmonary system:**
   - Acute respiratory failure requiring ventilatory support
   - Pulmonary emboli with hemodynamic instability
   - Patients in an intermediate care unit, who are demonstrating respiratory deterioration
   - Need for nursing/respiratory care not available in lesser care areas such as floor or intermediate care unit
   - Massive hemoptysis
   - Respiratory failure with imminent intubation.
3. **Neurological disorders:**
   - Acute stroke with altered mental status
   - Coma, metabolic toxic or anoxic
   - Intracranial hemorrhage with potential for herniation
   - Acute subarachnoid hemorrhage
   - Meningitis with altered mental status or respiratory compromise
   - Central nervous system or neuromuscular disorders with deteriorating neurological or pulmonary functions

- Status epilepticus
- Brain dead or potentially brain dead patients, who are being aggressively managed, while determining organ donation status
- Severe head injured patients.

4. **Drug ingestion and drug overdose:**
   - Hemodynamically unstable drug ingestion
   - Drug ingestion with significantly altered mental status with inadequate airway protection
   - Seizures following drug ingestion.
5. **Gastrointestinal disorders:**
   - Life-threatening gastrointestinal bleeding including hypotension, angina, continued bleeding or with comorbid conditions
   - Fulminant hepatic failure
   - Severe pancreatitis
   - Esophageal perforation with or without mediastinitis.
6. **Endocrine:**
   - Diabetic ketoacidosis complicated by hemodynamic instability, altered mental status, respiratory insufficiency or severe acidosis
   - Thyroid storm or myxedema coma with hemodynamic instability
   - Hyperosmolar state with coma and/or hemodynamic instability
   - Other endocrine problems, i.e. adrenal crises.
7. **Hemodynamic instability:**
   - Severe hypercalcemia with altered mental status, requiring hemodynamic monitoring
   - Hypermagnesemia or hypomagnesemia with hemodynamic compromise or dysrhythmias
   - Hypokalemia or hyperkalemia with dysrhythmias or muscular weakness
   - Hypophosphatemia with muscular weakness
   - Hyponatremia or hypernatremia with seizures, altered mental status.
8. **Surgical:** Postoperative patients requiring hemodynamic monitoring/ ventilatory support or extensive nursing care.
9. **Miscellaneous:**
   - Septic shock with hemodynamic instability
   - Hemodynamic monitoring
   - Clinical conditions requiring ICU level nursing care
   - Environmental injuries (lightning, near drowning and hyporthermia/ hyperthermia)
   - New/Experimental therapies with potential for complications
   - Any patient at risk for a precipitous, life-threatening event.

Chapter 2 Management of Client with Shock

Shock is a complex clinical syndrome that may occur at any time and in any place. It is a life-threatening condition often requiring team action by many healthcare providers, including nurses, physicians, laboratory, technician, pharmacists and respiratory therapists.

DEFINITION

Shock is defined as failure of the circulatory system to maintain adequate perfusion of vital organs, leading to inadequate tissue perfusion results in decreased oxygenation at the cellular level. This inadequate oxygenation results in anaerobic cellular metabolism. If not treated, cell death and organ death occurs.

CLASSIFICATION OF SHOCK

Hypovolemic Shock

Hypovolemic shock is due to inadequate circulating blood volume resulting from hemorrhage with actual blood loss. Burns with a loss of plasma, proteins and fluid shifts or dehydration with a loss of fluid volume, it is the most common type of shock.

Etiology

Hemorrhage: Clinical manifestations indicative of hypovolemic shock may begin to appear a blood volume deficit of 15–25% or about 500–1,500 mL in an adult with a normal circulating volume.

Burns: Hypovolemic shock produced by burns, occur most often in persons with large partial-thickness or full-thickness burns. There is a shift of plasma from the vascular space into interstitial space. The client may have cardiac dysfunction due to presence of myocardial depressant factor.

Dehydration: Shock occurs from either reduced oral fluid intake or significant losses of fluid. For example, excessive urine output, prolonged vomiting or diarrhea, exercise causing fluid loss from sweating and hot environment.

Cardiogenic Shock

Cardiogenic shock is due to inadequate pumping action of the heart because of primary cardiac muscle dysfunction or mechanical obstruction of blood flow caused by myocardial infraction (MI), valvular insufficiency due to disease or trauma, cardiac dysrhythmias or an obstructive condition, such as pericardial tamponade or pulmonary embolism (PE). Cardiogenic shock occurs in 15–20% of all the clients following MI and has at least 80% mortality rate. Cardiogenic shock after an MI, usually occurs when 40% or more of the myocardium has been damaged.

Etiology

Cardiogenic shock results primarily from an inability of heart muscle to function adequately or mechanical obstruction of blood flow to or from the heart.

Myocardial infarction: Impaired heart muscle action is most often caused by MI. The area of dead or dying tissue that occurs with infarction impairs contractility of the myocardium and the cardiac output decreases. It may occur in blunt cardiac trauma, cardiomyopathy and congestive heart failure.

Obstructive conditions: Mechanical obstruction to blood flow causing cardiogenic shock includes a large PE, pericardial tamponade and tension pneumothorax.

Pericardial tamponade: It is an accumulation of blood or fluid in the pericardial space.

Tension pneumothorax: It is the significant amount of air in the pleural space.

Other causes: Cardiac valvular insufficiency from trauma or disease, myocardial aneurysms (previous MI), rupture of a ventricle, aortic stenosis and mitral regurgitation.

Obstructive Shock

In obstructive category, shock develops in conditions that lead to sudden obstruction of blood flow. These problems include cardiac tamponade, tension pneumothorax and PE.

Distributive Shock

Distributive shock is due to changes in blood vessel tone that increase the size of the vascular space without an increase in circulating blood volume.

Acute Allergic Reaction (Anaphylactic Shock)

Anaphylactic shock occurs as a result of an acute allergic reaction from exposure to a substance to which the client has been sensitized. Common sensitizing agents are penicillin and its derivatives, bee stings, chocolate, strawberries, peanuts, snake-venom, iodine-based contrast for X-ray and non-steroidal anti-inflammatory drugs (NSAIDs).

Spinal Cord Injury (Neurogenic Shock)

Neurogenic shock occurs from sever central nervous system (CNS) damage. As it results in low blood pressure (BP), occasionally with a slowed heart rate, i.e. attributed to the disruption of the autonomic pathways within the spinal cord.

Infection (Septic Shock)

Sepsis shock is the systemic response to infection. The process begins with the growth of various microorganisms at the site of infection.

STAGES OF SHOCK

Based on Progression

Non-progressive Stage

Body's compensatory mechanisms can maintain BP within a normal to below normal range.

Progressive Stage

Body begins to decompensate, systemic circulation no longer works, results in decreased circulation.

Irreversible Stage

The shock state becomes progressively more severe.

Based on Compensation

- Early compensation stage
- Decompensation stage.

RISK FACTORS

- Trauma
- Heart muscle injury
- Allergen
- Impaired skin category
- Invasive procedures
- Exposure to pathogens.

CLINICAL MANIFESTATIONS

- Restlessness and anxiety
- Decreased level of consciousness
- Irritability, dry mouth and thirsty
- Cyanosis, cold and clammy skin
- Nausea and vomiting
- Rapid thready pulse, slow capillary refilling and collapse
- Diaphoresis
- Tachycardia

- Hypotension
- Oliguria
- Decreased oxygen saturation
- Decreased systolic BP more than 20 mm Hg with heart rate increased more than 20 beats per minute.

DIAGNOSTIC ASSESSMENT

- The 12-lead electrocardiogram (ECG)
- Complete blood count (CBC)
- Arterial blood gases (ABGs) analysis
- Pulse oximetry
- Spirometry
- Central venous pressure (CVP) measurement
- Pulmonary artery or Swan-Ganz catheter measurement.

MANAGEMENT

Medical Management (Emergency Care)

As prescribed by the concerned physician, which may include as per type of shock:

- Stop external bleeding, transfuse with fresh whole blood/packed cells, fresh frozen plasma
- Start intravenous (IV) fluids, various fluids are given to correct specific problems
- Dopamine/Dobutamine infusions
- Begin to compensate for acid-base imbalance. Positive-end expiratory pressure may be added when the client is being mechanically ventilated
- Elevate the leg side of the bed (in modified Trendelenburg position), in lower extremities are elevated 30°–45°.

Drug Choice

1. If one sure that it is septic shock, then use norepinephrine.
2. If it is anesthesia related or spinal shock, then use phenylephrine.
3. If it is cardiogenic shock, then use dobutamine and norepinephrine.
4. If it is anaphylactic shock, then use epinephrine.
5. If the patient is with bradycardia and hypotensive, then use epinephrine.
6. If one do not know what is causing the shock, then use epinephrine or dopamine.
7. Maintain adequate perfusion.

Vasoconstriction

Vasoconstriction elevates the BP by constricting peripheral arterioles.

Vasodilators

Vasodilators may be helpful during shock, when vasoconstriction is severe and persists even though fluids have been infused in adequate amounts for fluid replacement.

Improving Oxygenation

Supplemental oxygen is administered to protect against hypoxemia. Endotracheal tube or tracheostomy may be performed to rest an exhausted client during severe or prolonged shock and to correct respiratory failure (if the client not ventilated).

Assisting Circulation

Mechanical devices that assist circulation or decrease the heart workload, may be used as temporary measures. For example, medical antishock trousers (MAST) and intra-aortic balloon pump.

Providing Autotransfusion

It involves collecting and retransfusing blood into the same client. It is used in prevention or treatment of existing hypovolemic shock caused by hemorrhage. It is common in the treatment of chest injuries.

Evaluating Fluid Replacement

It can be evaluated by CVP monitoring. If CVP is low, i.e. below 4 cm H_2O/2 mm Hg, continue infusion of fluids or blood. When CVP is higher than normal, i.e. above 15 cm H_2O/mm Hg, benefit cannot be expected from the continued infusion of fluids or blood beyond maintenance amounts.

Monitoring Urinary Output

Impaired kidney function may result from inadequate renal tissue perfusion. In any attempt to prevent acute renal damage, the urinary output is monitored with an indwelling catheter and diuretics (e.g. furosemide) may be given. If tubular necrosis is present peritoneal dialysis/hemodialysis may be needed until regeneration of functioning renal tubular epithelium occurs.

Preventing Gastrointestinal Bleeding

An early physiological response to shock is a decrease in splanchnic circulation. This reduces the blood supply to the stomach and bowel, causing inadequate gastrointestinal tissue perfusion and delayed gastric emptying;

thus vomiting with aspiration of gastric contents into the lungs may occur. For this reason and for diagnostic purposes, nasogastric suction is often used during treatment of shock.

Non-invasive Techniques

Non-invasive techniques can be performed rapidly and relatively easily. They require little equipment and are readily observable. The first step in assessing a person in shock is a general overview, giving attention to the airway, breathing and circulation (ABC). Once the airway is patent, air exchange is adequate, a pulse is present and the cervical spine is immobilized, perform a rapid, initial head-to-toe physical assessment. The goal is to identify major problems and gross abnormalities. The following observations should be made:

1. **Airway patency:** Noisy respirations and obstructions.
2. **Breathing:** Respiration rate and efforts.
3. **Respiratory pattern:** Chest wall expansion, chest wall bulges or deflates.
4. **Circulation:** Pulse, BP, skin color and temperatures.
5. **Level of consciousness:** Orientation to place, time and person; ability to move extremities; sensation in all extremities; pupils, size and reaction to light.
6. Monitor hydration and perfusion of the skin.
7. Monitor circumference of abdomen and extremities, and peripheral pulses.
8. Presence of lacerations, contusion and bone deformities.
9. Palpation of radial and brachial pulses.
10. Doppler instrument usage.
11. **Temperature monitoring (core temperature):** An indwelling flexible rectal probe connected to a continuous display monitor is more accurate and less traumatic than intermittent rectal temperature measurements. Core temperature can also be obtained if the client has a thermodilution (Swan-Ganz) catheter in place.
12. **Cardiac monitoring:** For assessment and evaluation purposes, the electrical activity of the heart needs to be continuously monitored in all clients in shock, regardless of age. Frequent ECGs are must.

Invasive Techniques

Hemodynamic monitoring

Measurement of CVP: It is one of the hemodynamic technique that may be used in initial shock management, especially with hypovolemic shock. The CVP measurements are used to determine the amount of fluid needed to fill the enlarging vascular space. The rate of fluid replacement is adjusted to maintain the desired CVP. It is serious if the CVP continues to fall, in spite of fluid replacement.

Peripheral arterial catheters: There are used to measure arterial BP and to obtain blood samples for chemical and blood gas analysis.

Swan-Ganz catheter: By the use of this catheter pulmonary artery and pulmonary capillary wedge pressure (PCWP) measurements are monitored to assess left-sided heart function and to guide fluid administration. If PCWP rises with cardiogenic shock, it may indicate left-sided heart failure. A low value may indicate that volume replacement is needed.

Mixed venous oxygen saturation monitoring (SvO_2): Depending on the type of Swan-Ganz catheter used, additional measurements may be obtained. Some catheters have a fiberoptic tip that allows measurement of oxygen saturation of hemoglobin in the venous blood. The normal range is 60–80%. When it falls below 60%, it has either decreased arterial oxygenation or increased tissue oxygenation demand; if it is more than 80%, the indication in relation to shock is that oxygen is unable to either reach the issue or to be extracted by the tissues.

Monitoring cardiac output: This may be used to determine cardiac output by a thermodilution technique. A fourth lumen opens at the level of the right atrium and CVP measurements (preload) can be obtained for this lumen. Cardiac output is measured in liter per minute and is the amount of blood pumped by the left ventricle in the aorta, each minute. During shock, cardiac output may be decreased because of myocardial damage resulting from an MI or in hypovolemic shock from inadequate volume replacement. This measurement assesses the overall cardiac function and the function of the left ventricles. Most Swan-Ganz catheter have a thermistor bead just proximal to the balloon.

Monitoring urine output: An indwelling catheter is a simple means of monitoring a client during shock. It is important to know about peripheral blood flow and kidney function. Minimal 30 mL/or less than 40 mL in 8 hours or absence urinary output indicates treatment is not successful.

Monitoring BP: When client is in shock, it is difficult to auscultate with a standard stethoscope. To obtain BP measurement, palpate the radial or brachial pulse during deflation of the BP cuff and use of Doppler instrument.

Monitor level of consciousness: Using Glasgow coma scale; using person, place and time; sensation in all extremities.

Nursing Management

1. Initiate a flow sheet containing all pertinent data in an easily read format. This flow sheet must accompany the client at all times.
2. At the bedside, immediate laboratory assessments are essential in treating shock.
3. Blood chemistries, blood gases, oxygen saturation and electrolytes need to be determined frequently and reported promptly, so therapy can be adjusted to the clients with rapidly changing physiological status.

4. Do not administer narcotics to a client suffering from acute, multiple traumas without first knowing if the blood volume is adequate. Narcotic administration causes vasodilation, which results in severe hypotension or shock. When narcotics are appropriate for a client in shock, they are most effective if administered IV in small doses.
5. Restlessness is a common assessment finding, especially in trauma victims and is frequently due to hypoxia.
6. Even though a person in shock may feel cold and may be hypothermic, do not apply heat to the skin.
7. The environment has to be kept warm.

Surgical Management

Surgical functions that can help in shock state are limited. However, they may be very useful in trauma situations, in hypovolemic shock states due to trauma and can be performed in an attempt to control source of bleeding. Once bleeding has been controlled, interventions aimed at restoring adequate fluid volume are more effective.

Chapter 3 Therapeutic Management of Cardiovascular System

NURSING ASSESSMENT OF CARDIAC SYSTEM

Nursing History

The history collection and recording is detailed in Box 3.1.

Box 3.1: History collection

Demographic data

Name of the patient:	Inpatient number..
Age:	Gender: ....
Marital status:	Nationality: ....
Language spoken:	Religion: ....
Occupation:	Home town/City: ....
Education:	Income: :...
Date of admission:	Treatment received on arrival to hospital:
Provisional diagnosis:	....

Name of the doctor who is treating the patient: ....
Unit: ....

Reason for visit: ....
When did the symptoms start? ....
General status of health: ....
Was the onset sudden or gradual? ....
How often the problem occurs? ....
Has the problem occurred before? ....
Document the progression of the first manifestation: ....

Chief complaint

History of present illness: ....
Ask any or all of the following as appropriate and write a summary ....
....

Rely on objective testing (laboratory values)
Chest pain is one of the most common manifestations of cardiac disease (expanded cardiac assessment)

Onset of chest pain

Location: ....
Duration: ....
Characteristics: ....

Associated manifestations

- Gastrointestinal disorders such as burning colic, aching and tightness
- Musculoskeletal disorders such as aching
- Neurological disorders such as aching/constant burning and needle sharp

Contd...

Contd...

- Psychogenic states such as vague burning/diffuse
- Chest pain, typical pressure, burning/heaviness/gradual onset

Worsened by
- Exertion
- Eating
- Emotion
- Cold
- Deep breathing
- Position changes

Relieved by
- Rest
- Nitroglycerin
- Pain pills
- Spontaneously

Palpitation

Specific review of systems

Past medical history: ....

- Thyroid disease
- Valvular heart disease
- Heart murmur
- Rheumatic heart disease
- Childhood infectious disease
- Immunizations
- Hospitalizations
- Major illness/Infectious disease
- Prior history of rheumatic fever
- Streptococcal infection
- Congenital abnormalities
- Previous hospitalization
- Outcome treatment

Medication prescription/Cold medications/Nasal spray/Habits illicit drug use/ Caffeine intake: ....

- Central/Peripheral/Unilateral/Bilateral
- Congenital heart disease
- Pulmonary disease
- Tobacco use

Allergies
- Environmental
- Food
- Medication
- Iodine or contrast dye

Medication history
- Prescription
- Over-the-counter medication:
  - Vitamins: ....
  - Herbal: ....

Contd...

Contd...

- Aspirin: ....
- Nitroglycerin: ....
- Laxatives: ....
- Nasal spray: ....

Dietary habits
- Restriction advised: Yes/No
- Cholesterol/Salt/Fluid/Sugar/Caffeine intake

Family history
- Cardiovascular disease
- Hypertension
- Diabetes mellitus
- Stroke
- Renal disease
- Liver disease
- Relationship to member affected and treatment provided: ....

Physical examination

Assessment proceed from head to toe

General appearance
- Does the client lie: Quietly/Restless
- Position: Lie flat/Upright/Erect
- Respiratory distress/Cyanosis/Pallor/Dyspnea

Patient general level of consciousness
- Client behavior appropriate for surroundings
- Fear/Depression/Anger
- Identify significant others
- Identify time

Vital signs

Temperature: ....

Respiration: ....

Breath easily/Does the client have to sit-up to breathe easily: Yes/No

Weight:

Blood pressure (BP), while client:
- Lying: ....
- Sitting: ....
- Standing: ....

Pulse
- Apical: ....
- Radial: ....
- Tachycardia [100 beats per minute (bpm)]
- Bradycardia (60 bpm)
- Irregular pulse/Bounding pulse/Absent pulse/Tachypnea

Head and neck
- Eyes: A light gray ring around the iris (possibly caused by cholesterol deposits)
- Examine ear lobes normal: Yes/No
- Lips and buccal mucosa normal: Yes/No

Contd...

Contd...

Neck vein assessment

- Jugular vein: Engorges/Slight provocation/Distention absent with client at 45° angle

Abdomen

- Ascites, hyperactive/hypoactive bowel sounds

Skin

- Central cyanosis/Peripheral cyanosis/Decreased turgor/Warm to touch/Cool to touch/Edema

Nail

- Clubbing/Splinter hemorrhage

Diagnostic testing

Diagnostic procedures are both noninvasive and invasive; nursing responsibilities for these various tests include:

- Scheduling the procedures
- Explaining the purpose, procedure and answering any question
- Procure consent
- Providing prescribed medication for preprocedure
- Providing physical and psychological support
- Providing postprocedure care

Name of the test	*Test result*
Non-invasive tests	
• Electrocardiography test	....
• Holter monitoring	....
• Exercise testing (treadmill test)	....
• Echocardiography	....
• Upright tilt-table test	....
• Radiographic cardiac test	....
• Chest X-ray	....
• Computed tomography (CT) angiography	....
• CT scan pulmonary embolism protocol	....
• Magnetic resonance imaging (MRI)	
• Magnetic resonance angiography (MRA)	....
• Visibility scan (positron emission tomography)	....
Invasive cardiac test	
• Transesophageal echocardiography	....
• Cardiac catheterization	....
• Left heart catheterization	....
• Right heart catheterization	....
• Electrophysiological studies	....
• Coronary angiography	....
• Hemodynamic monitoring	....
• Arterial BP	....
• Pulmonary artery pressure	....
• Pulmonary artery wedge pressure (PAWP)	....

Contd...

Contd...

Cardiovascular assessment	
Criteria	*Remarks*
• Obtains a baseline heart rate (HR) and BP	....
• Obtains and interprets a baseline cardiac rhythm strip	....
• Auscultates the heart sounds for the following:	....
– S_1, S_2	....
– S_3, S_4	....
– Murmurs	....
– Pericardial friction rub	
• Assesses the skin for color, temperature, turgor, edema and diaphoresis	....
• Inspect the nail bed for capillary refill after temporary compression	....
• Palpates the peripheral arterial pulses for rhythm, amplitudes and bilateral equality	....
• Inspects the internal jugular veins for distension with the patient at a 45° angle	....
• Assesses for the presence of central and peripheral intravenous (IV) lines	....
• Assesses the hemodynamic waveforms and measurements of the arterial central or pulmonary artery catheter	....
• Identifies the presence of a permanent or temporary pacemaker; if a temporary pacemaker is present, note the type and settings (milliamperes, sensitivity, mode and rate)	....

CORONARY ARTERY DISEASE

Terminology

Arteriosclerosis: It is commonly called hardening of the arteries, which includes a variety of conditions that cause the artery walls to thicken and lose elasticity.

Atherosclerosis: It is a form of arteriosclerosis in which the inner layers of artery walls become thick and irregular because of the deposits of a fatty substance. As the interior walls of arteries become lined with layer of these deposits, the arteries become narrowed and flow of blood through the arteries is reduced.

Coronary artery disease (CAD): It is the presence of atherosclerosis in the coronary arteries.

Coronary heart disease (CHD): It is CAD and the presence of symptoms as manifested by angina (specific chest pain) or a history of acute myocardial infarction (AMI). The term atherosclerotic heart disease is synonymous with CHD.

Ischemic heart disease: It is a more general term that includes all causes of myocardial ischemia (poor blood supply to the heart muscle).

Pathology and Natural History

Atherosclerosis is a slow progressive disease that may have its beginning early in life. Significant disease may be present before the age of 20 and long before the function of the heart muscle is impaired. There is an asymptomatic period when risk-factor modification may halt or reverse the process. The inner portion of the arterial wall becomes thickened with deposit of fats (lipid and cholesterol) and eventually calcium. The result is gradual narrowing of the arterial lumen. When the blood flow is severely reduced by atherosclerosis, a clot can form as blood trickles and sludges through the narrowed vessels causing a sudden, complete stoppage of blood flow. Injury to the heart muscle occurs because of this decrease or interruption of blood flow, creating an imbalance between the demand of the heart muscle for oxygen and the ability of the narrowed coronary artery to meet the demand. Atherosclerosis is a generalized disease process that may involve arteries in different areas such as heart (leading to a heart attack), brain (leading to a stroke) or legs (leading to pain precipitated by walking or leg cramps during exercise).

Clinical Manifestation of Coronary Heart Disease

A person with CAD may show no signs or signals of heart disease (asymptomatic) or have a sign that suggests CHD (symptomatic). In a person with asymptomatic CAD, coronary artery narrowing progresses overtime. This is the period before enough decrease in blood supply occurs to produce symptoms of heart disease. Symptomatic CHD can manifest as chest discomfort (angina pectoris), a heart attack (MI) or sudden death, which are discussed in detail here. Occasionally some people, especially those with diabetes may have severe CHD on testing, but otherwise have no symptoms. This is known silent ischemia, such as patients are more likely to die or have a heart attack (as compared with those without silent ischemia).

ANGINA PECTORIS

Angina pectoris is a common symptom of CHD, is a transient pain or discomfort due to temporary lack of adequate blood supply to the heart muscle. The pain may be located in the center of chest or it may be more diffuse, i.e. through front of the chest. It is usually described as being crushing, pressing, constricting, oppressive or heavy. It may spread to one (more often the left) or both shoulders and/or arms or to neck, jaw, back or epigastrium without anterior chest discomfort may also be a manifestation of angina. It is a steady discomfort often brought on by any factor that increases the heart rate, including exercise, unusual exertion and emotional or psychological stress. It commonly lasts from 2 to 15 minutes. The most frequent causes of angina is coronary atherosclerosis. As the severity of the coronary narrowing increases, the amount of exertion needed to bring on angina decreases. Angina is usually promptly relieved by rest or nitroglycerin. With severe CHD few days or weeks before a heart attack, angina may occur at rest or may even awaken someone from sleep.

Types of Angina

Unstable Angina

Unstable angina is a clinical syndrome that is characterized by rapidly worsening angina (crescendo angina), angina on minimal exertion or angina at rest. An acute coronary syndrome (ACS) may present as a new phenomenon or against a background of chronic stable angina.

Chronic Stable Angina

Chronic stable angina refers to a chest pain that occurs intermittently over a long period with a same pattern of onset.

Nocturnal Angina and Decubitus

Nocturnal angina and decubitus occurs only at night. Angina decubitus is chest pain that occurs only, while the person is lying down and is usually relieved by standing or sitting.

Prinzmetal's Angina or Vasospastic Angina

Prinzmetal's angina or vasospastic angina is caused by coronary artery spasms and occurs at or with exercise, rest. The pain may occur during rapid eye movement, when myocardial oxygen consumption increases.

Diagnosis

- History and assessment of chest pain
- 12-lead electrocardiography (ECG)
- Chest X-ray
- Exercise stress test
- Echocardiography
- Positron emission tomography
- Coronary angiography
- Creatine kinase-muscle bone (CK-MB)
- Cardiac troponin
- Myoglobin
- Lipid profile.

Management

Patient should be admitted urgently to hospital, because there is a risk of death or acute MI during the unstable phase and appropriate medical therapy can reduce the incidence of adverse events. Bedrest, antiplatelet therapy (Aspirin 300 mg followed by 75–325 mg daily long term).

Drug Therapy for Chronic Stable Angina

Short-acting nitrates: Nitrates dilating coronary artery, increasing blood flow to the ischemic area of the heart. Sublingual nitroglycerin will usually relieve pain in 3 minutes.

Statins: Lower cholesterol level.

Beta blockers: Decrease pulse, BP and cardiac output, prevent release of renin.

Angiotensin-converting enzyme (ACE) inhibitors: Reduces peripheral arterial resistances.

Nursing Management

- Assess anginal pain/history of chest pain, type, location and pain radiation to other areas
- Obtain vital signs, BP, apical pulse, respiration and oxygen saturation
- Administer medication as prescribed
- Administer sublingual nitroglycerin as ordered
- Notify physician after any vital sign changes chest pain unrelieved by nitrates
- Reassess patient condition support emotionally
- Inform physician, if any changes in ECG
- Teach patient regarding medication, dosage and side effect
- Discuss lifestyle modification including modifiable and non-modifiable risk factors
- Teach patient to report the healthcare facilities, if they notice any changes in chest pain, increased diaphoresis
- Instruct the patient to carry nitroglycerin at all times
- After taking nitroglycerin pain is not relieved, report immediately to emergency department or near healthcare center.

ACUTE MYOCARDIAL INFARCTION (ACUTE CORONARY SYNDROME)

A heart attack occurs when an area of the heart muscle is deprived of blood (oxygen) for a prolonged period (usually > 20–30 min). It is usually results from severe narrowing or complete blockage of a diseased coronary artery and result in death of the heart muscle cells supplied by that artery. Myocardial infarction is also known as a Q wave MI, usually caused by a complete blockage of the artery. MI can occur at any age; silent ischemia occurs without pain and carries great risk. The people with hypertension or diabetes are most often noted to have silent ischemia.

Causes

- Due to the formation of occlusive thrombus at the site of rupture or erosion of atheromatous plaque in a coronary artery
- Prolonged ischemia can produce cellular damage.

Signs and Symptoms

- Chest pain is the classic symptoms of MI, crushing, vise-like chest pain with radiation to arm, shoulder, neck, jaw or back
- More common locations are substernal, retrosternal or epigastric areas
- The chest discomfort is similar to angina in location, character and radiation, but is usually more intense, lasts considerably longer, and is not relieved by rest or nitroglycerin
- Sweating, nausea or shortness of breath, dizziness
- Indigestion or gas pain
- Client often denies that they are having an MI because their symptoms are similar to other mild conditions, e.g. indigestion
- Silent ischemia occurs without pain and carries greater risk.

Diagnosis

- Patient history
- Electrocardiography findings, changes during MI include ST-segment elevations, segment inversion and necrosis large Q wave, and it is usually helpful in confirming the diagnosis
- Lactate dehydrogenase (LDH) elevates 14–24 hours after onset of myocardial damage
- Troponin level, increase 7–14 hours after myocardial injury
- Plasma biochemical markers are creatine kinase (CK), CK start to rise at 4–6 hours, peak at about 12 hours and falls to normal within 48–72 hours
- The CK-MB and cardiac specific proteins, troponins T and I, which are released within 4–6 hours and remain elevated for up to 2 weeks
- The C-reactive protein (CRP) levels are elevated in the presence of inflammation
- Magnesium levels are also checked
- Myoglobin is rapidly released when myocardial injury takes place and can be detected within 2 hours
- Prothrombin time (PT) and partial thromboplastin time (PTT)
- Leukocytosis is usually reaching a peak on the 1st day

- The erythrocyte sedimentation rate (ESR) becomes raised and may remain so for several days.

Early Management

Immediate Measure

1. Client should seek within 5 minutes for any unrelieved chest pain.
2. Client with AMI must receive immediate treatment in less than 30 minutes; thrombolytic therapy should start within 30 minutes.
3. Delay may increase damage to the heart and reduce the chance of survival.
4. Provide high-flow oxygen.
5. Intravenous (IV) access keep vein open (KVO).
6. 12-lead ECG monitor.
7. Analgesic morphine sulfate IV, as prescribed to relieve severe distress, reduce pulmonary and systemic vascular resistance.
8. Sublingual nitroglycerin as prescribed.
9. Antiplatelets Aspirin, oral administration of 75–300 mg first dose should be given within first 12 hours.
10. Vital signs including pulse oximetry is monitored.
11. Monitor dysrhythmias.
12. Obtain baseline blood work, e.g. cardiac markers.
13. First-line thrombolysis therapy (as per institutional policy) leads to perfusion with relief of pain, resolution of acute ST elevation as immediately as possible (within the first few hour) and streptokinase 1.5 million units in 100 mL of saline given as an IV infusion over 1 hour. Alteplase other choice of drugs as prescribed.
14. Beta blockers as prescribed.
15. Anticoagulants as prescribed. Subcutaneous heparin given in addition to oral Aspirin may prevent reinfarction after successful thrombolysis and reduce the risk of thromboembolic complications.
16. Vasodilators as prescribed.
17. Observe continuous monitoring.
18. Antidysrhythmic medication should be on hand.
19. Heparin is contraindicated in clients with known bleeding conditions or recent stroke.

Note: If perfusion is not attained or if the client is contraindicated for thrombolytic therapy, then primary angioplasty, stenting of coronary artery bypass grafting (CABG) may be performed as decided by clinician.

Nursing Management of Patient with Myocardial Infarction

Nursing Diagnosis

- Acute pain related to decreased coronary blood flow
- Ineffective tissue perfusion related to altered blood flow to myocardial tissue

- Decreased cardiac output related to cardiac ischemia
- Anxiety and fear-related threat of death, changes in lifestyle, chest pain
- Risk for activity intolerance related to imbalance between oxygen supply and demand
- Risk for constipation related to bedrest, pain medications
- Ineffective health maintenance related to disease condition, medical regimen and lifestyle.

Nursing Intervention

- Assess location, duration, intensity and radiation of chest pain
- Monitor 12-lead ECG as ordered
- Administer:
  - Pain medication as prescribed
  - Aspirin as prescribed
  - Nitrate sublingually as prescribed
  - Oxygen as prescribed and maintain continuous oximetry
  - Thrombolytic therapy as directed.
- Attach the client to cardiac monitor and explain the patient function of monitor
- Notify clinician regarding client response of pain medication
- Send blood specimen for laboratory as instructed
- Administer other medication as per frequency and maintain drug flow chart
- Report any changes in ECG
- Limit visitors and maintain calm environment
- Keep ready intubation and ventilator by side
- Keep ready defibrillator at the bedside
- Maintain intake and output
- Maintain IV fluid as prescribed and IV line patent
- Observe for any signs of pallor, cyanosis, coolness and diaphoresis
- Monitor hemodynamic status, if initiated
- Report to clinician if any changes in client condition
- Observe output, if output less than 0.5 mL/h inform clinician
- Monitor arterial blood gases (ABGs) levels and report
- Inform the family members regarding client progress
- Inform client and significant other about treatment plan
- Place the patient in Fowler's position or as required usually 35°–45° head elevated
- Record weight
- Reassure the client
- Provide bedpan/commode in time in bedside

- Discuss with patient not to strain during defecation
- Assist the patient with activities of daily living (ADL), until he/she is able to do these for themselves
- Encourage self-care as soon as it tolerated
- Provide calling with calling bell for getting nursing assistance, when needed
- Teach client about medication, dosage, route, duration, side effect of each medication and investigation required
- Encourage active and passive exercise as tolerated
- Provide opportunities for the client to express feelings about oneself and the illness
- Help the client identify strength and areas of control
- Encourage early ambulation
- Progressive physical activity should be balanced with a period of rest in between the activity, all activities should be supervised
- Before discharge from the hospital, the patient and significant others should be taught about the heart disease and make the patient to accept the therapeutic regime
- Teach about lifestyle modification; how he/she can bring modification in his/her lifestyle, food, rest activities, smoking, alcohol, obesity and managing associated disease.

Complications

- Dysrhythmias
- Cardiogenic shock
- Heart failure/Pulmonary edema
- Rupture of muscles or valves of the heart, septal rupture
- Pericarditis.

MANAGEMENT OF PATIENTS WITH CARDIAC MONITOR

Cardiac Monitor as a Diagnostic Tool

Cardiac monitor (Fig. 3.1) is one of the most valuable diagnostic tools in general medicine and is essential to recognize disorders of the cardiac rhythm. It can also help with diagnosis and alert healthcare staff to changes in a patient condition. However, cardiac monitor must be carried out meticulously. Poor technique can lead to misinterpretation of an ECG, a mistaken diagnosis, wasted investigation and management of patient.

The phrase cardiac monitoring generally refers to continuous monitoring of the heart activity, generally by ECG with assessment of the patient's condition relative to their cardiac rhythm. It is different from hemodynamic monitoring, which monitors the pressure and flow of blood within the circulatory system. The two may be performed simultaneously on critical heart patients.

Purpose of Cardiac Monitor

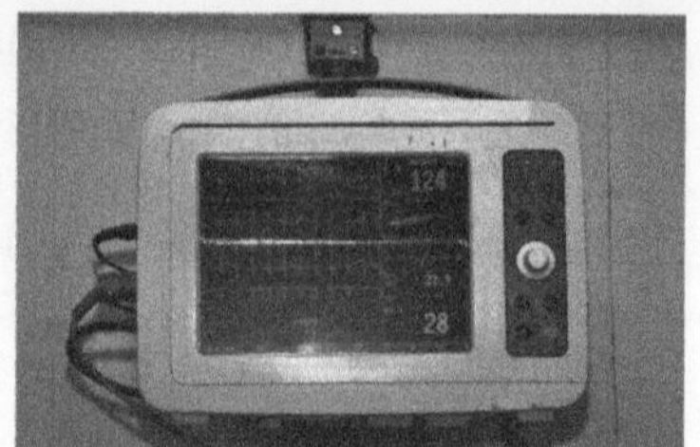

Fig. 3.1: Cardiac monitor (*Courtesy:* Anil Baghi, Multispecialty Hospital, Ferozepur, Punjab)

1. Early detection of disorders of rhythm and conduction. Continuous display of the ECG on a screen permits instant detection and prompt treatment of cardiac rhythms.
2. Prevention of lethal life-threatening rhythms by early detection and prompt treatment.
3. Cardiac monitoring is required in a variety of clinical situations including:
   - Chest pain
   - Myocardial infarction
   - Shock
   - Heart failure palpitations
   - History of syncope
   - During cardiopulmonary resuscitation (CPR).

Basic Components of Cardiac Monitor

The components of a particular monitoring system may differ and can vary widely according to the design and manufacture of the machine. These components and the operating details are described in the manual that accompanies each instrument. The purpose here is to describe the basic features of any cardiac monitor, although cardiac monitor differ in design, most of them have certain basic features in common.

Oscilloscope

Oscilloscope is the screen on which electrocardiographic pattern appears. This screen (television type) provides instantaneous and continuous representation of electrical activity of the heart. The oscilloscope screen also displays pulse, respiratory rates, oxygen saturation levels and hemodynamic parameters, if it is connected to the appropriate cables.

Rate Indicator

Rate indicator is a moving needle, which shows the heart rate. A built in machismo averages the number of ventricular contractions or heart beats per minute and the rate is shown on the indicator by a needle and flashing light. The rate indicator is integrated with alarm system, so that if pulse goes above or below the present limits, it triggers an alarm. These limits are set on the rate indicator by two needles. The limits vary, but they are usually based on sensitivity of the electrodes and condition of the patient. Thus, the alarm may be triggered to go off at either 20 beats above or below. An individual patient's normal heart rate is set automatically to go on at a high rate of 150 or low rate of 50 beats per minute (bpm).

Alarm

When the heart falls above or below the present levels, audio and visual alarms alert the nurse each time an alarm is triggered. The nurse must observe identity and take a prompt note regarding the cardiac rhythm.

Sweep Speed

The rate at which the electronic beam sweeps across the screen, this can be regulated. It can be set at trace speed of 25 mm/s, which means that the beam sweeps across the screen in 6 seconds or at 50 mm/s (second position). The 6 seconds position is generally used in cardiac monitoring, a sit allows a quick on the heart rate. The 3 seconds position is used for interpretation of rhythm.

Central Console

The individual bedside monitors in some coronary care units (CCUs) are connected to a central console the nursing station. This permits continuous visualization of the electrocardiographic pattern from all the monitors from one spot, single or multiple channel display is commercially available. Additional features or complementary parts can be added to the basic monitoring system as desired.

Electrocardiography Write Out

Electrocardiography write out feature allows a rhythm strip to be obtained automatically during preset alarm situation or any time by turning on the appropriate switch.

Memory Loop

Memory loop makes it possible to have a record of the abnormal cardiac rhythm, which even though missed by the observer on the oscilloscope or misinterpreted can be played back on the ECG recorder.

Problems

Artifacts

Electrical wave forms distort complexes and interrupt the rhythm often due to loose electrodes or to the movement of patient.

False Alarm

- May be due to poor electrode contact, movement of patient, shivering and trembling of patient
- Electrical interference
- Electrical current from outer sources create interference with monitor signals.

Poor Electrocardiography Signals

Defective pattern may result from:

- Poor contact electrodes
- Poor connection of cable
- Malfunction of monitor
- Too much paste or jelly
- Too little paste or jelly
- Profuse sweating.

Skin Irritation

Patient may show skin reaction if they are allergic to tape used to secure monitoring electrodes, electrodes paste or jelly may also cause irritation.

Electrical Hazards

The threat of current passing accidentally from the monitor to the patient should be recognized, especially when more than one electrical system is used. Efficient grounding can reduce the hazard grounding; serve as the reference for measurement of all voltage. In addition, the ground electrodes provide a path of least resistance for currents within the machine, in providing this drain for the current it eliminates the shock hazards and reduces the possibility of artifacts. For adequate grounding, the ground electrodes must be properly connected. No ungrounded equipment should be used in the monitoring area and patient monitor cable must be kept away from other power cable.

Operation of Cardiac Monitors

Electrodes

The electrodes pick up the heart's electrical signals at the surface of the skin and transfer this current to the monitor. Nurses need to know that this transmission must be efficient, otherwise the rest of monitoring will have little meaning and electrodes are of great importance for successful monitoring.

Types

There are three basic types of electrodes.

Direct contact electrodes: These are metal plates placed directly on the skin surface. Electrodes are anchored to the skin by means of adhesive tapes after conducting jelly is applied.

Floating or disk type electrodes: Conductive jelly fills the little space between the electrodes and skin. These electrodes are also attached to the skin by an adhesive.

Needle electrodes: These are small gauge 25 gauge long, which can be inserted directly under the skin. No electrode jelly is required. Electrical interference is minimal, but patients find this uncomfortable and are difficult to keep them in position.

Electrocardiography electrode placement

The standard left/precordial leads are:

1. **V1:** Fourth intercostal space, right sternal border.
2. **V2:** Fourth intercostal space, left sternal border.
3. **V3:** Diagonally between V2 and V4.
4. **V4:** Fifth intercostal space at left midclavicular line.
5. **V5:** Anterior axillary line (same level as V4).
6. **V6:** Midaxillary level (same level as V4 and V5).

The placement of electrodes depends with the type of technology that is appropriate and available for a standard 12-lead ECG, 10 electrodes (6 on the chest and 4 on the limbs) are placed on the body.

Reasons for using chest for placement of the electrodes

1. Motion artifact is reduced because the electrodes are on the chest instead of the moving limb.
2. The patient is less aware of being wired up with chest placement of the electrodes than he/she would be with limb placement.
3. Muscle artifact is reduced since the chest has fewer skeletal muscles.
4. Higher ECG signals can be expected because the electrodes are close to the heart.

Procedure for attachment of electrodes

1. Skin area should be cleaned thoroughly and prepared for electrodes placement.
2. Shaving of excessive hair may be necessary (hair, sweat and oily skin).
3. Allow skin to dry thoroughly.
4. Apply electrode jelly to the skin and attach electrodes to the skin adhesive tape, when using direct contact or floating electrodes.
5. Wires from skin electrodes should be oriented toward a common direction.
6. Electrodes wire is inserted into patient cable, which is coded:
   - 'R' for right electrodes
   - 'L' for left electrodes
   - 'G' for ground electrode.
7. Monitor end of the cable is inserted into appropriate socket. A secure contact is essential. After electrode placement and connection of cable, the monitor is ready for use. The power switch is turned 'on' rate meter,

alarm system and oscilloscope are adjusted for effective functioning. Use manufacturer's manual of instruction for learning detailed instructions for different design.

General rules

1. Once the electrodes are attached and machine is turned on, observe the ECG pattern on the oscilloscope. Care should be taken to select the lead, which best displays the upright QRS complex. Distinct P waves and a distinct artifact is a pacemaker used in pacing the patient's heart, if the waves are very low and cannot be increased by adjusting the controls. Position of the electrodes may have to be adjusted for a better signal.
2. If there is electrical interference, the electrode sites should be checked.
3. The limits of the high- and low-rate alarms must be adjusted to the patient's existing condition and modified as clinical picture changes.

Major Responsibilities of the Nurse

1. Continuous assessment of patient's cardiac status. The nurse must be aware of normal heart rhythm and be able to distinguish significant arrhythmias. Much of the success in the coronary care system is dependent upon the ability of the staff.
2. Direct observation of the patient. The information on the ECG must be correlated with other signs and symptoms, which may give a more correct picture and actual cardiac performance.
3. Explain the monitoring system to the patient. This procedure may be unfamiliar to many patients and frightening to some.
4. Proper preparation of the designated skin areas for electrode placement.
5. Assist with the operation of monitoring the equipment.
6. It should always be remembered that the use of monitoring system is no substitute for good clinical observation data from a cardiac monitor and cannot be treated in isolation. It must be combined with other information from the patient to provide the most complete base for care.
7. Assisting the patient to go off the monitor.

Going off the Monitor

Many patients would have developed a strong dependence on their monitor. Despite what they are told, they often continue to believe that the monitor makes their heartbeat. Many patients believe that if they are removed from the machine, their hearts will stop. Other patients, who appreciate that the monitor only portrays their heart rhythm, fear that once the instrument is discontinued they will develop a dangerous arrhythmia and no one will know. These fears should be anticipated and removed. The nurse should therefore give the patient every encouragement to discuss the interpretation of the order to discontinue monitoring. Does he/she consider it a step toward recovery or does he/she understand that the order is not written till his/her cardiac status is stable? How does the family view development? The idea that heart will stop beating when the monitor is discontinued can be corrected before it develops. With the physician permission, the monitor should be temporarily turned off and the patient instructed to feel his/her pulse still beating, also want to assure the apprehensive.

CARDIAC ARRHYTHMIAS

A cardiac arrhythmia can be defined, as any ECG rhythm that deviates from the normal sinus rhythm (NSR). Cardiac arrhythmias are generally classified into one of two group's arrhythmias that result from a disturbance in impulse formation and those that result from a disturbance in impulse conduction. Although this classification is helpful, it is also limited because some arrhythmias have a disturbance in both impulse formation and conduction.

Disturbance in Impulse Formation

Cardiac arrhythmias can be categorized in relation to their site or origin and the mechanisms of the disturbances.

Site of Origin

Sinoatrial (SA) node (sinus rhythms): For example, sinus bradycardia and sinus tachycardia.

Atria-atrial rhythm: For example, atrial premature, atrial fibrillation.

Atrioventricular (AV) junction (junctional rhythms): For example, junction rhythm.

Ventricles-ventricular rhythms: For example, ventricular premature, ventricular tachycardia (VT).

Dysrhythmias

Dysrhythmias are disorders of the formation of conduction of the electrical impulses within the heart. These disorders can cause disturbances of the heart rate, heart rhythm or both.

Normal Electrical Conduction

The electrical impulse that stimulates and passes the cardiac muscle normally originates in the SA nodes, located near the superior vena cava in the right atrium. The electrical impulses quickly travel from the sinus nodes through the atria to the AV node. This process is known as conduction. The electrical impulses then travel very quickly through the bundle of his to the right- and left-bundle branches, and Purkinje fibers located in ventricular muscle. The electrical stimulation of the muscle cells of the ventricles in turn causes the mechanical contraction of the ventricles (systole). The cells repolarize and the ventricles then relax (diastole). The electrical stimulation is called depolarization and electrical relaxation is called repolarization.

Normal Sinus Rhythm

Normal sinus rhythm occurs when the electrical impulses start at a regular rate in the sinus node.

Characteristics: Rate 60–100/min in adult.

Sinus Bradycardia

Impulse occurs lower than normal.

Characteristics: Heart rate less than 60 bpm in adult.

Sinus Tachycardia

The sinus nodes create impulse at faster than normal rate.

Characteristics: Heart rate 100–120 bpm.

Sinus Arrhythmias

Sinus arrhythmias occur when an impulse at an irregular rhythm rate usually increases with inspiration.

Characteristics: Heart rate 60–100 bpm.

Atrial Dysrhythmias

Premature atrial complex: It occurs when an electrical impulse starts in atrium before the next normal impulse. Heart rate depends on the underlying rhythm.

Atrial flutter: Occurs because of a conduction defect in the atrium.

Characteristics: Heart rate 250–400 bpm.

Atrial fibrillation: It is an uncoordinated atrial electrical activation that causes rapid disorganized and uncontrolled twitching of atrial musculature.

Characteristics: Heart rate 300–600 bpm. PR intervals cannot be measured.

Ventricular Dysrhythmias

Premature ventricular complex (PVC): It is an impulse that starts in ventricles and is conducted through the ventricles.

Ventricular tachycardia: Defined as three or more PVC in a row.

Characteristics: Heart rate exceeding 100 bpm.

Ventricular fibrillation (VF): Rapid disorganized ventricular rhythms.

Characteristics: Heart rate more than 300 bpm.

Ventricular systole: Commonly called flat line.

Characteristics: Absent QRS complex.

Conduction Abnormalities

Heart Block

First-degree AV block: Atrial impulses are conducted through the AV nodes into the ventricles at slower rate than normal.

Second-degree AV block: Each atrial impulse takes place a longer time for conduction than one before. PR intervals become longer.

Third-degree AV block: In this, two impulses stimulate the heart one stimulate ventricles represented by QRS complex and one stimulate atria represented by P waves having two impulses stimulate the heart result in condition called AV dissòciation.

If the medication is needed for treating heart rate condition and no effective alternative is available, pacemaker implantation may be indicated.

Pacemaker Therapy

A pacemaker is a medical device that uses electrical impulses, delivered by electrodes contacting the heart muscles, to regulate the beating of heart (or artificial pacemaker, so as not to be confused with the heart's natural pacemaker). Nursing care for pacemaker therapy is given in Table 3.1. Pacemakers and implantable cardioverter defibrillators (ICD) has been around for more than two decades for the treatment of cardiac arrhythmias.

The decision to implant a pacemaker in a patient with abnormal AV conduction depends on the presence of symptoms related to bradycardia or ventricular arrhythmias and their prognostic implications. Permanent pacing improves survival in patients with complete AV block, especially if syncope has occurred frequently.

Indication

- Symptomatic third-degree AV block is a class I indication for permanent pacing
- Asymptomatic third-degree AV block is a class II indication
- More recently, it has been recognized that type II second-degree AV block
- Patients with left ventricular dysfunction and markedly prolonged PR interval may benefit from pacing
- Bradyarrhythmia or tachyarrhythmia in the setting of heart disease
- Symptomatic bradycardia is the most common indication.

Living with Pacemaker

Once the pacemaker is implanted, it is periodically checked to ensure the device is operational and performing appropriately. Depending on the frequency set, device can be checked as often as it is necessary, routine pacemaker though depending upon patient/device status and remote monitoring availability.

Table 3.1: Nursing care for patient requiring temporary cardiac pacemaker support

Sl No.	Competency statement/Criteria	Remarks
1.	Identifies the indications for temporary cardiac pacemaker support	
2.	Defines the following terms pertinent to pacemaker therapy are output (milliamperes), capture, stimulation threshold, sensitivity, sensitivity threshold and crosstalk	
3.	Identifies the routes used for insertion of temporary internal pacemakers	
4.	Differentiates between unipolar and bipolar electrodes	
5.	Identifies and measures the following intervals in milliseconds on the electrocardiography (ECG); VV intervals, atrioventricular (AV) intervals and ventriculoatrial (VA) interval	
6.	Differentiates among the following pacing modes, atrial asynchronous, arterial demand, atrial overdrive, ventricular asynchronous, ventricular demand and dual-chamber pacing	
7.	Identifies and intervenes appropriately when the following complications occur, failure to pace and failure to capture and sense	
8.	Changes the dressing over the insertion site according to hospital guidelines and whenever it is moist or soiled using sterile technique; assess the site for inflammation, drainage and discoloration	
9.	Initiates appropriate electrical safety precautions	
10.	Changes the pacemaker battery routinely every 6 week or after 48 hour of continuous use	
11.	Performs an atrial electrocardiogram (AEG) with the atrial epicardial wires as ordered by physician	
12.	Documents all pertinent information	

Threshold: This test confirms the minimum amount of energy both volts and pulse required to reliably depolarize (capture) the chamber being tested.

Lifestyle considerations: Consider the following:

1. A patient's lifestyle is usually not modified to any great degree after insertion of a pacemaker. There are a few activities that are unwise such as full contact with sports and activities that involve intense magnetic fields.
2. Everyday actions need to be modified. For instance, vehicle seat belt may be uncomfortable, if the harness should fall across the pacemaker insertion site. Take precaution to avoid the belt.
3. Any kind of an activity that involves intense magnetic fields should be avoided, e.g. MRI machine.
4. The patient should inform all medical personnel that they have a pacemaker.

DEFIBRILLATION

Principles of Early Defibrillation

Early defibrillation is critical for clients of sudden cardiac arrest for the following reasons:

1. The most common initial rhythm in witnessed sudden cardiac arrest is VF. When VF is present, the heart quivers and does not pump blood.
2. The most effective treatment for VF is electrical defibrillation (delivery of a shock to stop the VF).
3. The probability of successful defibrillation decreases quickly overtime.
4. Ventricular fibrillation deteriorates to asystole, if not treated.
5. The earlier defibrillation occurs, the higher the survival rate. When VF is present, CPR can provide a small amount of blood flow to the heart and brain, but cannot directly restore an organized rhythm. Restoration of a perfusing rhythm requires immediate CPR and defibrillation within a few minutes of the initial arrest.
6. Without bystander CPR, the chance of survival from VF cardiac arrest declines by 7–10% per minute without defibrillation. Bystander CPR improves survival from VF cardiac arrest at most defibrillation intervals.
7. The use of automated external defibrillators (AEDs) increases the number of people (lay rescuers and healthcare providers), who can perform CPR and attempt defibrillation. Thus, shortening the time between collapse and defibrillation.

Structure and Function of AED

Automated external defibrillators are computerized devices that are attached to a pulseless client with adhesive pads, they will recommend shock delivery only if the client's heart rhythm is one that a shock can treat. The AEDs give rescuers visual and voice prompts to guide rescuer actions. The word automated actually means semiautomated, because most commercially available AEDs will 'advice' the operator that a shock is needed, but will not deliver a shock without an action by the rescuer (i.e. the rescuer must push the 'shock' button).

A small number of fully automated AEDs are now in use, if a fully automated defibrillator detects a rhythm that a shock can treat, it will deliver a shock without operator intervention. Adhesive electrodes attach the AEDs to the patient. Most AEDs operate in the same way and have similar components.

Automated External Defibrillators Operation

Use AEDs only if clients have the following three clinical findings:

- No response
- No breathing
- No pulse.

The patient in cardiac arrest may demonstrate agonal gasps. Agonal gasps are not effective breathing. A client who has agonal gasps and does not respond and has no pulse is in cardiac arrest. Remember that agonal gasps are not effective breaths.

Universal Automated External Defibrillator

Common steps to operate all AEDs are the following (Table 3.2):

1. Once the AED arrives, put it at the client's side, next to the rescuer who will operate it. This position provides ready access to the AED controls

Table 3.2: Universal steps for operating an automated external defibrillators

Steps	Action
1	Power on the automated external defibrillator (AED): This activates voice prompts for guidance in all subsequent steps: • Open the carrying case or the top of the AED • Turn the power on (some devices will power on automatically when you open the lid or case)
2	Attach electrode pads to the client's bare chest: • Choose correct pads (adult verses child) according to size/age of client; use child pads or child system for children < 8 years of age, if available • Do not use child pads or child system for clients above 8 years and older • Peel the backing away from the electrode pads • Quickly wipe the client's chest if it is covered with water or sweat • Attach the adhesive electrode pads to the client's bare chest • Place one electrode pad on the upper right side of the bare chest to the right of the breast bone, directly below the collarbone • Place the other pad to left of the nipple, a few centimeter below the left arm pit • Attach the AED connecting cables to the AED box (some are preconnected)
3	'Clear' the client and analyze the rhythm: • Always clear the client during analysis; be sure that no one is touching the client not even the person in charge of giving breaths • Some AEDs will tell patient to push a button to allow the AED to begin analyzing the heart rhythm; others will do that automatically • The AED may take about 5–15 second to analyze • The AED then tells, if a shock is needed
4	If the AED advises a shock, it will tell the examiner to be sure to clear the client: • Clear the client before delivering the shock and be sure no one should touch the client to avoid injury to rescuers • Loudly state clear the patient message such as 'I am clear, you are clear, everybody clear or simply clear' • Perform a visual check to ensure that no one is in contact with the client • Press the shock button • The shock will produce a sudden contraction of the client's muscles
5	• As soon as the AED gives the shock, begin cardiopulmonary resuscitation (CPR) starting with chest compressions
6	• After 2 min of CPR, the AED will prompt to repeat steps 3 and 4

and easy placement of electrode pads. It also allows a second rescuer to perform CPR from the opposite side of the client without interfering with AED operation.

2. The AED are available in different models. There are small differences from model-to-model, but all AEDs operate in basically the same way.

Using an Automated External Defibrillator on a Child

For unwitnessed, out-of-hospital cardiac arrest in children, perform five cycle or 2 minutes of CPR before using and attaching the AED. For any in-hospital cardiac arrest of a child or for any sudden collapse of a child out of hospital, use a AED as soon as it is available.

Choosing the AED pads or AED child system

Some AED systems have been designed to deliver both adult and child shock doses. If one uses an AED on a child and that AED can deliver a child shock dose, follow the AED instructions to select the lower (child) shock dose. There is need to turn a child key/switch or use child-size pads or both to reduce the shock dose. One must be careful not to deliver the child shock dose for client over 8 years of age because the smaller dose may not be effective for the larger or older client. Client need to be familiar with their AED.

While using an AED for a child 1–8 years of age and the AED does not have a child pads or child key/switch, one may use the adult pads and deliver the adult dose. If an AED has optional child pads or key, or switch to enable the child dose to be delivered, it is important to select the pads and settings that are correct for the client.

Outcomes and Actions after Shock Delivery

'Shock Indicated' Message: Recurrent VF

After AED delivers a shock to the client, follow the steps given in Table 3.3.

Table 3.3: Steps to be followed after automated external defibrillator delivers a shock to the client

Steps	Action
1	Immediately resume cardiopulmonary resuscitation (CPR) beginning with chest compression; do not delay CPR to check the patients pulse even if a displayed rhythm looks normal
2	After 5 cycle (about 2 min) of CPR, allow the automated external defibrillator (AED) to analyze the heart rhythm, if a shock is not advised, resume CPR (beginning with chest compressions) for 5 more cycles (about 2 min)
3	Continue until advanced care providers take over or the client starts to move; advanced care providers will indicate when a pulse check or other therapies are appropriate

'No Shock Indicated' Message: Pulse and Breathing Absent

If the AED does not detect a rhythm requiring a shock, the AED will prompt one to resume CPR, beginning with chest compressions. Do not recheck to see if there is a pulse. The AED may voice prompts and continues until advance care providers take over or the client starts to move. Advanced care providers will indicate when a pulse check or other therapies are appropriate.

Implantable Cardioverter

An ICD treats dangerously fast rhythm disorders called VT and VF in the lower chambers of the heart. The ICD sends a shock to the heart muscle to interrupt the rhythm disorder and allow the heart to resume its normal rhythm.

An ICD corrects rapid, abnormal heart rhythms. It constantly watches the heart and delivers treatment to stop an abnormally fast rate such as VT and VF, ICDs can treat slow rhythms as well. They do this by sending tiny electrical impulses to the ventricle, the atrium or both and it sends electrical pulses to the heart muscle through the leads. The electrical pulses slow the heart, therefore restoring a more normal rate.

Implanted Defibrillators and Pacemakers

Clients who have a higher risk for sudden cardiac arrest may have implanted defibrillators/pacemakers that deliver shocks directly to the myocardium. One can immediately identify these devices, because they create a hard lump beneath the skin of the upper chest or abdomen. The lump is half the size of a deck of cards with a small overlying scar, while placing an AED electrode pad directly over an implanted medical device, the device may block delivery of the shock to the heart. If any identifications are implanted defibrillator/pacemaker:

- Place the AED electrode pad at least 2.5 cm to the side of the implanted device
- Follow the normal steps for operating an AED.

Occasionally, the analysis and shock cycles of implanted defibrillators and AEDs will conflict; if the implanted defibrillator is delivering shocks to the patient (the patient muscle contract in a manner that observed after an AED shock) allow 30–60 seconds for the implanted defibrillator to complete the treatment cycle before delivering shock from the AED.

Transdermal Medication Patches

Do not place AED electrodes directly on top of a medication patch (e.g. patch of nitroglycerin, nicotine, pain medication, hormone replacement therapy or antihypertensive medication). The medication patch may block the transfer of energy from the electrode pad to the heart and may cause small burns to the skin. To prevent the medication patch from blocking delivery of energy, remove the patch and wipe the area clean before attaching the AED electrode pad. Nursing care for patient requiring cardiac monitoring is given in Table 3.4.

Table 3.4: Nursing care for patient requiring cardiac monitoring

Sl No.	Competency criteria	Remarks
1.	Prepares skin before electrodes placement by clipping the hair and cleaning the skin with alcohol swabs	
2.	Attaches electrodes in a lead II monitoring pattern or a lead designated by unit protocol	
3.	Uses the modified chest lead V1 [midclavicular line (MCL)], monitoring pattern; when needed	
4	Obtains and interprets a rhythm strip every 8 hour or more frequently; if needed	
5.	Sets alarm limits according to hospital policy	
6.	Institutes advanced cardiac life support (ACLS) algorithms for life-threatening dysrhythmias according to institutional policies	
7.	Obtains a 12-lead electrocardiography (ECG); if an acute dysrhythmia or change in the ST segment or T wave develop	
8.	Distinguishes artifact an electrical (60 cycle) interference from the patient's rhythm	
9.	Documents all pertinent information	

NURSING CARE OF THE PATIENT WITH CENTRAL VENOUS PRESSURE

Central venous pressure (CVP) is the measurement of pressure in the right atrium of the heart and is measured in 'cm H_2O'. The pressure recorded reflects the circulatory fluid volume and assessment of this may be required for critically ill patients, where close monitoring of fluid is needed. It is influenced by number of factors including cardiac output, respiratory activity, contraction of skeletal muscle (particularly legs and abdomen), sympathetic vasoconstrictor tone and hydrostatic force (i.e. gravity).

Indications

- Preoperative monitoring of patients with hemorrhage/trauma/shock
- Postoperative monitoring following major surgery
- Patients who are severely dehydrated/hypovolemia
- Patient in cardiogenic hypovolemia shock
- Patient with cardiac problem

- Patient with renal problem
- To evaluate the adequacy of circulating blood volume
- To give high volume of fluid quickly in seriously ill patient
- Drugs that is too hypertonic to be given safely by the peripheral route
- Administer long-term chemotherapy.

Purposes

- The measurement reflects the relationship between blood volume and cardiac competence
- The CVP line gives direct access to active circulation and serves as a route for infusion and medications
- It can be used to give total parental nutrition in patients who have extensive bowel surgery, severe burns, renal or hepatic failure and pancreatitis or severe sepsis.

Articles Required

- Venous pressure apparatus with water manometer
- Cut-down tray with IV catheter
- Infusion solution and infusion set
- A 3-way stopcock
- Intravenous pole attached to bed, arm board and adhesive tape
- Antiseptic solution to prepare the area.

Description

Route

- Femoral vein
- Internal jugular vein (IJV)
- Subclavian vein
- Brachiocephalic vein.

Types of Central Venous Pressure Lines

- Single lumen
- Double lumen
- Triple lumen
- Quadruple lumen
- Non-antibiotic coated
- Antibiotic coated
- Anticoagulant heparin coated.

Designations for Port Usage

When using a triple lumen catheter, the following designations are examples for port usage and do not represent the only way the lumens can be used:

1. **Proximal:**
   - Blood sampling
   - Medications
   - Blood administration.
2. **Medial:**
   - Total parenteral nutrition (TPN)
   - Medications (only if TPN use is not anticipated).
3. **Distal:**
   - The CVP monitoring
   - Blood administration
   - High volume or viscous fluids
   - Colloids
   - Medication.

Three Points to Consider

- Insertion
- Care and maintenance
- Removal.

Insertion and Position of the Patient

Anatomy

1. **Two major sites:**
   - *Subclavian vein:* Patient lies supine with his/her arms by the side, the head of the bed is lowered to 10° (Trendelenburg position)
   - *Internal jugular vein:* Patient lies supine, neck is extended and head away from the site, head of bed is lowered to 10°.
2. **Two minor sites:**
   - External jugular vein
   - Median cephalic vein.
3. **Patient lies supine:** Arms are extended with the palm upwards and elbow supported.

Preparation of the Patient

1. Explain the procedure to the patient. This will allay the patient's fears and elicit better cooperation.

2. Place the patient in the Trendelenburg position that is in supine with head down. This will engorge the large veins and aid insertion of the cannula. It will also prevent air embolism.
3. Place a rolled towel vertically between the patient shoulder blades; this will manipulate the patient's anatomy to aid insertion of the cannula.
4. Ideally, the patient should be connected to an ECG monitor; this is because the passage of the catheter can cause cardiac arrhythmias.
5. Ask the patient to turn his/her head away from the insertion site.

Inserting the Catheter

The physician will scrub wear, gown mask and gloves. The nurse assisting should have clean hands and also wear a mask. The physician will then clean the area of insertion with Betadine, drape the area and administer an anesthetic. After waiting for this to take affect, he/she will then insert a large bore needle into the vessels, while aspirating all. When he/she is satisfied that the needle is in the lumen of the intended vessels, he/she will then insert the sledging wire through the needle whilst keeping an eye on the ECG monitoring to ensure that the wire is not causing any arrhythmias, while holding the wire in place. The needle is withdrawn and a dilator is passed down the wire and vein insertion site is dilated after making a small skin nick. The dilator is then removed leaving the wire in place after flushing the lumen of catheter. The catheter is passed over the wire and inserted to the desired levels. The wire is then withdrawn and catheter lumen flushed with the heparinized saline and bunged off. The catheter is then stitched, a dressing is applied and a chest X-ray is ordered. When the chest X-ray shows that the catheter is in desired place, the infusion fluid can be started. During this procedure, nurse should reassure the patient and carry out the order of physician regarding the positioning of patient.

Procedure

- Explain the procedure to the patient and reassure him/her
- Collect all articles required
- Make the patient to lie flat
- Prepare the site
- The IV catheter (about 60.90 cm long size, 14–16 gauze) is passed through median, basilic, subclavian or jugular vein
- Attach the manometer to the IV pole with the zero point of the manometer on the level with the patient right atrium
- The CVP catheter is connected to a 3-way stopcock, which communicates with the manometer an open IV system
- Catheter is secured by a suture to prevent accidental removal
- Apply dressing.

Measurement of Central Venous Pressure

The CVP is measured with the patient lying flat; it is expressed in 'cm H_2O' above a point level with the right atrium. Normally, CVP may range from 5 to 12 cm H_2O. Any significant (especially if it occur suddenly) should be carefully noted and investigated. Elevated CVP occurs in congestive heart failure (CHF) and in conditions of circulatory overload as in excessive fluid infusion. A low CVP occurs in hypovolemic state due to fluid loss and in some cases of cardiogenic shock.

Factors Contributing to Increased Central Venous Pressure

- Decreased cardiac output
- Increased blood volume (occurs in renal failure)
- Venous constriction
- Arterial dilation
- Forced expiration (as occurs with a valsalva maneuver).

Catheter Maintenance

The CVP catheter is invasive devices that predispose the patient to complications that are costly in financial terms as well as in patient morbidity and mortality. Methods used in the cure and maintenance of the catheter during insertion, while indwelling can have a significant effect upon the catheter related complications. Hence, every intensive care unit (ICU) should have a protocol for insertion and maintenance (i.e. dressing material used, antimicrobial ointments, redressing, etc.). The catheter should be observed for signs of damage and the IV site for signs of infection. This is best done on a regular basis and can be incorporated.

Dressing Material

The classic IV dressing has consisted of gauze secured with tape, however, the introduction of transparent, semipermeable dressing has initiated a controversy as to which dressing material is superior. Each has its advantage and disadvantage (Table 3.5).

Various Antimicrobial Ointments

1. Bacitracin (Neosporin), neomycin, polymyxin (BNP) ointment:
   - Effective in reducing colonization or infection caused by gram-positive organisms
   - Not effective in gram-negative or fungal infections.
2. Povidone iodine is best for CVP lines due to broader spectrum of activity.

Redressing Interval Universally Accepted

- When a dressing is no longer adherent or occlusive
- Dressing becomes soiled.

Redressing Procedure Guidelines

- Hands must be washed thoroughly prior to the dressing
- Universal precaution must be observed
- To prevent cutting the catheter when removing old dressing, do not use scissors or sharp instruments
- Turn patient's head away from dressing site or have patient wear a mask
- Visually examine insertion site at least daily or with each dressing change for erythema, drainage, tenderness, suture integrity and catheter position
- Use circular motion to cleanse the area around the catheter, working from the site out in concentric circles and under the catheter hub
- Document dressing change with the date and initials of person redressing.

Maintaining Patency

When a catheter lumen is linger used for continuous infusion (Table 3.6), it should be cupped and locked.

Flushing/Locking Guidelines

- Use aseptic technique
- Heparinized salines are commonly used

Table 3.6: Nursing care for patient requiring a continuous medication infusion

Sl No.	Competency statement/criteria	Remarks
1.	Identifies the mode of action, indications, contraindications and adverse reactions of the medication infusion	
2.	Calculates the proper concentration and rate of infusion states the therapeutic range of the medication infusion and documents the dose hour	
3.	Administers the medications via volumetric infusion pump and if the medication has vasoconstructive properties into a central venous access	
4.	Monitors the patient's hemodynamic response continuously by electrocardiography (ECG) and arterial pressure	
5.	Titrates the medication infusion to obtain the desired results	
6.	Determines compatibility of medications before administering concurrently through the same intravenous (IV) access	
7.	Monitors the serum concentrations of certain medication infusion or by products of their metabolism to prevent toxicity	
8.	Documents all pertinent information	

- About 10 mL or more depending upon the length of catheter, so that the lumen is filled
- Monitor clotting factors during heparin use
- Always aspirate before one flushes the catheter to make sure that a clot in the lumen is not pushed into the circulation.

Management of Occlusions

Catheter occlusion is a frequently encountered problem, guidelines for declotting are:

- Prior to declotting, verify catheter tip placement by chest X-ray
- Rule out mechanical occlusion first
- Use a 10 cc syringe or larger to avoid excessive pressure
- Do not exceed catheter lumen filling volume
- Make sure the catheter is completely flushed out prior to trying another declotting agent.

Thrombolytic Agents Used for Declotting

- Urokinase 5 U/mL
- Streptokinase.

Instill a volume sufficient to fill the lumen, keep it for almost 15–20 minutes and then aspirate the cloth at regular time. Sometimes, the occlusions can be chemical, which can be dissolved by:

- Sodium bicarbonate ($NaHCO_3$) 8.4% solution
- Instill volume equal to the catheter lumen
- Allow it for 20 minutes
- Aspirate.

Note: Lipid sludge occlusions can be treated with $NaHCO_3$.

Significant Complications

A number of complications can occur at the time of insertion or show up later on these can include:

- Arterial puncture
- Air embolism
- Fluid overload
- Hemothorax
- Pneumothorax
- Pericardial tamponade
- Clot formation and pulmonary embolism
- Infection.

Air embolism can occur if the patient is not correctly positioned at the time of insertion or air is introduced to the line during bottle change, etc.

If air embolism is suspected, the patient should be placed in the left lateral position with a head-down tilt and help sought.

Nursing Management for the Patient with Catheter

Establish a systematic method for assessment (Box 3.2).

Box 3.2: Nursing care for patient requiring central venous pressure (CVP) monitoring

Competency statement/Criteria
• Identifies the indications for CVP monitoring • Assembles the necessary equipment for insertion of CVP catheter • Assists the physician with the procedure • Ensures that a chest radiography is performed and interpreted after catheter insertion • Positions the patient supine or with the head of bed elevated to measure the CVP; placing the zero reference of water manometer or air fluid interface of the transducer system at the phlebostatic axis • Balance or zero the transducer to atmospheric pressure at least every 4 hour or according to manufacturer's specifications (if using the transducer method) • Obtains CVP readings at end expiration either by the water manometer method, recognizing proper fluctuation or by the transducer method, recognizing a normal wave form • States the normal CVP reading • States the potential causes of abnormal readings • Assesses for blood return from the catheter every 4 hour • Changes the intravenous (IV) or heparinized normal saline flush solution, tubing and dressing according to hospital guidelines; inspects the site for signs of infection; disconnects the IV tubing from the catheter during the positive expiratory phase of respiration • Monitors the patient for inadvertent line disconnection or the development of a venous air embolism during catheter placement or tubing changes; places the patient in the left lateral decubitus position if an air embolism is suspected • Documents all pertinent information

Monitor

- Zero balance and level the transducer at least every 8 hours and when needed
- Zero balance with each new setup
- Zero balance prior to insertion of catheter
- Level the transducer at the phlebostatic axis with each zero balance.

Transducer

- Eliminate any air bubbles by flushing the transducer with the irrigation system
- If the blood has backed up in the transducer, change the entire flush system.

Catheter

- Inspect insertion site for potential kinks in the catheter
- Observe the oozing of fluid from the catheter or insertion site.

Line Setup Tubing

- Trace tubing for potential kinks, loose connections, obstructions, presence of blood or air bubbles
- Keep all connection sites visible to observe for potential bleeding.

Flush Solution

- Note approximate amount of fluid in the flush solution at least 50 cc of fluid should be present
- Ensure pressure bag is pumped to 300 mm Hg.

Air Embolism

1. Always use closed IV fluid system connected to CVP to prevent entry of air into veins. Always expel the air from the tubing before connecting them to the IV catheter.
2. If any air bubbles enters into the catheter, immediately turn the patient onto his/her left side and adjust the bed to Trendelenburg position. This should help to trap the air bubbles into the atrium and allow it to be absorbed.

Complications

- Catheter-tip embolism or thrombotic embolus
- Bleeding
- Hematomas formation
- Arterial cannulation
- Pneumothorax
- Hemothorax
- Air embolism
- Arrhythmias
- Infection.

Care of Central Venous Line (Nurses Responsibility)

- Always keep 3-ways stopcock capped
- After aspiration of blood, flush line with flushing fluid
- No blood should be visible in central venous line when not in use
- Before applying cap, 3-way connector shall be cleaned with spirit swab

- Lines should be changed after 72 hours
- Lines should be inspected daily for any signs of infection such as redness, edema or any discharge
- Lines should be dressed daily aseptically.

HEMODYNAMIC MONITORING

Hemodynamic studies provide rich information reflecting the earliest changes in the circulatory system. Direct pressure monitoring system diagnosis and manage the critical condition.

Types

Common Types of Monitoring

- Arterial pressure monitoring arterial line
- Pulmonary artery pressure monitoring: Pulmonary artery (PA) catheter, 'Swan-Ganz'
- Pulmonary artery wedge pressure (PAWP)
- Right atrial pressure (RAP) monitoring: RAP/CVP
- Central venous pressure
- Intra-arterial blood pressure monitoring.

Less Common Type of Monitoring

- Left arterial pressure monitoring.

Principles

- Blood pressure = Flow [Cardiac output × Resistance (Lumen size)]
- Circulatory system is continuous circuit
- Liquids flow from areas of higher pressure to lower pressure.

Components of Hemodynamic Monitoring

Arterial catheter is introduced into the appropriate blood vessels or heart chamber; it is connected to the pressure monitoring system that has several components:

- Transducer
- Converse, physiological events into electrical signals (e.g. pressure and temperature)
- An amplifier or monitor, which increase the size of the electrical signals for display on a oscilloscope
- Pick up electrical signals and transmits to display through cable
- Monitor display.

Reliable Measurement

- Pressure monitor kept patent and free of air bubble
- Balance—zero reference (negates atmosphere pressure) in order to ensure system is properly functioning
- Calibration—numerical accuracy
- Nurse check the stopcock is positioned at the level of atrium, this refer to as level phlebostatic (fourth intercostal space, midaxillary line)
- System setup and maintained properly
- A flush system composed of IV solution, which may include heparin.

Pulmonary Artery Pressure Monitoring

The procedure can be carried out in operation theater (OT) or cardiac catheterization room or bedside in critical care area (Box 3.3). Fluoroscopy may be used during insertion to visualize progression of the catheter:

1. A pulmonary artery catheter and pressure monitoring system are used, pulmonary artery catheter are balloon-tipped flow-directed catheter that have distal and proximal lumens.
2. The distal lumen has a port that opens into pulmonary artery; it is used to measure continuous pulmonary artery pressures.

Box 3.3: Nursing care for patient requiring arterial pressure monitoring

Competency statement/Criteria
• Identifies the indications for arterial pressure monitoring • Assembles necessary equipment for insertion of an arterial catheter • Perform Allen test • Assists the physician with the procedure by supporting the patient's hand and dorsiflexing the wrist • Places the air-fluid interface of the transducer system at the level of the cannulated artery, which is usually level with the heart or the phlebostatic axis • Balances or zeros the transducer to atmospheric pressure at least every 4 hour or according to the manufacturer's specifications • Identifies the normal arterial waveform and troubleshoots deviations as necessary • Compares the direct arterial pressure measurements with the indirect sphygmomanometer measurements • Assesses pulse, color, sensation and temperature distal to the insertion site every 2–4 hour • Observes the skin at the site and distally for balancing during irrigation • Changes the flush solution, tubing and dressing according to hospital guidelines, inspects the site for signs of infection • Take blood samples from the arterial catheter using the proximal stopcock • Discontinues the arterial catheter by removing the sutures and holding direct pressure over the site for 5–10 min • Documents all pertinent information

3. The proximal lumen has a port that open into the right atrium, it is used to administer IV medication and fluids or to monitor RAP.
4. A syringe is connected to the hub, which is used to inflate or deflate balloon with air.
5. Thermodilution catheter measures the cardiac output.

Pulmonary Artery Catheter

- Swan and Ganz developed flow-directed pulmonary artery (PA) catheter 1970 (Swan-Ganz is a brand)
- It reflects left heart pressure.

Types

- Four/Five (VIP) lumen
- Continuous cardiac output (CCO)
- Saturation venous oxygen (SvO_2)/CCO
- Right ejection fraction
- The SvO_2 catheter.

Sites

- Subclavian
- Jugular
- Femoral.

Description

- Balloon tipped
- Measures PA systolic, mean and wedge [pulmonary capillary wedge pressure (PCWP), PAWP and pulmonary artery occlusion pressure (PAOP)]
- Multilumen:
  - Proximal [rheumatoid arthritis (RA)]
  - Proximal injectate
  - Distal (PA)
  - Balloon.

Insertion

- Provide explanation and obtain informed consent
- Site usually subclavian or internal jugular
- Incision-guidewire introducer, catheter sheath
- Flush lumens
- Inserted with balloon down selected inflation to get into PA
- Wave form changes as catheter progresses

- Check for proper wedging
- Secure and dress site.

During insertion
- Monitor pressure in each chamber
- Record values
- Assess for complications, dysrhythmias and pneumothorax/hemothorax.

Pulmonary Artery Values

- Normal is 25–10 mm Hg with mean is 15
- Systolic 15–30 mm Hg
- Diastolic 4–12 mm Hg
- The PCWP 6–12 mm Hg.

Diastolic reflects PCWP unless pulmonary hypertension present (mitral valve open during end diastole, therefore open circuit).

Catheter passed into the vena cava and right atrium, in the right atrium the balloon tip is inflated, then passed through tricuspid valve into the right ventricles through pulmonic valve and to the branch of the PA and balloon is deflated when measuring PAWP inflating the balloon tip.

Interpretation

- Increased PA pressure: Volume overload, CHF
- Decreased PA pressure: Volume depletion.

Complications

- Infection
- Dysrhythmias
- Air embolism
- Thromboembolism
- PA rupture
- Pulmonary infarction.

Critical Thinking

1. What nursing intervention can assist in preventing complications associated with PA catheter?
2. Why is a chest X-ray done after the insertion of PA catheter?
3. What symptoms might indicate a pulmonary infarction?

Intra-arterial Monitoring

Indications

- Continuous BP monitoring
- Blood drawing.

Sites

- Radial (Allen test for circulation)
- Brachial
- Femoral.

Equipment

- Pressurized flush solution with transducer
- A line catheter (Angiocath).

Nursing Intervention

- Monitor waveform
- Compare values with cuff
- Arterial line should be more accurate reading
- Check connections in system
- Check site and circulation to extremities
- Set alarm.

Complications

- Air embolism
- Hemorrhage (keep connection tight)
- Thrombosis.

Critical Thinking

1. How much blood should be withdrawn from an A line?
2. What are strategies for blood conservation when withdrawing blood samples?

Right Atrial Pressure

Catheters that Measures Right Atrial Pressure

- Pulmonary artery catheter (proximal port)
- Central line (e.g. triple-lumen catheter)
- Peripherally inserted central catheter (PICC) line.

Measurement

- Measured via pressure system
- Normal value is 0–8 mm Hg
- Recorded as mean value.

Nursing Implications

- Zero level/balance
- Positioning patient
- Respiratory cycle.

Complication of Insertion

- Pneumothorax
- Heart perforation
- Dysrhythmias.

Critical Thinking

1. What assessment should be done during insertion and immediately after insertion?

Chapter 4 Nursing Management of Unconscious Patient

CONSCIOUSNESS

Capable of responding to sensory stimuli awake, alert, aware of one's external environment in part of psyche or mental functioning on which thoughts, ideas, emotions and other matter as content are in complete awareness. A clear state of awareness of self and the environment in which attention is focused are immediate matter as distinguished from mental activity of a subconscious nature.

UNCONSCIOUSNESS

A state of complete or partial unawareness or lack of response to sensory stimuli as a result of hypoxia resulting from respiratory insufficiency or shock from metabolic or chemical brain depressants such as drug, poisons, ketones or electrolytes imbalance or form of brain pathology condition such as trauma, seizures, cerebrovascular accident, brain abscess, hemorrhage, tumor or infection, etc.

Coma

A state of profound unconsciousness characterized by the absence of spontaneous eye movement, response to painful stimuli and vocalization, the person cannot be aroused; coma may be the result of trauma, hematoma, toxic condition, acute infection diseases with encephalitis, vascular disease, poisoning diabetic and intoxication.

Causes of Unconsciousness

- Head injury
- Skull fracture
- Asphyxia
- Fainting
- Concussion
- Compression
- Extremes of body temperature
- Cardiac arrest
- Blood loss
- Cerebrovascular accident
- Epileptic fits

- Infantile convulsions
- Hysteria
- Hypoglycemia
- Hyperglycemia
- Drug overdose
- Hypothermia
- Poisonous substances and fumes.

Clinical Manifestation of Unconsciousness

- Decreased level of consciousness
- Confusion and decreased attention
- Headache
- Sensory motor deficit
- Aphasia
- Visual loss or seizures
- Specific manifestations are related to specific area of brain that is affected.

Diagnostic Procedures

- Lumbar puncture
- Computed tomography (CT)
- Electroencephalography
- Magnetic resonance imaging (MRI).

Laboratory Test

- Blood glucose
- Electrolyte
- Serum ammonia
- Blood urea nitrogen level (BUN)
- Calcium level
- Prothrombin time
- Serum ketones and alcohol.

Pathophysiology

Masses within the brain alter the functioning of the brain in many ways. Masses or lesions may place a pressure on the brain because the brain is encased in the cranium, there is no space within the skull for expanding brain pressure. The pressure slows as blood and cerebrospinal fluid (CBF) flow out of the brain and reduces cerebral function. The level of consciousness and the ability to move purposefully are affected. The pressure reaches the brainstem vitals and respiration is affected.

Initial Assessment

Initial assessment of the comatose patient includes:

- Level of consciousness
- Pattern of respiration
- Pupil size and reactivity
- Deep and superficial reflexes
- Responses to painful stimuli
- Examine ear for ruptured ear drum or otorrhea
- Determination of serum oxygenation, blood alcohol, blood urea nitrogen, ammonia and glucose level if manifestations suggest metabolic disorders
- History from significant others
- Glasgow coma scale assessment.

If available, the history from relatives or ambulance staff will often give all the necessary clues needed to make a provisional diagnosis of the cause of unconsciousness. However, if they are apyrexial, depressed epileptic diabetic that has been unwell recently. Making a diagnosis is important, because it will direct appropriate therapy.

Evaluation

The comatose patient should be physically examined for any helpful signs, such as lumps on the head and non-blanching rashes. The system, which will be examined most intently (and often provides the least information) is the nervous system. There are certain parts of the central nervous system (CNS), which are easy to examine, including the eyes and reflexes, but other information is provided by the posture and muscle tone, and the respiratory pattern. The eyes do give useful information about pupil size and equality, and direction of gaze. A truly comatose patient is deeply unconscious, with no response to pain. However, it is often found that patients are not completely unconscious and so can be categorized onto a point on a 'coma scale.' Here is an example of a simple 5-point scale.

- Fully awake: 1
- Conscious, but drowsy: 2
- Unconscious, but responsive to pain with purposeful movement, e.g. flexion/withdrawal: 3
- Unconscious, but responding to pain by extension: 4
- Unconscious and unresponsive to pain: 5.

This scale gives a simple measure of the degree of unconsciousness, but disregards other information that may be available. The most commonly used complex scale, using three groups of observations, is the Glasgow coma scale, which was originally suggested for the assessment of head injury patients.

Points

Best Motor Response

- Movement in response to command: 6
- Localizes pain: 5
- Withdraws from pain: 4
- Flexes in response to pain: 3
- Extends in response to pain: 2
- No response: 1.

Best Verbal Response

- Fully orientated: 5
- Confused: 4
- Inappropriate words: 3
- Incomprehensible sounds: 2
- No response: 1.

Best Eye Response

- Eyes open spontaneously: 4
- Eyes open to command: 3
- Eyes open in response to pain: 2
- Eyes remain closed: 1.

Continue to Observe

- Airway
- Respirations
- Circulation
- Bleeding.

Emergency Care

Initial Care

Initial care of an unconscious patient include:

1. Clearing the airway immediately and loosing all tight clothing especially around the neck, never move recently injured or unconscious patient without stiff collar until cervical injury diagnostic test determined.
2. Remove and store any artificial denture, these could cause airway obstruction or could be broken and swallowed.
3. Remove any obstruction if present.

4. Place the patient in semi prone or lateral position to facilitate drainage of pulmonary secretion and prevent tongue falling back.
5. Patient airway, ventilation and circulation must be maintained. A nasal or airway may be inserted for a short time or endotracheal intubation.
6. If required patient may be put into ventilator to reduce partial pressure of arterial carbon dioxide ($PaCO_2$).

Immediate Intervention

1. Monitoring the airway, establish an adequate airway and ensure ventilation. Obstruction of the airway is a risk for unconscious patient because the epiglottis and tongue may relax occluding the oropharynx or patient may aspirate vomits or nasopharyngeal secretions.
2. Elevate the head of the bed to a 30° angle, helps to prevent aspiration of secretions.
3. The patient requires frequent suctioning and oral hygiene.
4. The nurse must maintain the patency of endotracheal tube or tracheostomy.
5. Monitor airway, breathing and circulations (ABCs) and maintain ventilator settings.
6. Chest physiotherapy and postural drainage are initiated to promote pulmonary hygiene.
7. Frequent and systematic, and objective nursing assessment, including neurological status is essential.
8. Periodically assess the entire body observing laceration, bruises, ulcerations, fractures, dislocation and contractures also note skin closure, texture and temperature.
9. Inspect dressing frequently for purulent or bloody drainage.
10. Following intervention appropriate for all unconscious patient regardless of the cause of unconsciousness/coma as under.
11. Easy access to:
    - Ambu bag with valve and mask or intubation (and tracheostomy) equipment
    - Neurological observation chart and tray containing vital signs and emergency medication.

Nursing Management

Nursing management of unconscious patient are listed in Table 4.1.

Table 4.1: Nursing management

Nursing action	Rationale
The room or ward area should be warm and well lit and adequately ventilated with easy access to patient	To facilitate rapid assessment of the patient at a glance. For example: • Color of the skin: Cherry red after carbon monoxide poisoning, frost in uremia, yellow in hepatic failure, blue in cyanosis • Smell: Alcohol, toasted almonds after cyanide poisoning, the sickly sweet of diabetic ketoacidosis
Nurse the patient in bed with a firm base, a detectable bed head (and cot as needed)	To facilitate cardiac massage and intubation if required, to prevents self-injury to the restless patient
Place patient in lateral or semiprone position (if condition allow) *Note:* If a patient's in uries or other conditions prevent him/her from being nursed from side to side or prone, then a nurse should be in attendance at all times, while there is an airway hazards	To prevent occlusion of airway by tongue falling back against the pharyngeal wall; to encourage drainage of respiratory secretions and prevent of same in throat
Pass nasogastric tube if indicated	To empty gastric contents, paralytic ileus occurs frequently in the unconscious patient and this may lead to aspiration of stomach contents
Place the patient body as follows: • Head: Put the patient's head on pillow • Trunk: Keep the spine straight and place the pillow at the patient's back • Upper limbs: Bring the upper most arm forward in front of the patient bend the elbow slightly, but keep the wrist extended, support the arm on a pillow and bring the bottom arm alongside the face facing upwards • Lower limbs: Flex the upper most leg and bring it forward and support it in pillows keep the lower leg extended straight and in line with the spine; make sure the patients uppermost leg does not rest on the lower leg • Consult with physiotherapist and anesthetist about positioning exercise to enhance pulmonary function	To promote comfort and maintain proper alignment of the body To prevent edema by inappropriate pressure on venous flow To prevent internal rotation of the hip To avoid pressure ulcer Optimal respiratory function and gaseous exchange

Contd...

Contd...

Nursing action	Rationale
• Institute passive physiotherapy exercise and observe color, temperature and pulses of limbs • Apply antiembolism stockings as ordered	To prevent deep vein thrombosis formation to recognize early signs of limb deformity To aid venous return to the heart
Remove all dental prosthesis and note loose teeth, bleeding gums, etc. Clean patient nostrils, insert an airway (either oral or nasal) as appropriate	To obtain and maintain clear airway
Perform neurological assessment as frequently as patient condition dictates	To note changes in condition and act on changes as appropriate
Strict asepsis must be maintained when carrying out procedures involving puncture site of cannula or sterile end of intravenous infusion sets	To prevent infection, local or systemic
Maintain feeding regime either by nasogastric tube or parental feeding	To maintain metabolic status To prevent weight loss
Call the patient by name, introduce yourself, explain each procedure before starting, talk to the patient, tell the patient data, time, etc.	Hearing often remains intact in the unconscious patient to prevent sensory deprivation
Touch the patient gently and describe boundaries and environment, e.g. place patient hand on the bed, side blankets, lockers and explain what each item is describe the room environment	Through touch, individuals establish and maintain their body boundaries and relationships with others, and their environment, being denied opportunities to touch can impair physiological, psychological and social development
Give the patient daily bath or as required	To ensure patient skin is kept clean, dry and supple
Carry out eye care, the eye may be cleansed with cotton balls, moistened with sterile normal saline to remove debris and discharge	The blink reflex is absent during unconsciousness or the patient eye's may be open all the time this may lead to corneal drying, irritation and ulceration
Carry out mouth care, inspect for dryness, infection and presence of crusting oral care is given a thin coating of petroleum on the lips	To maintain a clean moist condition, to prevent the accumulation of oral postnasal secretion and to prevent the development of mouth infections
Observe the patient for signs of bladder distensions or urinary by	To prevent urinary complication In males an external sheath may be used and

Contd...

Contd...

Nursing action	Rationale
pass of catheter urinary catheterization read catheter information carefully perform regular catheter care	catheterization may be done immediately if necessary To prevent over distention To prevent infection
Carry out bowel care inspect for bowel care, inspect for bowel distention and sounds	To prevent constipation and/or diarrhea
Change the patient position every 2 hour or as required	To relieve pressure areas To prevent respiratory complications for allowing postural drainage and for each side of the chest, to receive a period free of compression by body weight when it can expand fully
Keep relatives and friends informed of changes in the patient's conditions and involve them in caring for the patient as appropriate	To help family and friends, adjust to the situation and depending on prognosis, and to prepare anticipated grief

Nursing Precaution

Nursing precaution to manage unconscious patient are listed in Table 4.2.

Table 4.2: Nursing are precaution

Problem	Cause	Suggested action
Restlessness/ Confusion	A degree of restlessness may indicate that the patient is regaining consciousness during this time there may be a clouding of consciousness with confusion, aggression uncooperative behaviors and disorientation; restlessness may also indicate brain damage cerebral anoxia (when there is a partially obstructed airway) a full bladder, or bowel pain or discomfort	Ascertain, where possible, the cause of the discomfort and rectify as appropriate, summon help if the patient becomes aggressive or violent, ensure the patient does not inflict self-injury
Seizures	An unconscious patient is a potential candidate for seizures	Maintain a clear airway; protect the patient from self-injury observe the patient during the seizures; record observations on the chart; administer prescribed drugs

Contd...

Contd...

Problem	Cause	Suggested action
Cerebrospinal fluid leakage through nose or ears	The unconscious patient is prone to develop ear or nose leakage (due to head injury) or damage due to medulla oblongata	Do not plug the ear, nose collect fluid for laboratory investigation
Vomiting	The unconscious patient is prone to paralytic ileus	Maintain clear airway, keep stomach empty
Distended bladder	Urinary catheterization if required	Keep ready the catheterization set

Special Consideration

- Padded side rails are provided and raised at all times
- Physical restrain should be avoided as possible
- Fluid are never given by mouth to the patient who cannot swallow
- The patient is assessed for hydration status of the mucous membrane are examined and the skin is assessed for tissue turgor
- Maintaining correct body position so that contracture are prevented
- Use of splint or foot board aid in prevention of foot drops.

Chapter 5 Preparation of Drug Infusion

PREPARATION

Responsibility

Nurse in-charge of the case is responsible for preparation of drug infusion. Preparation of drug infusion is the responsibility of nurse in-charge.

Prepare Infusion as per the Instruction

1. Dobutamine/Dopamine/Lignocaine:
   - Add 3 mg of drug × body weight in kg/50 mL of fluid
   - Add 6 mg of drug × body weight in kg/100 mL of fluid.
2. Adrenaline/Isoprenaline/Noradrenaline/Phenlylephrine:
   - Add 0.03 mg of drug × body weight in kg/50 mL of fluid
   - Add 0.6 mg of drug × body weight in kg/100 mL of fluid.

Other Instructions

1. Always mark the name of the drug clearly on the burette or syringe and point of attachment of infusion with the three way stopcock near the patient.
2. Always mark the strength of the drug on the burette or syringe.
3. In case exact amount of drugs calculated, above could not be added to the infusion mark, the multiple amount of drug used as 'strength' on the burette.
4. Always prepare infusion after wearing gloves and face mask on a trolley or tray covered by sterile towel.

EMERGENCY/CRASH TROLLEY AND DRUG TRAY

Responsibilities

The following critical areas are handled by nurse in-charge.

Drug Tray

Under mentioned drugs should be kept readily available at patients' bed side in concentration given against each drug in prefilled syringes, when indicated:

1. **Adrenaline:**
   - 1 mg in 1 mL (1:1,000)
   - 1 mg in 10 mL
   - 5 mg in 5 mL, 1 mg/mL.

2. **Atropine:**
   - 1 mg in 1 mL
   - 1 mg in 10 mL (diluted).
3. **Calcium chloride:** 1 g in 10 mL (10%).
4. **Lignocaine:** 200 mg in 10 mL (2%).
5. **Sodium bicarbonate:** 1 mEq/mL (25 mL).
6. **Nalbuphine:** 1 mg/mL (20 mL).
7. **Morphine:** 1 mg in 10 mL.
8. **Pancuronium:** 4 mg in 10 mL.
9. **Midazolam:** 1 mg/1 mL (5 mL).
10. **Atracurium:** 10 mg/mL (2.5 mL).

Five extra ampules or vials of the above drugs will also be present in the tray.

DRUG INFUSION GUIDELINES

Adrenaline Infusion (Table 5.1)

Table 5.1: Adrenaline infusion

Adrenaline 3 mg/50 mL (60 µg/mL)		
Syringe driver	• Use adrenaline 1 mg in 1 mL ampules • Dilute 3 mg (3 mL) up to 50 mL with normal saline or 5% dextrose • Commence at 2 µg/min (2 mL/h) and adjust rate according to clinical response	
50 mL syringe	*Dose range*	*Rate of infusion through syringe driver*
	2 µg/min	2 mL/h
	5 µg/min	5 mL/h
	10 µg/min	10 mL/h
	20 µg/min	20 mL/h
Adrenaline 3 mg/500 mL (6 µg/mL)		
Infusion pump	• Use adrenaline 1 mg in 1 mL ampules • Dilute 3 mg (3 mL) with normal saline or 50% dextrose • Commence at 2 µg/min (20 mL/h) and adjust rate according to clinical response	
500 mL bag	*Dose range*	*Rate of infusion through infusion pump*
	2 µg/min	20 mL/h
	5 µg/min	50 mL/h
	10 µg/min	100 mL/h
	20 µg/min	200 mL/h

Indications

Management of shock (after hypovolemia has been excluded), status asthmaticus.

Precautions and Side Effects

1. Correct hypovolemia.
2. Administer via central venous line or into a large peripheral venous line (extreme caution with concentrated solution in a peripheral vein because the risk of vasoconstriction, ischemic pain and local necrosis).
3. Monitor electrocardiogram (ECG) and blood pressure (BP) closely.
4. Side effects include pulmonary edema, arrhythmias, tachycardia, myocardial ischemia, anxiety, palpitations, hypertension and peripheral ischemia.

Special Notes

1. Infusion should be titrated to achieve desired clinical endpoint, e.g. systolic BP 80–100 mm Hg. Usual range between 1 and 70 μg/min in adult.
2. Double strength solution may be needed on some occasions should only be administered on a doctor accompanied flight unless under exceptional circumstances (with standing order).

Amiodarone Infusion (Table 5.2)

Table 5.2: Amiodarone infusion

Amiodarone 600 mg/50 mL (12 mg/mL)			
Syringe driver	• Use amiodarone 150 mg in 3 mL ampules • Dilute 600 mg (12 mL) up to 50 mL with 5% dextrose • In an emergency give 150–300 mg over 1–2 min, otherwise commence with a loading dose of 5 mg/kg over 20 min [e.g. 350 mg (29 mL) for a 70 kg adult] • Follow this with an infusion of 0.4–0.7 mg/kg/h for the next 24 h [e.g. 28–50 mg/h (2.3–4.2 mL/h) for a 70 kg adult]		
50 mL syringe	*Dose range*	*Rate of infusion through syringe driver*	
	Loading dose over 20 min (70 kg patient)	350 mg (29 mL)	87 mL/h for 20 min only
	Maintenance dose (70 kg patient)	28–50 mg/h	2.3–4.2 mL/h
Amiodarone 600 mg/500 mL (1.2 mg/mL)			
Infusion pump	• Use amiodarone 150 mg in 3 mL ampules • Dilute 600 mg (12 mL) up to 500 mL with 5% dextrose		

Contd...

Contd...

Amiodarone 600 mg/500 mL (1.2 mg/mL)			
Infusion pump	• In an emergency give 150–300 mg over 1–2 min otherwise commence with a loading dose of 5 mg/kg over 20 min [e.g. 350 mg (290 mL) for 70 kg adult] • Follow this with an infusion 0.4–0.7 mg/kg/h for the next 24 h [e.g. 28–50 mg/h (23–42 mL/h) for a 70 kg adult]		
500 mL bag	*Dose range*	*Rate of infusion through syringe driver*	
	Loading dose over 20 min (70 kg patient)	28–50 mg/h	23–42 mL/h

Indications

Treatment and prophylaxis of serious arrhythmias refractory to other treatment, including ventricular arrhythmias, atrial tachyarrhythmias and junctional tachycardia.

Precautions and Side Effects

1. Infuse via large or central vein.
2. Contraindicated in second or third degree atrioventricular (AV) block (without pacemaker) and in pregnancy.
3. Caution with use in patients on beta blockers, verapamil or diltiazem (increased risk of bradyarrhythmias) and in patients with thyroid or hepatic disease.
4. Side effects include nausea and vomiting (especially, while loading), headache, dizziness, fatigue, photosensitivity, bradycardia, AV block, torsades de pointes and liver dysfunction.

Special Notes

Should only administered on a doctor accompanied flight unless under exceptional circumstances (with standing order).

Dopamine Infusion (Table 5.3)

Table 5.3: Dopamine infusion

Dopamine 200 mg/50 mL (4,000 μg/mL)	
Syringe driver	• Use dopamine 200 mg in 5 mL ampules • Dilute 200 mg (5 mL) up to 50 mL with normal saline • Commence at a low dose (e.g. 2.5 μg/kg/min) and adjust rate to obtain desired blood pressure and urinary output > 0.5 mL/kg/h (1 mL/kg/h in children)

Contd...

Contd...

Dopamine 200 mg/50 mL (4,000 µg/mL)						
50 mL syringe	*Dose range*	*Rate of infusion (mL/h) through syringe driver*				
	–	40 kg	60 kg	70 kg	80 kg	100 kg
	2.5 µg/kg/min	2	2	3	3	4
	5 µg/kg/min	3	5	5	6	8
	10 µg/kg/min	6	9	10	12	15
Dopamine 200 mg/500 mL (400 µg/mL)						
Infusion pump	• Use dopamine 200 mg in 5 mL ampules • Dilute 200 mg (5 mL) up to 500 mL with normal saline • Commence at a low dose (e.g. 2.5 µg/kg/min) and adjust rate to obtain desired blood pressure and urinary output > 0.5 mL/kg/h (1 mL/kg/h in children)					
500 mL bag	*Dose range*	*Rate of infusion (mL/h) through infusion pump*				
	–	40 kg	60 kg	70 kg	80 kg	100 kg
	2.5 µg/kg/min	15	23	26	30	38
	5 µg/kg/min	30	45	53	60	75
	10 µg/kg/min	60	90	105	120	150

Indications

- Management of shock (where hypovolemia has been excluded)
- Improvement in renal blood in oliguria.

Precautions and Side Effects

1. Hypovolemia must be fully corrected prior to administration.
2. Administer via a central venous line or into a large peripheral venous line (extreme caution with concentrated solution in a peripheral vein because of the risk of vasoconstriction, ischemic pain and local necrosis).
3. Side effects include ectopic beats, tachycardia, angina, palpitations, nausea, vomiting, headache and dyspnea.

Special Notes

1. Low doses (2.5–5 µg/kg/min) are used to improve urinary output; higher doses (5–10 µg/kg/min) have an additional inotropic effect. Doses greater than 10 µg/kg/min are rarely indicated. If additional effects are required adrenaline, noradrenaline or dobutamine are more effective inotropic agents.
2. Most of all patients are not requiring dopamine for a medical escort on board.

Dobutamine Infusion (Table 5.4)

Table 5.4: Dobutamine infusion

	Dobutamine 250 mg/50 mL (5,000 mg/mL)					
Syringe driver	• Use dobutamine 250 mg in 5 mL ampules • Dilute 250 mg (5 mL) up to 50 mL with 5% dextrose • Commence at a low dose (e.g. 2.5 µg/kg/min)					
50 mL syringe	*Dose range*	*Rate of infusion (mL/h) through syringe driver*				
	–	40 kg	60 kg	70 kg	80 kg	100 kg
	2.5 µg/kg/min	2	2	2	2	3
	5 µg/kg/min	4	4	4	5	6
	10 µg /kg/min	5	7	8	10	12
	Dobutamine 250 mg/500 mL (500 µg/mL)					
Infusion pump	• Use dobutamine 250 mg in 5 mL ampules • Dilute 250 mg (5 mL) up to 500 mL with 5% dextrose • Commence at a low dose (e.g. 2.5 µg /kg/min)					
500 mL bag	*Dose range*	*Rate of infusion (mL/h) through infusion pump*				
	–	40 kg	60 kg	70 kg	80 kg	100 kg
	2.5 µg/kg/min	12	18	21	24	30
	5 µg/kg/min	24	36	42	48	60
	10 µg/kg/min	48	72	84	96	120

Indication

Management of shock (where hypovolemia has been excluded), especially cardiogenic shock.

Precautions and Side Effects

1. Hypovolemia must be fully corrected prior to administration.
2. Administer via a central venous line or into a large peripheral venous line (extreme caution with concentrated solution in a peripheral vein because of the risk of vasoconstriction, ischemic pain and local necrosis).
3. Side effects include ectopic beats, tachycardia, angina, palpitations, nausea, vomiting, headache and dyspnea.

Special Notes

1. Stocked by regional hospitals.
2. Predominantly a β-1 stimulant of the myocardium.
3. Infusion should be titrated to achieve desired clinical end point, e.g. systolic BP 80–100 mm Hg. Usually dose range is 2.5–10 µg/min. Discuss with receiving intensive care unit before use.
4. Should only be administered on a doctor accompanied flight.

Glyceryl Trinitrate Infusion (Table 5.5)

Table 5.5: Glyceryl trinitrate infusion

Glyceryl trinitrate 50 mg/mL (1,000 μg/mL)		
Syringe driver	• Use glyceryl trinitrate 50 mg in10 mL ampule • Dilute 50 mg (10 mL) up to 50 mL with 5% dextrose • Commence at 25–50 μg (1.5–3 mL/h) • Increase by 1 mL/h every 5–10 min according to response	
50 mL syringe	*Dose range*	*Rate of infusion through syringe driver*
	50 μg/min	3 mL/h
	100 μg/min	6 mL/h
	150 μg/min	9 mL/h
	200 μg/min	12 mL/h
Glyceryl trinitrate 50 mg/mL (1,000 μg/mL)		
Infusion pump	• Use glyceryl trinitrate 50 mg in 10 mL ampule • Dilute 50 mg (10 mL) up to 100 mL with 5% dextrose, preferably in a glass bottle • Commence at 25–50 μg/min (3–6 mL/h) • Increase by 2 mL/h every 5–10 min according to response	
100 mL bag	*Dose range*	*Rate of infusion through syringe driver*
	50 μg/min	6 mL/h
	100 μg/min	12 mL/h
	150 μg/min	18 mL/h
	200 μg/min	124 mL/h

Indications

- Ischemia, chest pain or unstable angina not adequately relieved by oral, sublingual or transdermal nitrates
- Acute left ventricular failure
- Acute hypertension.

Precautions and Side Effect

1. Up to 80% of active agent may be absorbed by giving sets or intravenous (IV) fluids bags absorption increases with increased concentration and increased exposure time to the plastic. Plastic syringes and minimum volume tubing reduce absorption, but the dose may still need to be gradually increased. Use clinical response rather than calculated dose to get a dose that is appropriate for the patient.
2. Headache is common, other CNS effects can include restlessness, dizziness apprehension, vomiting. Cerebrovascular system (CVS) side effects include hypotension, reflex tachycardia, palpitations and circulatory collapse.

3. Usual starting dose is 50 μg/min, but some patients, particularly those with low BP or pulmonary edema, may require a lower starting dose.

Noradrenaline Infusion (Table 5.6)

Table 5.6: Noradrenaline infusion

Noradrenaline 4 mg/50 mL (80 μg/mL)		
Syringe driver	• Use noradrenaline 1:1,000 (2 mg/2 mL) ampules • Dilute 4 mg (4 mL) up to 50 mL with 5% dextrose • Commence at 1 μg/min (0.8 mL/h) and adjust rate according to clinical response	
50 mL syringe	*Dose range*	*Rate of infusion through syringe driver*
	1 μg/min	1 mL/h
	5 μg/min	4 mL/h
	10 μg/min	8 mL/h
	20 μg/min	15 mL/h
Noradrenaline 4 mg/500 mL (8 μg/mL)		
Infusion pump	• Use noradrenaline 1:1,000 (2 mg/2 mL) ampules • Dilute 4 mg (4 mL/h) and adjust rate according to clinical response • Commence at 1 μg/min (8 mL/h) and adjust rate according to clinical response	
500 mL bag	*Dose range*	*Rate of infusion through infusion pump*
	1 μg /min	8 mL/h
	5 μg/min	37 mL/h
	10 μg/min	75 mL/h
	20 μg/min	150 mL/h

Indication

Management of shock (after hypovolemia has been excluded).

Precautions and Side Effects

1. Correct hypovolemia prior to administration.
2. Administer via a central venous line or into a large peripheral venous line (extreme caution with concentrated solution in a peripheral vein because of the risk of vasoconstriction, ischemic pain and local necrosis).
3. Monitor ECG and BP closely.
4. Side effects include pulmonary edema, arrhythmias, tachycardia, myocardial ischemia, anxiety, palpitations, hypertension and peripheral ischemia.
5. Incompatible with normal saline.

Special Notes

1. Infusion should be titrated to achieve desired clinical endpoint, e.g. systolic BP 80–100 mm Hg. Usual doses is between 1 and 70 µg/min discuss with receiving intensive care unit before use.
2. Should only be administered on a doctor accompanied.

Octreotide Infusion (Table 5.7)

Table 5.7: Octreotide infusion

Octreotide 0.1 mg/50 mL (2 µg/mL)		
Syringe driver	• Use octreotide 0.1 mg/mL in 1 mL ampules • Dilute 0.1 mg (1 mL) up to 50 mL with normal saline or 5% dextrose • Commence at 25 µg/h (10 mL/h)	
50 mL syringe	*Dose range*	*Rate of infusion through syringe driver*
	25 µg/h	12.5 mL/h
	50 µg/h	25 mL/h
Octreotide 0.1 mg/500 mL (0.2 µg/mL)		
Infusion pump	• Use octreotide 0.1 mL ampules • Dilute 0.1 mg (1 mL) up to 500 mL with normal saline or 5% dextrose • Commence at 25 µg/h (125 mL/h)	
500 mL bag	*Dose range*	*Rate of infusion through infusion pump*
	50 µg/h	125 mL/h
	5 µg/min	250 mL/h
	10 µg/min	75 mL/h
	20 µg/min	150 mL/h

Indication

First line control of acute variceal bleeding.

Precautions and Side Effects

1. Blood glucose should be monitored regularly during administration.
2. At low doses (< 100 µg), there are generally no side effects. Greater doses may cause nausea, delayed abdominal pain and diarrhea.
3. A loading bolus of 25–50 µg may be given.
4. Increase infusion rate is 50 µg/h, if bleeding is not adequately controlled.
5. Check ampule concentration carefully. May be supplied to 0.05 mg/mL, 0.1 mg/mL or 0.5 mg/mL.

Isoprenaline Infusion (Table 5.8)

Table 5.8: Isoprenaline infusion

Isoprenaline 1 mg/50 mL (20 µg/mL)		
Syringe driver	• Use isoprenaline hydrochloride 1 mg in 5 mL ampules • Dilute 1 mg (5 mL) up to 50 mL with 5% dextrose • Give 20 µg (1 mL) repeated according to clinical response followed by an infusion at 1–4 µg/min (3–12 mL/h)	
50 mL syringe	*Dose range*	*Rate of infusion through syringe driver*
	1 µg/min	3 mL/h
	2 µg/min	6 mL/h
	4 µg/min	12 mL/h
Isoprenaline 1 mg/500 mL (2 µg/mL)		
Infusion pump	• Use isoprenaline hydrochloride 1 mg in 5 mL ampules • Dilute 1 mg (5 mL) up to 500 mL with 5% dextrose • Give 20 µg (10 mL), repeated according to clinical response, followed by an infusion at 1–4 µg/min (30–120 mL/h)	
500 mL bag	*Dose range*	*Rate of infusion through infusion pump*
	1 µg/min	30 mL/h
	2 µg/min	60 mL/h
	4 µg/min	120 mL/h

Indication

- Bradycardia with poor perfusion
- Most commonly complete heart block.

Precautions and Side Effect

1. Side effects include palpitations, headache, flushing of the skin, angina, nausea, vomiting, tremor, dizziness, weakness and sweating.
2. If heart rate exceeds 80 beats per minute or patient develops chest pain or other arrhythmias decrease dose or temporarily discontinue infusion.
3. Administer with caution in the elderly, diabetic, hyperthyroid, patients with ischemic heart disease or concurrently with other inotropes.
4. Administer via a central venous line or into a large peripheral venous line (extreme caution with concentrated solution in a peripheral vein because of the risk of vasoconstriction, ischemic pain and local necrosis).

Special Notes

1. Required response usually achieved at less than 3 µg/min, though may increase up to 20 µg/min, if necessary to obtain required response.
2. Should only be administered on a doctor accompanied.

REPLACEMENT OF POTASSIUM

Responsibility

The responsibility of nurse in-charge are given below.

To Replace Potassium

- Keep potassium above 4.0 mmol/L
- If less than 2.5 mmol/L replace the deficit
- Calculate deficit by formula:
- 0.4 × Body weight (kg) × (5.0 – Laboratory value)
- Time, give in 30–45 min IV infusion
- Do not give more than 1 mmol/kg in 30 minutes
- Adults should not be given more than 25 mmol in 1 hour
- Always give it through central venous line because it causes pain if given in peripheral line
- Always mark the burette clearly as potassium infusion
- Always give potassium through syringe pump/drip counter/dial—a flow, which could give higher accuracy and there is no danger to run the potassium in
- Never give potassium in an uncontrolled drip
- Danger, patient can be killed if potassium is given faster than recommended rate.

Chapter 6

Therapeutic Management of Respiratory System

ACUTE RESPIRATORY DISTRESS SYNDROME

The alveolocapillary membrane become inflamed and damaged either by direct contact with an inhaled irritant or by chemical mediators that is released when systemic injury occurs. Alveoli collapse (atelectasis) and fibrotic changes take place. In combination with edema and atelectasis, reduce gas exchange and result in hypoxia.

Respiratory system is unable to supply the oxygen (O_2) or eliminate carbon dioxide (CO_2) result in respiratory failure. Acute failure may be hypoxemic or ventilatory failure and caused by pulmonary edema, near drowning, adult respiratory distress syndrome (ARDS) or problem such as pneumonia, bleeding into chest or lungs, resulting in central nervous system (CNS) depression to sustain breathing.

Causes

- Pneumonia
- Trauma
- Shock
- Narcotic overdose
- Inhalation of irritants
- Aspiration.

Signs and Symptoms

- Dyspnea
- Respiratory alkalosis
- Labored breathing
- Patient become cyanotic
- Respiratory acidosis.

Laboratory Test

- Arterial blood gases (ABGs)
- Chest X-ray
- Electrocardiography (ECG)
- Blood test.

Medical/Nursing Management

- Assess patient respiratory status
- Monitor patient mental status, including restlessness, confusion and level of consciousness
- Oxygen therapy
- Monitor ABGs
- Assist and monitor intubation and ventilator care
- Administer diuretics as prescribed
- Administer intravenous (IV) fluids as prescribed
- Monitor intake and output
- Monitor O_2 saturation and vital signs
- Monitor/Assist hemodynamic status
- Administer antibiotic as prescribed
- Administer and monitor total parenteral nutrition, if ordered
- Monitor/Report the laboratory result.

PULMONARY EMBOLISM

Pulmonary embolism (PE) is the obstruction of the pulmonary artery that originates somewhere in the venous system. Deep vein thrombosis (DVT) and PE collectively make up the condition. Thrombus formation in the deep vein is usually in the calf or thigh.

Risk Factors

- Trauma
- Major abdominal surgery
- Prolonged immobilization, sitting and standing
- Hypercoagulability
- Increase platelets count
- Prolonged postoperative time
- Advanced age.

Signs and Symptoms

Symptoms depend on size of the thrombus and area of the pulmonary artery occluded by the thrombus. Signs and Symptoms of PE are as follows:

- Sudden substernal pain
- Dyspnea and tachypnea
- Chest pain

- Tachycardia
- Hemoptysis
- Substernal pain
- Pain similar to angina pain
- Anxiety
- Fever
- Cough
- Syncope
- Diaphoresis
- Weak pulse
- Sudden death
- After onset of symptoms, within few hours sudden death may take place.

Diagnostic Study

- Chest X-ray
- Electrocardiography
- Arterial blood gases
- Ventilation/Perfusion scan
- Pulmonary angiography
- Computed tomography (CT) scan.

Medical Management

Pulmonary embolism is medical emergency. Managements are given below:

- Anticoagulation therapy
- Provide 100% O_2, nasal O_2 immediately to relive hypoxemia
- Keep vein open for administration of emergency medication and IV fluids
- Hemodynamic measurement
- Continuous monitoring of ECG
- Monitoring ABGs
- Dobutamine as prescribed to treat hypotension
- Cardiac monitoring continuously
- Digitalis, diuretics, administration as prescribed
- Monitor electrolytes imbalance
- Monitor elimination needs as required
- Careful administration of sedative, if prescribed to reduce anxiety
- Monitor endotracheal intubation, if present
- Monitor and take care if the patient on ventilator
- Use of antiembolic stockings to reduce venous stocking
- Elevating the leg (above the level of heart).

Pharmacological Therapy

1. Anticoagulant therapy, heparin warfarin to manage DVT. Observe for bleeding precaution because major side effect of bleeding anywhere in the body and anaphylactic reaction resulting in shock or death.
2. Initially heparin, a potent anticoagulant medication, is administered via continuous IV infusion.
3. Warfarin sodium (Coumadin), an oral anticoagulant, is used for at least 3–6 months following PE to prevent recurrence and also can use in to prevent risk factors.
4. Heparin never given intramuscularly.

Thrombolytic Therapy

1. Thrombolytic therapy resolves the thrombi or emboli and restore normal hemodynamic functioning, the pulmonary circulation and improving perfusion.
2. Commonly used drugs are:
   - Urokinase
   - Streptokinase
   - Alteplase.

Before thrombolytic therapy is started confirm the laboratory values of the following:

- Partial thromboplastin time (PTT)
- Hematocrit
- Platelet count
- Stop all anticoagulant therapy
- Avoid invasive procedure as much as possible
- Blood transfusion, if required.

Nursing Management

Preventing Thrombus Formation

- Nurse encourages active and passive leg exercise to prevent venous stasis in patient, who required long term bed care
- Explain the patient and family causes leading to DVT and PE
- Assess the patient for respiratory distress
- Continuous monitoring of ECG
- Discuss importance and side effect and precaution, while patient on anticoagulant and thrombolytic therapy
- Avoid use of sharp instruments
- Use soft brush
- Do not take aspirin

- Explain importance of wearing antiembolism socking
- Advise the patient not to sit or lie in bed for prolonged periods, not to cross the legs
- Monitor regularly anticoagulant therapy
- Not to wear constructive clothing
- Catheter, IV and central venous pressure (CVP) should not be left for long period
- Avoid invasive procedure
- Assess extremities for warmth, redness
- Administer analgesics as prescribed
- Monitor pulse oximetry, nebulization therapy
- Manage postural drainage, if required
- Encourage deep breathing exercise.

PLEURISY

Pleurisy is an inflammation of pleura. The most common causes are pneumonia, tuberculosis (TB), chest trauma, pulmonary infraction and neoplasm. The inflammation usually subsides with adequate treatment of primary diseases. The pain of pleurisy is typically abrupt and sharp in onset, and is aggravated by inspiration. Treatment of pleurisy is aimed at treating the underline diseases and providing pain reliefs splinting an affected site may provide relief.

PLEURAL EFFUSION

The accumulation of serous fluid within the pleural space is termed pleural effusion. Accumulation of frank pus (emphysema) or blood (hemothorax). In general, pleural fluid accumulates as a result of either increased hydrostatic pressure or decreased osmotic pressure (transudative effusion as seen in cardiac, liver or renal failure) or from increased microvascular pressure due to disease of the pleural surface itself or injury in the adjacent lung (exudative effusion).

Clinical Assessment

- Insidious onset
- Breathlessness
- Cough and tachypnea
- Absent breath sounds and vocal resonance
- The causes can usually be identified through history, examination and relevant investigation
- A dull sound is heard, when the affected area is percussed
- Lung sounds are decreased or absent.

Diagnosis

- Chest X-ray
- Computed tomography scan
- Ultrasonography (USG) is more accurate than plain X-ray.

Etiology

Transudative effusions may result heart failure, liver disorders or kidney disorders. Exudative effusion more commonly occur with lung cancer, infection or inflammation.

Management

Bedrest is recommended to enhance spontaneous resolution of the effusion. If symptoms are severe, a therapeutic thoracentesis is done to remove the excess fluid from the pleural space and relieve the patient of dyspnea; chest tube might be placed to continuously drain the pleural space.

Pleural Aspiration and Biopsy

Pleural aspiration and biopsy is necessary to sample fluid unless atypical features are present, simple aspiration provides information on the color and texture of fluid and on appearance alone may immediately suggest an empyema or chylothorax.

EMPHYSEMA

Emphysema is a pleural effusion, which contains pus. It is caused by condition such as pneumonia, TB, lung abscesses and infection of surgical wound of chest. A complication of emphysema is fibrothorax. Clinical manifestations are progressive dyspnea, decreased movement of chest wall and pain, develop pleural effusion, fever night sweat, cough and weight loss. A thoracentesis reveals an exudate containing thick pleural material.

Treatment

Treat the cause by sodium restriction, diuretics, chest tube drainage and antibiotics.

OXYGEN ADMINISTRATION

How Body Works?

Every part of body needs O_2 to survive, when there is not enough O_2 cells in body may be damaged or die. When breathe O_2 from the air enters, lungs and then to blood; the blood and O_2 is then pumped by heart throughout the body.

Heart is a hollow muscle about the size of the first. It is in the chest behind the lower part of the breast bone. The heart is a two-sided pump. The right side of the heart receives blood from the body and sends it through the lungs, where waste, i.e. CO_2 is removed and fresh O_2 is added. The left side of the heart receives the oxygenated blood from the lungs and sends it through large vessels (arteries) to the rest of the body. With each beat of the heart, blood rushing through the arteries creates a pulse that you can feel. The pulse varies according to the age, fitness and level of activity. Each time of breathing lung fills with fresh air containing O_2. When breathe out, waste, e.g. CO_2 is removed. The air that enters into the lung contains about 21% O_2. Air that breathes out contains about 16% O_2 and about 5% CO_2. So, the air breathes out still has enough O_2 to help a person, who has stopped breathing.

The brain cells stop functioning very quickly, when O_2 is not available. A person may lose consciousness and stop breathing, if the brain goes without O_2 for 4-6 minutes some parts may be permanently damaged. The O_2 transport system consists of the lungs and cardiovascular system. Delivery depends on the amount of O_2 entering the lungs (ventilation), blood flow into the lungs and tissue (perfusion) rate of diffusion and O_2 carrying capacity. Chemical regulation, maintains appropriate rate and depth of respiration, based on changes in the blood's CO_2, O_2 and hydrogen (H) concentration.

Factors Affecting Oxygenation

Physiological Factors

Any cardiopulmonary disorders affect the O_2 demand of the body, anemia, any infection, pregnancy, toxic inhalant, high altitude, dehydration and pulmonary disease.

Developmental Factors

Infants and children are risk for upper respiratory tract infection, unhealthy diet, lack of exercise, stress and substance abuse.

Lifestyle Factors

Acquiring healthy behavior reduces the risk for developing respiratory problems. Malnourished children experience respiratory problems; children who are obese, increasing CO_2 load. They are encouraged to have healthy food practice high in potassium, calcium, fruit, vegetables, protein and fiber-rich diet. Physical exercise program has many benefits.

Environmental Factors

The environment also influences oxygenation, pollution, dust and airborne fibers creating lung diseases.

Oxygen Therapy

A deficiency of O_2 leads to a lowered O_2 tension of blood plasma.

Indications for Administering Oxygen

- Correct hypoxemia (anoxemia)
- Increase the O_2 tension
- Restore the oxyhemoglobin in the red blood cells.

Oxygen given in higher concentration than it present in the air. Usually, it is given in concentrations from 40 to 60%. Although, even 100% may be given through the face mask technique. Oxygen should be warmed to room temperature and humidified before it is given to prevent chilling of the child and drying of secretions in the respiratory tract.

Method of Oxygen Administration in Children

Oxygen can be administered by following methods.

Oxygen mask: This can be simple face mask, venture mask or partial rebreathing mask, permits easy access to the child mobility of the child and high consistent flow rate of O_2. Children may not cooperate when this technique is used.

Nasal cannula: It is a simple, comfortable device for delivering O_2 to client. The two tips of the cannula about 1.5 cm (0.5 inch) long, protrude from the center of a disposable tube and are inserted into the nostrils. O_2 is delivered via the cannula with a flow rate up to 5–6 L/min. Higher flow rates dry airway mucosa and do not increase inspired O_2 concentration. The nurse must know what flow rate produces a given percentage of fraction of inspired oxygen (FiO_2), these O_2 percentage will vary, depending on the rate and depth of the client breathing (Table 6.1).

A nasal cannula is an effective mechanism for O_2 delivery. It allows the client to breathe through the mouth or nose, is available for all age groups and is adequate for short-term or long-term use. Cannula is inexpensive, disposable, generally comfortable and easily accepted by most clients. Checklist for application of nasal cannula is given in Table 6.2.

Oxyhood or face tent: Permits easy access to the child without loss of O_2 and efficient delivery of O_2. Children generally accept an oxyhood without loss of O_2 and efficient delivery of O_2 should not blow directly on the child face. The edges of the hood should not rub against the child's chin, neck or shoulder. Some O_2 hoods may be open at the top.

Table 6.1: Approximate flow rate and inspired oxygen concentration

Flow (L/min)	Concentration (flow)
1	21–24.5%
2	24–28%
3	28–32%
4	32–36%
5	36–40%
6	40–44%

Table 6.2: Performance checklist during application of nasal cannula

Steps	S	U	Comments
Implementation			
Washed hands			
Attached nasal cannula to oxygen (O_2) tubing and to humidified O_2 source			
Adjusted O_2 flow rate to prescribed dosage			
Placed tips of cannula into clients nares and adjusted cannula to clients comfort; allowed sufficient slack on O_2 tubing and secured to clients clothing			
Check cannula every 8 hour, keeping humidification jar filled at all times			
Followed the advice of the physician if arterial blood gases (ABGs) were necessary			
Evaluation			
Reassessed client to determine response to O_2 administration via nasal cannula			
Observed client's nares and ears for skin breakdown			
Checked physician order each shift			
Assessed adequacy of cannula each shift			
Identified unexpected outcomes			
Recording and reporting			
Record in nurses notes respiratory assessment; findings before and during O_2 therapy, method of O_2 therapy, delivery, flow rate, patency cannula, client's response, adverse reaction and any change in physician order			

Invasive method: In this method O_2 given by orotracheal, nasotracheal or tracheostomy route and nasopharyngeal catheter, nasal cannula or prong.

Oxygen tent or canopy: This is comfortable for children beyond the age of infancy, when a child has facial injuries or for any other reason cannot tolerate an O_2 mask, then this method can be used. The tent is first flooded with O_2 and then flow of 4–5 L/min is given. This will maintain a service of 40–50% in the tent. A tent is a most uneconomical and inefficient method of giving O_2 because of leakage, loss of O_2, whenever the tent is opened and a high liter flow needed to provide the required concentration. A cooling mechanism is used to maintain a comfortable temperature level within the tent.

Procedure (Table 6.3)

Table 6.3: Procedure of oxygen therapy

Sl No.	Steps	Rationale
1.	Explain to the client and family, what procedure entails and purpose of oxygen (O_2) therapy	Decreases client's anxiety and O_2 consumption, increases cooperation
2.	Place 'oxygen in use' signs at door at client's room and overhead bed	Provides client and staff safety; O_2 is combustible and can fuel a fire, even from cigarette sparks
3.	Wash hands	Reduces transmission of microorganisms
4.	Attach nasal cannula to O_2 tubing and to humidified O_2 source	Humidification prevents drying of nasal and oral mucous membranes, and airway secretions; humidification might not be used for < 3 min
5.	Adjust O_2 flow rate to prescribed dosage usually between 1 and 6 L/min; observe that water in humidifier is bubbling	O_2 flow rate > 6 L/min, may irritate nasal mucosa
6.	Place tips of cannula into client's nares and adjust elastic headband or plastic slide until cannula fits snugly and comfortably; allow sufficient slack on O_2 tubing and secure to client's cloths	Directs flow of O_2 into client's upper respiratory tract; client is more likely to keep cannula in place, if apparatus fits comfortably
7.	Check cannula in every 8 hour, keeping humidification jar filled at all times, if used	Ensures patency of cannula and O_2 flow, and prevents inhalation of dehumidified O_2
8.	Encourage physician to obtain arterial blood gases (ABGs) 5–10 min after initiating O_2 therapy or changing O_2 flow rate	ABGs provide objective data regarding blood O_2
9.	Wash hands	Reduces transmission of microorganisms
10.	Observe for decreased anxiety, improved level of consciousness and cognitive abilities, decreased fatigue, absence of dizziness, decreased pulse with regular rhythm, decreased respiratory rate, return to normal blood pressure, improved color	Determine that hypoxia is corrected or reduced
11.	Observe clients nares and superior surface of both ears for skin breakdown	O_2 therapy can cause drying of nasal mucosa; pressure on ears from cannula tubing or elastic can cause skin irritation

Contd...

Contd...

Sl No.	Steps	Rationale
12.	Observe pulse oximetry for O_2 saturation	Documents arterial O_2 saturation
13.	Assess adequacy of O_2 flow through nasal cannula each shift	Documents patent nasal cannula
14.	Unexpected outcomes that may occur include client experiences nasal irritation, irritation to posterior surfaces of ear, drying of nasal mucosa, sinus pain and epistasis	One or more of these signs indicates adverse response to method of O_2 delivery

Applying an Oxygen Mask

An O_2 mask is shaped to fit snugly over the client mouth and nose, and is secured in place with a strap. The two primary types of masks are the high- and low-concentration O_2 mask.

A simple face mask is a flexible, cone-shaped device with a metal strip to mold the mask to the nose, an adjustable head strap and multiple exhalation ports. The mask is contraindicated for client, who retains CO_2 such as clients with chronic obstructive pulmonary disease (COPD). A non-breathing mask is a flexible, cone-shaped device with a reservoir bag attached. A one-way flip valve is between the bag and mask to allow for inhalation of O_2 and prevent accumulation of expired CO_2. One-way flap valves cover the exhalation ports to prevent dilution of O_2 with room air. A non-breathing mask is used for severe hypoxia because high O_2 concentrations are obtained. When a flow rate of 10 minutes or more is used, the flow is 80–95%, depending on the client's respiratory rate, depth of respiratory rate and depth of respirations (Table 6.4). The reservoir bag should not collapse inspiration.

A partial rebreathing mask is a flexible, cone-shaped device with a reservoir bag attached. This mask differs from the non-breathing mask in that there are no one-way flip valves between the bag and the exhalation ports. The partial rebreathing bag delivers a flow of 60–90% as with the other reservoir bags, it use is indicated for clients with severe hypoxia.

A venture mask is a cone-shaped device with entrainment ports of various sizes at the base of the mask. The entrainment ports are adjustable to permit regulation of flow from 24 to 50%. This mask is useful, because it delivers a known concentration of O_2 to the client.

The face tent is a shield-like device that fits under the clients chin and sweeps around the face. O_2 concentration of 21–50% may be delivered. When higher O_2 concentration is desired, the flow rate should be set at 10 minutes.

Table 6.4: Approximate flow rate of oxygen face mask

Rate (L/min)	Percentage
5–6	40
6–7	50
7–10	60

Equipment

- Face mask or face tent
- Small bore O_2 tubing (if face tent is used, use large bore aerosol tubing)
- Humidifier
- Sterile water
- Oxygen source
- Flow meter
- Oxygen in use sign.

Assessment, nursing diagnosis and planning are as in the procedure of oxygen inhalation by nasal cannula (Table 6.5) and checklist given in Table 6.6.

Table 6.5: Procedure

Sl No.	Steps	Rationale
Implementation		
1.	Wash hands	Reduce transmission of microorganisms
2.	Attach face mask or tent to appropriate size of oxygen (O_2) tubing	Connects masks or tent to O_2 source
3.	Attach face mask or tent and O_2 tubing to humidified O_2 or gas source	Prevents drying or oral and nasal mucosa, and airway secretions, when compressed gas in used for room air, air should be humidified
4.	Adjust O_2 flow rate to prescribed dosage verify that water in humidifier is bubbling being moistened before delivery to client	Presence of bubbling distilled water in humidifier indicates that O_2 is humidifying
5.	Place face mask or tent on client and adjust to snug, but comfortable fit	Maintains prescribed concentration of inhaled O_2; if mask is too loose O_2 escape
6.	Observe for proper functioning of face mask or tent: • Non-breathing mask: Reservoir bag fill on exhalation and almost collapse on inhalation • Partial rebreathing mask: Reservoir should fill on exhalation and almost collapse on inhalation • Venture mask: Percentage of flow of O_2 should correlated with flow rate • Face tent: Mist should always be present	Ensures that specialized face masks are working properly
7.	Observe for moisture in reservoir bags or large bore O_2 tubing face tent is used; remove water from bag or tubing and discard; do not drain reservoir bag or tubing into humidifying device	

Table 6.6: Checklist for applying an oxygen mask

Sl No.	Steps	Comments
Implementation		
1.	Washed hands	
2.	Attached face mask to appropriately sized oxygen (O_2) tubing	
3.	Attached O_2 tubing to humidified O_2 or gas source	
4.	Adjusted O_2 flow rate to prescribed dosage and verified that water in humidifier was bubbling	
5.	Placed face mask or tent on client and adjusted to snug comfortably fit	
6.	Observed for proper functioning of non-breathing mask partial rebreathing mask; Venturi mask or face tent	
7.	Observed for presence of moisture in reservoir bag or O_2 tubing	
8.	Assessed humidity source every 4 hour and changed container every 24 hour	
9.	Observed for pressure necrosis with tightly fitting mask every 2 hour	
10.	Followed up with verifying need for arterial blood gases (ABGs)	
11.	Checked physician order every 4 hour	
12.	Observed for gagging, vomiting and removed mask when necessary	
13.	Washed hands	
Evaluation		
1.	Reassessed client to determine response to administration of O_2 by nasal cannula	
2.	Observed the client's nose and ears for skin breakdown	
3.	Identified unexpected outcomes	
Recording and reporting		
4.	Recorded in nurses notes respiratory assessment findings before and during O_2 therapy, method of O_2 delivery, flow rate, patency of airway, client response any adverse reactions or side effects, change in physician's orders	

Safety Alert

Oxygen in high concentration has a great combustion potential and readily fuels fire. Safety instructions are the following:

1. Place an 'oxygen in use' sign on the client door and in the client room.
2. Keep O_2 delivery system away from any open flames.
3. No smoking should be allowed on the premises.
4. When using O_2 cylinder secure them, so that they will not fall over.
5. Check that all electrical equipment in the room/ward is functioning properly grounded. An electrical spark in the presence of O_2 can result in a serious fire.
6. Check the O_2 cylinder level of portable tanks before transporting a client to ensure that there is enough O_2 in the cylinder.
7. In hospital, O_2 cylinder usually connects the regulator to the O_2 source.

Nursing Care (Table 6.7)

Table 6.7: Provided nursing care for the patient requiring oxygen therapy

Sl No.	Competency statement/Criteria	Remarks
1.	Identifies the indications for oxygen (O_2) therapy	
2.	Assembles the necessary equipment for O_2 therapy	
3.	Identifies the different devices for O_2 administration: • Low flow systems: – Nasal cannula – Simple face mask – Partial rebreathing mask • High flow systems: – Venture mask – Tracheostomy collar – Face tent	
4.	Assesses the effectiveness of O_2 therapy	
5.	States the safety precautions associated with patients suffering from chronic obstructive pulmonary disease (COPD)	
6.	Documents all pertinent information	

NURSING ASSESSMENT OF RESPIRATORY SYSTEM

Nursing History

The history collection and recording is detailed in Box 6.1.

Box 6.1: History collection

Demographic data

Name of the patient: .... Inpatient No.: ....
Age: .... Gender: ....
Marital status: .... Nationality: ....
Language spoken: .... Religion: ....
Occupation: .... Home town/City: ....
....
Education: .... Income: ....
Date of admission: .... Treatment received on arrival to hospital:
....
Provisional diagnosis: .... Name of the doctor who is treating the patient: ....
Unit: ....

Reason for visit: ....
When did the symptoms start? ....
General state of health: ....
Was the onset sudden or gradual? ....
How often the problem occurs? ....
Has the problem occurred before? ....
Document the progression of the first manifestation: ....

Chief complaint

History of present illness

Ask any or all of the following as appropriate and write a summary:

- Rely on objective testing (laboratory values)
- Breathing pattern changed
- Unexplained restlessness or irritability
- Dyspnea (shortness of breath)
- Wheezing
- Pleuritic chest pain
- Tachycardia
- Cough
- Sputum production
- Hemoptysis
- Voice change
- Cyanosis
- Diaphoresis
- Decreased urinary output

Respiratory history

Assessment

What type of breathing problems are you having? ....
Describe the problem you are having with your heart: ....
Does it occur a specific time of the day, during or after exercise, or all the time ....
....

Contd...

Contd...

How has your breathing pattern changed? ....
Are you having sputum with coughing? Is the different? ....
Are you having any chest pain? Does the pain occur with breathing? ....
When did you notice your sputum change in color and amount? ....
Have you been exposed to cold or flu? ....

Breathing pattern changes related to activities: ....

Cigarette smoking history
Are you smoking? Yes/No
If yes, how many cigarette each day? ....
Since how long? ....
Are you interested in stopping? Yes/No
Have you ever smoked any drugs? Yes/No
Breathlessness: Nothing at all/Very slight/Moderate/Severe/Very severe
Are you ever short of breath during exercise/at rest? Yes/No

Past medical history
- Childhood infectious disease: ....
- Immunizations: ....
- Hospitalizations: ....
- Major illness/Infectious disease: ....
- Prior history of rheumatic fever: ....
- Streptococcal infection: ....
- Congenital abnormalities: ....
- Previous hospitalization: ....
- Outcome treatment: ....

Allergies
- Environmental: ....
- Food: ....
- Medication: ....
- Iodine/Contrast dye: ....

Medication history
- Prescription: ....
- Over the counter: ....
- Vitamins: ....
- Herbal: ....
- Bronchodilators: ....
- Nasal spray: ....

Dietary habits
- Restriction advised? Yes/No
- Have you recently lost weight? Yes/No
- Do any particular foods affect your sputum production or breathing? ....

Family history
- Patient received immunization for influenza
- Any of the family member suffered with wheeze/strider/continuous musical sound constant pitch, absent breath sounds/chronic obstructive pulmonary diseases (COPD)/tuberculosis (TB)/lung cancer

Contd...

Contd...

Physical examination

Assessment proceed from head-to-toe

General appearance

- Does the client lie, quietly/restless
- Position: Lie flat/Upright/Erect position
- Respiratory distress/cyanosis/pallor/dyspnea

Patient general level of consciousness

- Client behavior appropriate for surroundings
- Fear/Depression/Anger
- Identify significant others
- Identify time

Vital Signs

Temperature: ....

Respiration: .... breath easily/does the client have to sit up to breath? Yes/No

Weight: ....

Blood pressure: While client, lying sitting .... standing

....

Pulse: Apical .... Radial .... Tachycardia > 100 beats per min .... Bradycardia < 60 beats min/irregular pulse/bounding pulse/absent pulse/tachypnea

Perform a respiratory assessment on admission and at least every 4 hour thereafter *Competency statement/Criteria*	*Remarks*
• Identifies the type of artificial airway and supplemental oxygen device, if present	....
• Inspects the patient's chest for depth, rhythm, rate and symmetry of respirations	....
• Observes the color, amount, consistency and odor of sputum	....
• Palpates the chest and neck area for the presence of subcutaneous emphysema	....
• Auscultate the lungs for equality of breath sounds and presence of adventitious sounds	....
• Assesses chest drainage systems for proper functioning	....
• Documents all pertinent information	

DIAGNOSTIC TESTS

Laboratory Test

1. **Blood test:** Complete blood count, ABG analysis.
2. **D-dimer:** This blood test measures fibrin degradation products, which are present if there is a blood clot in the body. It helps to diagnose the presence of a pulmonary embolism.
3. **Sputum culture and sensitivity:** To identify pathogens present in the sputum. The sensitivity test determines which antibiotics will be effective against those pathogens.

4. **Throat culture:** To determine the presence of viral or bacterial pathogen in the pharynx.
5. **Nasal culture and sensitivity:** To identify flu or other respiratory viruses to be accurate.
6. **Oxygen saturation:** To measure O_2 saturation.
7. **Capnography:** To measure persons exhaled CO_2 level.
8. Chest X-ray.
9. Computed tomography.
10. Ventilation/Perfusion scan.
11. **Pulmonary function studies:** Test is done to determine lung volume, capacity and flow rates.

ARTERIAL BLOOD GAS ANALYSIS

Arterial blood gas analysis is one of the most common tests perform in critical patients, which measure the effectiveness of gas exchange. Blood sample is usually taken from the radial artery in the wrist, by the trained technician or physician or nurse.

Acid-base Balance

The cells of the body functions are best, when the fluids and electrolytes are within a very narrow range. Hydrogen is an another ion that must stay within its normal limits. The amount of hydrogen determines whether a fluid is an acid or base. An acid is a substance that releases a hydrogen ion. The stronger the acid, the more hydrogen ions are released. A base is a substance that binds the hydrogen.

Sources of Acid and Bases

Acids and bases are formed in the body as a part of the normal metabolic processes. Acids are formed as end products of glucose, fat and protein metabolism, they are called fixed acid because they do not change once they are formed a weak acid. Carbonic acid can be formed when the CO_2 resulting from cellular metabolism combines with water, this acid can change to bicarbonate and hydrogen, therefore, it is not a fixed acid.

The extracellular fluid (ECF) maintains a delicate balance between acids and bases. The strength of acids and bases can be measured by pH (negative logarithm of the H^+ concentration). The pH of a solution can vary from 0 to 14, with 7 being neutral, 0-6.99 being acid and 7.01-14 being basic or alkaline. The normal serum pH level is 7.35-7.45, which slightly alkaline.

Control of Acid-base Balance

Body has several ways in which it lives to compensate from changes in the serum pH. Three major mechanisms are used:

1. Cellular buffers: These are the first to attempt a return of the pH to its normal range. For example, cellular buffers are proteins, hemoglobins, bicarbonate and phosphates. These buffers acts as a type of sponge to soak up extra hydrogen ions, if there are too many (too acidic) on release hydrogen ions, if there are not enough (too alkaline).
2. The lungs are the second line of defense to restore normal pH. When the blood is too acidic (pH is decreased), the lungs blow off additional CO_2 through rapid deep breathing. This reduces the amount of CO_2 available to make carbonic acid in the body. If the blood is too alkaline (pH increased), lungs try to conserve CO_2 through shallow respiration.
3. The kidneys are the slowest to respond in changes in serum pH, taking as long as 24–48 hours assist with compensation. The kidney helps in number of ways, including regulating the amount of bicarbonate (base) that is kept in the body. If serum pH lowers, it becomes too acidic. The kidneys reabsorb additional bicarbonate rather than excreting, so that it can help neutralize the acid, if the serum pH increases and becomes too alkaline, the kidneys excrete additional bicarbonate to get rid of the extra base. The kidneys also buffer pH by forming acids and ammonia (base).

Acid-base imbalance is caused by a number of acute and chronic illness or conditions. Patients with diabetes mellitus, COPD and kidney disease frequently develop acid-base imbalance. The pulmonary treatment for each of the imbalances is to manage the underlying the cause, which corrects the imbalance the role of nurse is to identify patients at risk and monitor laboratory test values for significant changes.

The laboratory tests that are used to evaluate acid-base balance are called ABGs, which is a blood test performed using blood from an artery with thin needle and syringe and drawing a small volume of blood. The most common puncture site is the radial artery, but sometimes the femoral artery in groin.

An ABG is a test that measures the arterial oxygen tension (PaO_2), arterial carbon dioxide tension ($PaCO_2$) and acidity (pH) of blood, and addition arterial hemoglobin saturation (SaO_2) can also be determined (Table 6.8). The ABGs testing are mainly used in pulmonology dealing with disease involving respiratory system.

Table 6.8: Normal arterial blood gas values

Features	Values
pH	7.35–7.45
$PaCO_2$*	35–45 mm Hg
HCO_3†	20–30 mEq/L
PaO_2	75–100 mm Hg
Oxygen saturation	96–100%
HCO_3	22–26

*PaCO2, arterial carbon dioxide tension; †HCO_3, bicarbonate; §PaO_2, arterial oxygen tension O_2.

Types of Acid-base Imbalance

The two broad types of acid-base imbalance are:

1. Acidosis:
   - Respiratory
   - Metabolic.

2. Alkaline:
   - Respiratory
   - Metabolic.

Each of these imbalances can occur suddenly, which is called acute imbalance or develop over a long period, referred to as a chronic imbalance.

Disorder of Acid-base Balance

The four general classes of acid-base imbalance are:
1. Respiratory acidosis.
2. Respiratory alkalosis.
3. Metabolic acidosis.
4. Metabolic alkalosis.

Sampling for Analysis of ABGs

Arterial blood gas analysis is usually drawn by a technician, a nurse or physician. Blood is most commonly drawn from radial artery because it is easily accessible, can be compressed to control bleeding and has less risk for occlusion, before drawing the blood from artery heparin is added to syringe to prevent coagulation.

Complications of Procedure

- Bleeding at punctured site
- Blood flow problems at punctured site
- Burning at punctured site delayed bleeding at punctured site
- Feeling of lightheadedness
- Infection.

Nursing Care (Table 6.9)

Table 6.9: Nursing care for patient requiring arterial pressure monitoring

Sl No.	Competency statement/criteria	Remark
1.	Identifies the indications for arterial pressure monitoring	
2.	Assembles necessary equipment for insertion of an arterial catheter	
3.	Perform Allen test	
4.	Assists the physician with the procedure by supporting the patient's hand and dorsiflexing the wrist	
5.	Places the air fluid interface of the transducer system at the level of the cannulated artery, which is usually level with the heart or the phlebostatic axis	

Contd...

Contd...

Sl No.	Competency statement/criteria	Remark
6.	Balances or zeros the transducer to atmospheric pressure at least every 4 hour or according to the manufacturer's specifications	
7.	Identifies the normal arterial wave form and troubleshoots deviations as necessary	
8.	Compares the direct arterial pressure measurements with the indirect sphygmomanometer measurements	
9.	Assesses pulse, color, sensation and temperature distal to the insertion site every 2–4 hour	
10.	Observes the skin at the site and distally for balancing during irrigation	
11.	Changes the flush solution, tubing and dressing according to hospital guidelines, inspects the site for signs of infection	
12.	Draws blood samples from the arterial catheter using the proximal stopcock	
13.	Discontinues the arterial catheter by removing the sutures and holding direct pressure over the site for 5–10 min	
14.	Documents all pertinent information	

PULMONARY FUNCTION TEST

Pulmonary function tests provide information about respiratory function by measuring lung volumes, lung mechanisms and diffusion capabilities of the lungs. Pulmonary function can measure respiratory volumes and capacities (Table 6.10); the result reveals obstructive and restrictive pulmonary disorders. Pulmonary function test is a procedure for determining the capacity of the lungs to exchange O_2 and CO_2 efficiently. There are two general kinds of respiratory function tests. One measures ventilation or ability of the bellows action of the chest and lungs to move gas in and out of alveoli. The other kind measures the diffusion of a gas across the alveolar capillary membrane and the perfusion of the lungs by blood. Efficient gas exchange in the lungs requires balanced ventilation/perfusion ratio, with area receiving ventilation and well-perused, and area receiving blood flow capable of ventilation.

Table 6.10: Pulmonary function parameters

Test	Definition
Inspiratory reserve (IRV)	Maximal volume that can be expired forcefully after normal expiration
Expiratory reserve (ERV)	The maximal volume that can be expired forcefully after normal expiration

Contd...

Contd...

Test	Definition
Forced vital capacity (FVC)	Maximum amount of air expired forcefully after maximum inspiration
Peak expiratory flow rate (PEFR)	Maximum flow of air expired during FVC
Tidal volume (TV)	Air inspired and expired in one breath
Residual volume (RV)	Air remaining in lungs after normal expiration
Functional residual capacity (FRC)	Air remaining in lungs after normal expiration

The patient is asked to use special mouthpiece to blow into a cylinder that is connected to a computer that show the result.

CHEST DRAINAGE

Trauma, disease or surgery can result in air or fluid leaking into the intrapleural space. Small leak are absorbed spontaneously. Occasionally, in emergency situation, a one-way valve is inserted through the chest wall to treat air leaks. This one-way wall allows air to exit from the intrapleural space on expiration, but prevents air from entry during inspiration. No drainage chamber is used with this simple device.

A chest tube is inserted after chest trauma or open chest surgery or in the case of a large intrapleural leak. A closed chest drainage system and possible suction are attached to the chest tube to promote drainage of air and fluid. Lung expansion occurs as the fluid or air is removed. The location of the chest tube indicates the type of drainage expected. Apical and anterior chest tube placements removal of air, which is necessary in the case of a pneumothorax, because air raises chest tubes are placed high, allowing evacuation air from the intrapleural space and allowing the lung to re-expand. A mediastinal chest tube is placed just below the sternum and is connected to the drainage system. This tube drains blood or fluid, preventing its accumulation around the heart.

A variety of disposable commercial chest drainage systems are available. The single bottle system is used primarily in the treatment of pneumothorax. It allow air from the pneumothorax to bubble out of the water seal and escape through the air outlet preventing air from re-entering the intrapleural space. It is not recommended for the evacuation of fluid because drainage would raise the level of the water seal liquid. One bottle commercial systems are available. However, most hospitals prefer to purchase a two- or three-chamber system, because it drains both hemothorax and pneumothorax effectively.

Two-chamber Water Seal System

One expiration, fluid or air is forced out of the intrapleural space and by gravity or suction is pulled down the chest tube into drainage collection chamber. Upon entering the drainage collection chamber, this fluid or air displaces the air present in the chamber by pushing it through the water seal and out of the system into the atmosphere.

Three-chamber Water Seal System

If suction is to be used the two-chamber water seal system is set up with the suction control chamber added. A prescribed amount of sterile fluid is poured into the suction control chamber, which is then attached to a suction source by tubing. The suction is turned up until the water in the suction control bottle exhibits a continuous gentle bubbling. This provides the prescribed amount of suction (negative pressure).

If the suction source delivers more negative pressure than the suction control chamber, water level allows there is no danger, because atmospheric air is pulled into the suction control chamber through an inlet, causing the excess suction to dissipate. The extra air pulled into the chamber causes vigorous bubbling, if this occurs, the suction source setting needs to be lowered to reduce noise and evaporation of the fluid. No bubbling indicates that no suction is exerted in the system. The suction setting should be raised to restore gentle bubbling.

Guidelines (Box 6.2)

Box 6.2: Chest drainage system guidelines

- Observe the water seal for intermittent bubbling from its 'U' tube or a rise and fall of fluid that is synchronous with respirations, constant bubbling in the water seal or a sudden unexpected stoppage of water seal activity is considered abnormal
- After 2–3 day, tidling or bubbling on expiration is expected to stop, indicating that the lung has re-expanded
- Know the type and amount of expected chest tube drainage
- Know the expected color of the drainage
- In the water seal system, observe for constant gentle bubbling in the suction control chamber when it connected to suction
- Add sterile water or saline to the water seal chamber, so that the U tube is submerged 2.5 cm or1 inch below the surface of the fluid; document in the nurses' notes
- A sudden decrease in the amount of chest tube drainage can indicate a possible clot or obstruction in the chest tube
- A sudden increase of more than 100 mL of drainage can indicate fresh bleeding from the thorax
- Set water seal or disposable system upright; encourage client to cough and deep breath, document in nurses' note
- Any changes, notify the physician

Nursing Care (Table 6.11)

Table 6.11: Nursing care for clients with chest tube connected

Sl No.	Assessment	Remark
1.	Obtain informed consent	
2.	Explain procedure to the patient	
3.	Gathered necessary equipment and supplies	
4.	Wash hand	
5.	Prepared prescribed drainage system	
6.	Correctly tapped all connections and checked system for patency	
7.	Turned off suction source and unclamped drainage tubing before connecting client to system	
8.	Positioned client correctly	
9.	Assisted physician in giving anesthetic medication	
10.	Assisted physician in connecting drainage system	
11.	Taped the tube connection between the chest and drainage tubes	
12.	Assessed patency of air vents in system	
13.	Coiled and secured excess tubing on matters next to client	
14.	Promoted drainage by correctly adjusting tubing to hang in straight line from matters to drainage chamber	
15.	Milked chest tube as necessary	
16.	Assisted client to comfortable position	
17.	Disposed soiled material	
18.	Removed gloves and washed hands	
19.	Checked chest tube insertion site and dressing	
20.	Checked chest tube drainage output at appropriate time intervals	
21.	Recorded client compliance to coughing, deep breathing	
22.	Follow-up activities: • Locate the source of external air leak, correct situation if is in the chest drainage system, notify physician and document, the nurse should immediately reinforce the dressing to make it as occlusive as possible • Monitor vital signs and mark drainage in write on column at 15–30 min • Correct kink occlusion or leaks in tubing, remove occlusion to air vent • Set water seal or disposable system upright; encourage client to cough and deep breath document • Make sure that the client is not lying on the drainage tubing and that it is not depressed or kinked	

Nursing Responsibility (Box 6.3)

Box 6.3: Nursing responsibility while removing chest tubes

- Identify lung expansion
- Clamp chest tube 12–24 hour before removal as per instruction by the doctor
- Administer premedication as prescribed
- Assisted client to correct position and support the client, while removing dressing and suture
- Ask the client to take deep breath and hold it or exhale completely
- Remain with client, while physician pulled out chest tube and applied occlusive dressing
- Assist client for comfortable position
- Remove article from bedside
- Washed hands
- Document the procedure

Removal of Chest Drains

Responsibility

The responsibility of a patient goes to nurse in-charge.

Removing Drains

While removing the drains ensure that:

- There is no drainage for last 2–3 hours (especially after change of posture and physiotherapy)
- Drains are removed in the presence of doctor or senior intensive care unit (ICU) nurse
- Patient be given prior analgesics
- It is carried out by two persons, so that sutures around incision are immediately tightened to prevent pneumothorax
- Aseptic dressing must be done afterwards
- X-ray must be repeated after removal of drains.

DEEP VEIN THROMBOSIS AND THROMBOEMBOLISM PROPHYLAXIS

Responsibility

Nurse in-charge of ICU.

Prophylactic Treatment

Following will receive prophylactic treatment:

- After surgery for more than 2 hours
- After orthopedic and neurosurgical patients

- Patients with prior history of myocardial infarction (MI), ischemic heart disease (IHD), diabetes mellitus (DM) and valvular heart disease
- Patient on anticoagulant therapy
- Patients requiring prolonged bedrest or more than 3 days
- Patients with increased risk factors such as advanced age, obesity, varicose veins, previous DVT, thrombophilia, cancer, heart failure, estrogen therapy and immobility
- Mechanical prophylaxis includes graduated elastic compression stockings (GECS) and international pneumatic compression (IPC)
- Drug prophylaxis includes low-dose unfractionated heparin (UFH), low-molecular-weight heparin (LMWH) and warfarin
- Mechanical prophylaxis given to those patients, who are at increased risk of bleeding or deranged coagulation profile such as head injury and severe sepsis.

PNEUMOTHORAX

Pneumothorax is an entry of air into the pleural space, air in the chest and lungs or visceral pleura is breached or negative pressure in pleura is not maintained.

Types of Pneumothorax

- Simple pneumothorax
- Traumatic pneumothorax
- Tension pneumothorax
- Spontaneous pneumothorax
- Open pneumothorax.

Simple Pneumothorax

Simple pneumothorax occurs as air enters the pleural space through rupture on the surface of the lung. A spontaneous pneumothorax occurs in absence of trauma due to rupture of air-filled bleb, allowing air to enter in pleural cavity.

Traumatic Pneumothorax

Traumatic pneumothorax may occur due to blunt trauma, e.g. rib fracture or invasive thoracic procedure. Traumatic pneumothorax often accompanied by hemothorax (collection of blood in the pleural space) and also hemopneumothorax after major trauma.

Tension Pneumothorax

Tension pneumothorax occurs when air enters the pleural space, but cannot escape with each breath; tension (positive pressure) is increased. This causes lung to collapse and the heart. Both respiration and respiratory functions are compromised resulting decreased cardiac output.

Spontaneous Pneumothorax

If no injury is present, the pneumothorax is considered spontaneous pneumothorax. This occurs mostly in tall and thin individual, patient with underlying lung disease, weakened lung tissue from lung cancer can lead to pneumothorax.

Open Pneumothorax

If air can enters and escape through the opening in the pleural space, it is considered an open pneumothorax.

Signs and Symptoms

- Pain
- Chest discomfort
- Anxious
- Dyspnea and air hunger
- Tachypnea
- Increased use of accessory muscles
- Central cyanosis.

Assessment

- Tracheal alignment
- Expansion of the chest
- Breath sounds
- Air hunger
- Agitation
- Increased hypoxemia
- Hypotension
- Tachycardia
- Diaphoresis.

Medical/Nursing Management

- Stopping the flow of air through the opening in the chest wall
- Chest tube is inserted near the second intercostal space
- Chest tube is connected to water seal drainage to remove air and fluid
- If hemothorax insert large diameter catheter and suction is applied
- Pressure dressing is applied
- Needle aspiration (thoracentesis)

- High concentration oxygen therapy
- Monitoring oxygen saturation by pulse oximetry
- Condition prolonged surgery may be required
- Re-establish the negative pressure and expand the lungs by removing the air and fluids.

HEMOTHORAX

Presence of blood in the pleural space, result of traumatic injury, lung cancer and pulmonary embolism.

Signs and Symptoms

- Dyspnea
- Chest pain
- Tachypnea and tachycardia
- Hypoxemic
- Bradycardia.

Laboratory Test

- Ultrasound (US)
- Chest X-ray
- Computed tomography scan
- Arterial blood gas.

Medical and Nursing Management

- Assessment of dyspnea and chest pain
- Administer and monitor O_2 therapy
- Assist pleural aspiration/needle aspiration
- Assist and monitor chest tube/water seal drainage system
- Assist and maintain patient position
- Administer antibiotic as prescribed
- Monitor pain management
- Assist for thoracentesis, if required
- Close monitor condition
- Monitor frequent assessment
- Monitor oxygen saturation
- Monitor vital signs and level of consciousness
- Monitor lung sounds
- Any changes in patient condition report to physician immediately.

TRACHEOSTOMY

Stoma is an opening through the neck into the trachea through which an indwelling tube may be inserted. The patient breathes through this opening by passing the upper airways (Fig. 6.1).

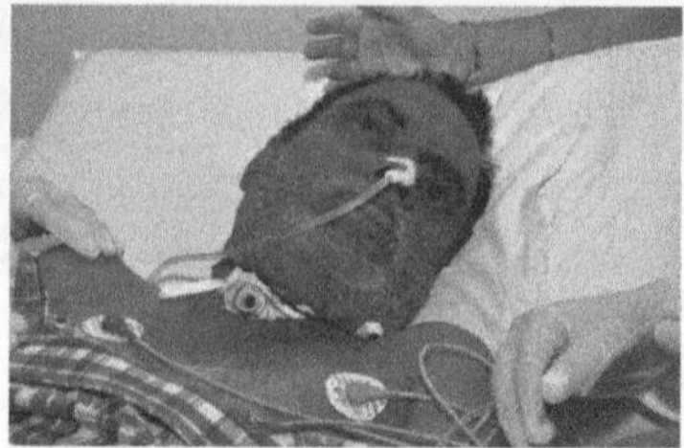

Fig. 6.1: Patient with tracheostomy (*Courtesy:* Anil Baghi, Multispecialty Hospital, Ferozepur, Punjab)

Indication for Tracheostomy

- Airways obstruction caused by trauma or tumor
- Difficulty in clearing secretions from the airway
- Prolonged mechanical ventilation
- Cancerous larynx removed.

After tracheostomy the patient chest is auscultated for breath sounds indicative of pulmonary congestion, mucous membranes and finger tips are observed for cyanosis and humidified oxygen is given directly into the tracheostomy tube. The patient is reassured that the tube is open and that air can pass through it. The tube is suctioned frequently to keep it free tracheobronchial secretion using suction catheter attached to a Y connector. The catheter is inserted 6–8 inches into the tube, the catheter is rotated and intermittent suction is applied for no longer than 5 seconds. The patient is taught to cough to move secretions up and out of the bronchi.

- Suction inner cannula, if necessary
- Clean tracheostomy, keep ready tracheostomy care kit
- If patient receiving O_2 keep mask intact, if mask must remove for care replace immediately
- Suction inner cannula, if necessary
- Reinsert new or cleaned inner cannula into the tracheostomy tube
- Apply sterile dressing
- Maintain aseptic technique
- Teach communication.

Nursing Responsibilities (Box 6.4)

Box 6.4: Nursing responsibilities for the patient with tracheostomy

- Clean tracheostomy according to institutional policy
- Assess lung sounds every 4 hour
- Encourage patient to deep breath and cough as possible
- Suction patient as required
- Maintain fluid and electrolytes balance
- Provide room humidifier
- Monitor oxygen saturation
- Monitor and report, if any signs and symptoms of infection

Contd...

Contd...

• Protect tracheostomy opening for foreign material, food, sprays and powder • Keep head elevated 30°–45° • Consult speech therapist • Give attention to patient communication, provide pen or pencil with paper for communication • Allow the patient to verbalize his/her concern about tracheostomy • Approach patient with an accepting attitude

Checklist (Table 6.12)

Table 6.12: Nursing checklist for the patient requiring tracheostomy

Sl No.	Competency/Criteria	Remarks
1.	Identifies the indications for tracheostomy	
2.	Assembles the necessary equipment for insertion of a tracheostomy	
3.	Assists the physician with the procedure by monitoring the patients airway, heart rate (HR), blood pressure (BP) and arterial saturation levels via pulse oximetry	
4.	Assesses for proper tube placement after insertion and obtain a chest radiography	
5	Identifies the different types of tracheostomy tubes: • Low-pressure cuff • High-pressure cuff • Fenestrated tracheostomy tubes	
6.	Assesses the tracheostomy site and performs tracheostomy care at least every 8 hour	
7.	Assesses the patient for cuff leak or rupture	
8	Assesses the patient for signs of tube obstruction	
9.	Ensures that an extra tracheostomy tube of the same size and the obturator are present at the bedside	
10.	Document all pertinent information	

ENDOTRACHEAL INTUBATION

Patients are unable to maintain adequate breathing because of airway obstruction or respiratory failure, these patient are intubated with a special endotracheal tube (ETT) through the mouth or nose into the trachea. Most intubated patient are mechanically ventilated, ETT is inserted in to the trachea via the mouth or nose. The ETT provides a stable airway and facilitates removal of secretions. Nursing care for this is given in Table 6.13.

Table 6.13: Nursing care for the patient requiring nasotracheal or endotracheal suctioning

Sl No.	Competency statement	Remarks
1.	Identifies the indications for nasotracheal or endotracheal suctioning	
2.	Assembles the necessary equipment for suctioning an endotracheal tube or performing nasotracheal suctioning	
3.	Performs hyperinflation and hyperoxygenation of the patient on the ventilator before and after suctioning	
4.	Instill normal saline before suctioning	
5.	Assesses the patient before, during and after suctioning	
6.	Document all pertinent information	

Indications

- Respiratory failure
- Hypoxia, hypercapnia, tachypnea or apnea, i.e. acute respiratory distress syndrome (ARDS), asthma, pulmonary edema, infection and COPD exacerbation
- Maintenance or protection of an intact airway.

Contraindications

Condition associated with difficult intubation:
- Congenital anomalies
- Infection in airway, retropharyngeal abscess epiglottitis
- Tumor in oral cavity or larynx.

Equipment Preparation (Fig. 6.2)

- Laryngoscope (Figs 6.3A and B)
- Laryngoscope blade (Fig. 6.4)

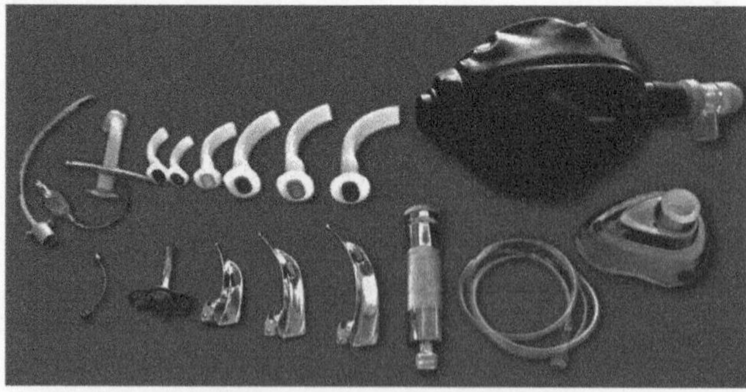

Fig. 6.2: Equipment preparation

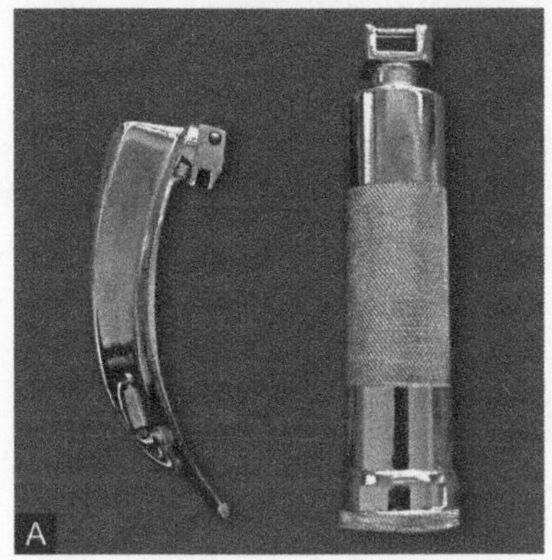

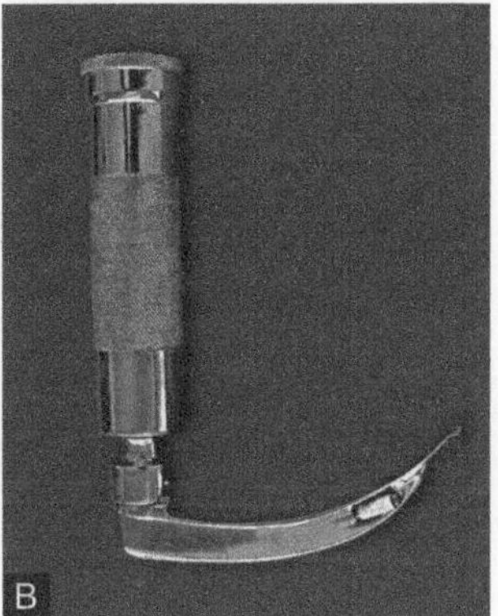

Figs 6.3A and B: Laryngoscope. **A** Two parts of laryngoscope; **B.** After fixing the blade.

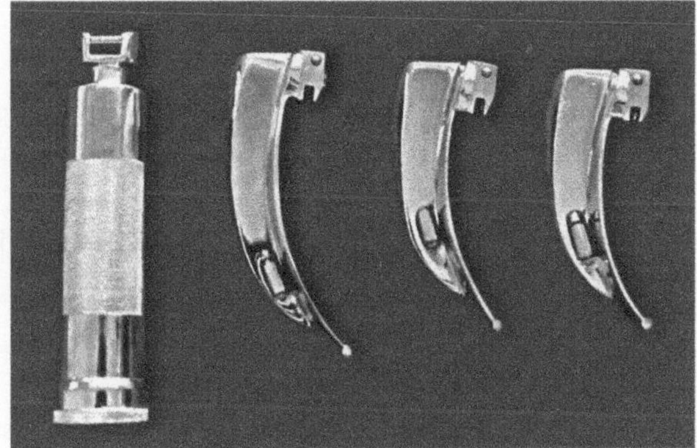

Fig. 6.4: Laryngoscope blade

- Oropharyngeal airway (Fig. 6.5)
- Endotracheal tube (Fig. 6.6).

Other Equipment

- Stylet (malleable)
- Oropharyngeal airway
- Suction catheter and machine
- Face mask and self-inflating bag
- Magill forceps
- Syringe
- Lubricating jelly
- Dynaplast/Tape is used to strap the endotracheal tube.

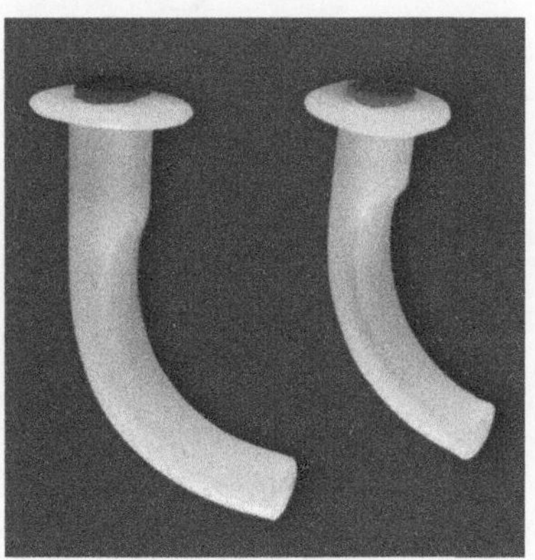

Fig. 6.5: Oropharyngeal airway

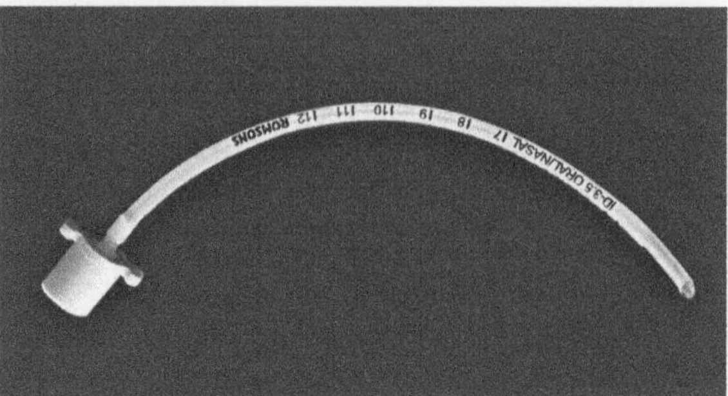

Fig. 6.6: Endotracheal tube

Preoxygenation

- Ventilate with 100% oxygen for approximately 3 minutes
- Position bed/table height
- Bring the patient's head to naval height.

Sniffing Position

Extension at atlanto-occipital joint flexion at lower cervical spine. Neck flexion is maintained by placing a few inches of padding behind the head (Fig. 6.7).

Bag Mask Ventilation (Fig. 6.8)

- Thumb and index finger of left hand in the shape of a 'C' press down
- The other three fingers at the inferior ramus of the mandible and lift the mandible up (jaw thrust) 'E' (Fig. 6.9).

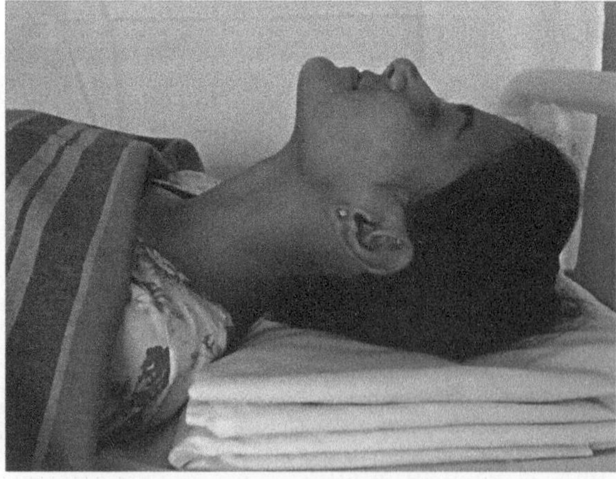

Fig. 6.7: Sniffing position

Intubation Technique

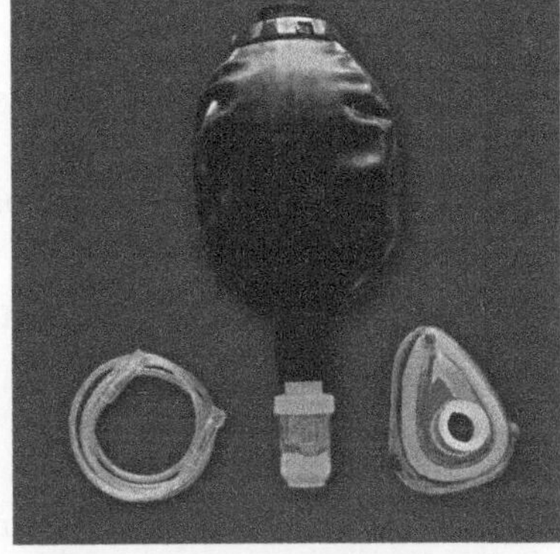
Fig. 6.8: Bag mask ventilation

- Introduce the blade into the right side of the patient's mouth
- Move the blade posteriorly and toward the midline, sweeping the tongue to the left and keeping it away from the visual path with the flange of the blade
- Ensure the lower lip is not being pinched by the lower incisors and laryngoscope blade
- Advance the laryngoscope until the epiglottis is in view
- Lift the laryngoscope upward and forward
- Insert the ETT from the right angle of mouth with its concave curve facing downward and to the right side of the patient
- Maneuver the ETT into the larynx, midway between the cricoid cartilage and the sternal angle
- Lifting up a laryngoscope, pull the blade forward and upward using firm, but steady pressure without rotating the wrist
- Avoid leaning on the upper teeth with the blade
- In most situations vocal cords should become visible
- If not exert gentle pressure over the cricoid area to help bring them into view.

Role of a Nurse

- To provide the ETT to the operators right hand
- To apply cricoid pressure

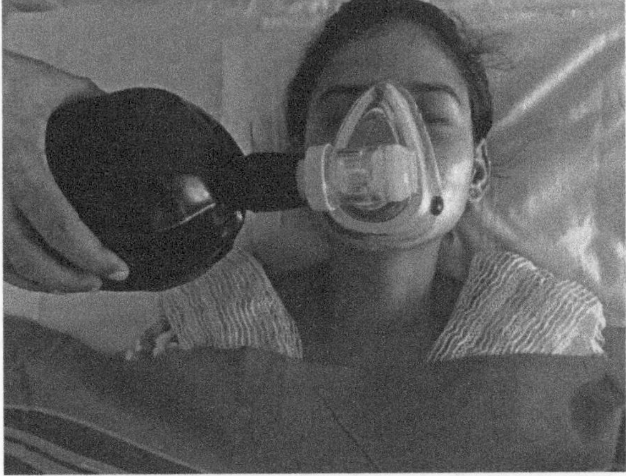
Fig. 6.9: Airway mask breathing unit (AMBU) bag

- Facilitate intubation using BURP maneuver (BURP stands for backward, upward and right ward pressure)
- Inflate the cuff and apply positive-pressure ventilation, while the assistant auscultate
- Secure the ETT in position after bilaterally (b/I) equal air entry is confirmed.

Complication of ET Intubation

During Intubation

- Trauma to lip, tongue or teeth
- Hypertension, tachycardia or arrhythmia
- Pulmonary aspiration
- Laryngospasm
- Bronchospasms
- Increased intracranial pressure
- Spinal cord trauma in cervical injury.

While Intubated

- Obstruction from kinking, secretion or over inflation of cuff
- Accidental extubation
- Pneumothorax, lip or nasal ulcer in case with prolonged period of intubation.

Endotracheal Tube Suctioning

Equipment

- A 5 mL syringe
- Non-sterile gloves
- Suction machine or wall suction setup
- Sterile gloves
- Large towel
- Sterile irrigation saline
- Suction catheter gown or protective apron
- Endotracheal tube holder
- Benzoin/Elastoplast
- Nasal/Oral care item
- Petroleum jelly
- Blood pressure (BP) apparatus.

Purposes

- Maintains open airway for breathing assistance
- Facilitates maximum clearance of secretions.

Procedure

The procedure, along with nursing action and its rationale are detailed in Table 6.14.

Table 6.14: Procedure for endotracheal (ET) suctioning

Sl No.	Nursing action	Rationale
1.	Explain procedure to the patient	Reduces anxiety
2.	Wash hands and organize equipment	Reduces microorganism transfer Promote efficiency
3.	If changing ET tube (ETT), prepare tape	Maintain proper tube placement
4.	Don glove	Protect nurse from contact with secretion
5.	Position client on side or back with head of bed elevated	Facilitates maximum breathing during procedure
6.	Turn suction machine on and place finger over end of tubing attached to suction machine	Tests suction machine pressure [should range from 50 mm Hg (in infants) to 120 mm Hg (in adults)]
7.	Open sterile irrigation solution and pour into sterile cup	Allows for sterile rinsing of catheter
8.	Place towel under client's chin	Prevent soiling of clothing
9.	Pick up suction catheter with sterile hand and attach suction control port for tubing to suction source (held with non-sterile hand)	Ensure correct attachment of catheter
10.	Lubricate 3–4 inches of catheter tip with irrigating solution	Facilitates passage of suction catheter in to ETT
11.	Set oxygen on airway mask breathing unit (AMBU) breathing bag to 100% and turn on full flow	
12.	Administer three to five deep ventilation or allow client to take three to five deep breaths, if able Remove AMBU bag	Provides additional oxygen to body tissue before suctioning
13.	Perform suction maneuvers	
14.	Encourage client to cough facilitates loosening and removal of secretions Suctioning should not be applied for > 10–12 second	Facilitates loosening and removal of secretions Prevents unnecessary mucosal injury from suction
15.	Place tip of suction catheter in sterile solution and apply suction for 1–2 second	Clears clogged suction catheter and tubing

Contd...

Contd...

Sl No.	Nursing action	Rationale
16.	If secretion are thick place 2–3 mL saline into ETT	Stimulates cough to loosen thick secretion for removal
17.	Repeat suction	Removes loosened secretion
18.	Allow client to take about five breaths, while you auscultate and assess, the status of secretion	Determine, if repeat suctioning is needed
19.	Deflate ETT cuff and repeat suctioning	Removes secretion
20.	Reinflate cuff to appropriate pressure	Prevent trauma to tracheal tissue from excessive pressure
21.	Suction oral airway and perform oral care	Removes pooled secretions
22.	Disconnect suction catheter from suction tubing and turn off suction machine	
23.	Position client with head of bed at 45°, side rails up	Maximize lung expansion
24.	Discard equipment appropriately	Promote clean environment

Box 6.5: Nursing care for the patient requiring endotracheal tube (ETT) management

Nursing action
• Identifies the indications for endotracheal intubation • Assembles the equipment required for insertion of an ETT • Assists the physician with the procedure by monitoring the patient's airways, heart rate (HR), blood pressure (BP) and arterial saturation levels via pulse oximetry • Assess for proper tube placement after insertion • Ensures that the endotracheal is properly secured and positioned • Maintains ETT placement • Assesses proper cuff inflation by the minimal occlusion volume technique or by measurement of cuff pressure • Perform oral care in every 8 hour and repositions the ETT to the opposite corner of the mouth daily • Identifies the criteria for endotracheal extubation • Assembles the equipment necessary for extubation • Assists the physician with extubation • Assesses the patient after extubation • Documents all pertinent information

Cuff Deflation

Endotracheal cuff should remain inflated at all times. If cuff deflation is required, suction the trachea and clean the area above the cuff of secretion by gently suctioning deep into the oropharynx, advance the suction catheter to the end of the ETT and deflate the cuff, while applying the suction to the suction catheter.

Box 6.6: Nursing care for the patient requiring nasotracheal or endotrecheal suctioning

Nursing activity
• Identifies the indications for nasotracheal or endotracheal suctioning • Assembles the necessary equipment for suctioning an endotracheal tube or performing nasotracheal suctioning • Performs hyperinflation and hyperoxygenation of the patient on the ventilator before and after suctioning • Instill normal saline before suctioning • Assesses the patient before, during and after suctioning • Documents all pertinent information

Complications During Extubation

- Laryngospasm
- Pulmonary aspiration
- Edema of upper airway.

Nursing Care

Nursing care for ETT management is given in Box 6.5 and nasotracheal/ endotracheal suctioning in Box 6.6.

Chapter 7 Managing Diabetic Emergencies

HYPOGLYCEMIA

Hypoglycemia is the one of the acute complication, it may due to or often referred as low blood sugar or insulin reaction. Too much or too little insulin, can be managed by food and exercise. A blood glucose level below 3 mmol/L is the most common side effect of insulin and sulfonylureas therapy. Hypoglycemia does not occur in patients treated only by diet and is rare in patients receiving metformin alone.

Precipitating Factors

- Missed meals or snacks, not enough food (carbohydrate)
- Increased physical activity/unaccustomed physical activity or exercise
- Errors of insulin dosage and oral drugs
- Delayed and variable absorption of subcutaneous insulin
- Change from animal insulin preparation to human insulin without dose reduction
- Excessive alcohol ingestion
- Effects of other drugs such as Aspirin, tetracycline, Inderal, Tenormin.

Signs and Symptoms

Mild: Hunger, giddiness, trembling, sweating, cool skin and palpitations.

Moderate: Headache, confusion, blurred vision, slurred speech, drowsiness and bad behavior in children, blood sugar level < 60–50 mg/dL, numbness and inability to concentrate.

Severe: Convulsion, loss of consciousness, coma, if untreated, may lead to death.

Management

1. Blood glucose measurement is needed to confirm the diagnosis, but it is not mandatory, clinical evidence or presumption is sufficient to initiate therapy.
2. If at home, the patient can be given orange juice or sugar candy or two spoon of honey to improve the blood sugar level. If the patient becomes drowsy of coma he/she can be shifted to the hospital.
3. In a conscious adult, give sweetened drink and repeat amounts, if necessary.

4. In an unconscious patient give 20 mL of 50% glucose intravenously, if this is not available, give 100 mL of 10% dextrose intravenously. Alternatively, especially in situations, where facilities for intravenous (IV) glucose are not available. Use 1 mg glucagon intramuscularly. Intravenous fluids of 25% dosage depends on clinical parameter.
5. Monitor glucose levels regularly until the patient is receiving an adequate alimentation.
6. In children, administer 25% of glucose, 2 mL/kg as an IV bolus, followed by IV infusion of 5% glucose in the rate of 5 mL/kg/h. The dose and rate of glucose infusion will be adjusted according to the blood glucose level.
7. When consciousness returns, give a short-acting carbohydrate (sweet drink) followed by a long-acting carbohydrate (bread, sandwich or biscuits).

Prevention of Hypoglycemia

1. The blood glucose should be monitored to determine the pattern of low blood sugar.
2. Consistency in insulin administration, dietary intake and activities are important.
3. There should be an adjustment of insulin and diet for variations in activity.
4. People with diabetes mellitus must avoid delaying meals for more than half-an-hour.
5. All people with diabetes mellitus, who depend on insulin/drugs should follow all the principles mentioned for diet, exercise.
6. Patients and family members should be informed about the signs and symptoms of hypoglycemia, and the necessary measures to be taken in case of severe reaction.
7. Advise persons with diabetes mellitus, who experience warning symptoms of hypoglycemia during driving, stop the vehicle and take an oral carbohydrate such as sweet drink, sugar lump then biscuits or sandwich and allow time for recovery.
8. While driving, an emergency supply of glucose or sweets should be kept in the vehicle, taking into consideration unexpected delay, breakdown, etc. On a long journey, the blood glucose should be monitored regularly and snacks should be taken at regular intervals.

DIABETIC KETOACIDOSIS (IN ADULT)

Diabetic ketoacidosis is a potentially lethal condition. However, the majority of cases can be prevented by avoiding precipitating factors. Early recognition and diagnosis are important, if mortality is to be reduced.

Ketoacidosis results from a combination of high blood sugar and buildup of fat breakdown products in blood. It is common in type 1 diabetes [insulin-dependent-diabetes mellitus (IDDM)]. Although, it may also occur in type II diabetes [non-insulin-dependent-diabetes mellitus (NIDDM)] during stressful situations.

Precipitating Factors

- Infection, especially urinary, respiratory and abscess
- Myocardial infarction and cerebrovascular accident
- Trauma and surgery
- Insulin withdrawal or inadequate treatment
- Unrecognized onset of insulin-dependent diabetes.

Signs and Symptoms

- Polydipsia
- Polyuria
- Nausea and vomiting
- Hyperventilation
- Tachycardia and hypotension
- Hypothermia
- Abdominal pains and muscle cramps
- Drowsiness and in severe cases, coma.

Diagnosis

- Urine test shows heavy glycosuria and ketonuria
- Blood glucose concentrations may range from slightly increased to extreme hyperglycemia
- Blood pH ranges from normal to 6.9 and the bicarbonate value is reduced
- Serum potassium levels may be normal or raised. Sodium is usually normal or reduced. Urea and creatinine may be raised because of dehydration.

Management

Saline infusion: In a case of ketoacidosis of average severity, start 0.9% saline at the following rates:

- 1,000 mL given over the first ½ hour
- 1,000 mL given over the next 1 hour
- 1,000 mL given over next 2 hours
- 1,000 mL given over next 4 hours
- 1,000 mL given over the next 8 hours.

Note: Above dosage will be decided by the clinician according to the patient condition. Be cautious in elderly patients and those with cardiovascular decompensation; in mild cases rehydration can be adjusted according to the patient's need.

NON-KETOTIC HYPEROSMOLAR HYPERGLYCEMIC COMA

Non-ketotic hyperosmolar hyperglycemic coma condition is characterized by absence of ketone, high osmolarity and marked dehydration. The absence of ketosis is likely to be due to residual insulin secretion, since all patients with this syndrome may be managed subsequently with diet alone or with diet and oral hypoglycemic agents.

Precipitating Factors

- Infection
- Treatment with antihypertensive drugs such as diuretics and steroids, phenytoin and cimetidine.

Diagnosis

- Urine glycosuria
- Negative test for ketonuria
- Markedly raised plasma glucose concentration
- Prerenal uremia
- Raised hematocrit.

Management

Treatment is similar to ketoacidosis. However, the patient may be hypernatremic and therefore half normal saline (0.45% NaCl) may be given instead of 0.9% NaCl. Cases with condition should always be referred to the diabetologist.

LACTIC ACIDOSIS

Metabolic disorder characterized by an increased content of lactic acid and in increased blood lactate/pyruvate ratio, it is feature of acidosis resulting from widespread tissue hypoxia.

Severe lactic acidosis in diabetic patients occurs as a feature of ketoacidosis and as a rare complication of biguanides. It is linked to the presence of other severe generalized disorders such as septicemia, renal failure, shock pulmonary embolism, myocardial infarction, hepatic cirrhosis and acute hepatic dystrophy.

Management

- When associated with ketoacidosis, lactic acidosis resolves with standard treatment of ketoacidosis
- In case of severe lactic acidosis to elevate arterial blood pH, administer IV bicarbonate
- Dialysis to avoid sodium overload
- Sodium dichloroacetate administration lowers lactic acid by stimulating pyruvate dehydrogenase
- All cases require immediate medical attention.

CHRONIC COMPLICATIONS OF DIABETES MELLITUS

Diabetic Retinopathy

Diabetic retinopathy is the most common microvascular complication of diabetes affecting the retina. Patients with hypertension are at greater risk of developing diabetic retinopathy. Pregnancy also causes deterioration of diabetic retinopathy. However, attention should also be given to other manifestations of diabetic eye disease such as cataract and glaucoma.

Prevention

To prevent retinopathy and visual loss, the followings are recommended:

- Promoting good glycemic control in all diabetic individual
- Controlling blood pressure
- Detecting and treating glaucoma at early stage
- Detecting and treating cataract
- Detecting and providing timely treatment of potentially serious retinal changes.

Management

In every case of eye assessment and management should include the followings:

- History of visual symptoms, glaucoma and cataract
- Physical examination such as visual acuity testing and ocular pressure
- Fundus examination by direct ophthalmoscopy (preferably after pupillary dilatation)
- Further assessment should be performed once every year.

Diabetic Nephropathy

Diabetic nephropathy is a major cause of death among people with diabetes and an important cause of morbidity and increased healthcare cost due to diabetes. It leads to end stage renal disease requiring dialysis or renal transplantation.

Prevention

Diabetic nephropathy complication may be prevented and progression can be slowed down by:

- Strict glycemic control
- Vigorous treatment of hypertension
- Avoidance of nephrotoxic drugs and early effective treatment of infection. The onset of clinical nephropathy is manifested by proteinuria (incipient < 300 mg/L, which requires special test to detect it and overt > 300 mg/L, which could be detected by chemical test).

Management

- Diabetes patient should have their urine test for protein at initial assessment and then periodically
- Collect urine of 24 hours and sent for protein and creatinine estimation
- Ensure optimal glycemic control
- Advise the patient to reduce protein and salt intake
- Strict adherence to antihypertensive drugs.

Hypertension in Diabetes

Hypertension is commonly associated with diabetes and may complicate it. Both conditions are important and independent risk factors for cardiovascular, renal, cerebral and peripheral vascular disease. Hypertension should be detected early and treated aggressively as it is contributing to increase morbidity and mortality along with diabetes, is to be avoided.

Management

1. Unless the blood pressure (BP) is severely elevated, diagnosis should usually be based on high BP measurement made at least three occasions.
2. Blood pressure is elevated, when the BP is persistently more than 140 mm Hg systolic and or more than 90 mm Hg diastolic.
3. Blood pressure should be examined in supine and standing position to detect postural changes.
4. The presence of target organ damage (e.g. retinal, renal or cardiovascular) should be evaluated.
5. Other modifiable cardiovascular risk factors should be checked.
6. In general, the goal of BP treatment should be to maintain BP at less than 140 mm Hg systolic and less than 85 mm Hg diastolic.
7. Treatment should be initially based on non-pharmacological therapy, namely weight reduction, dietary modification, increased physical activity and smoking cessation.

8. The aim of dietary therapy should focus on a low-salt intake (sodium intake of less than half tablespoon per day) and low saturated fat to reduce the risk of cardiovascular disease (CVD). For overweight individuals, calorie reduction to achieve gradual weight loss should be planned together with regular physical exercise. Alcohol increases plasma triglyceride levels. Excessive consumption can also lead to a further rise in BP.
9. Drug treatment should be considered only if the therapy targets are not reached with non-pharmacological measures. An exception to this recommendation is severe hypertension.

Drugs Used to Lower Blood Pressure in Diabetes

Thiazides: Used in small doses (12.5–25 mg hydrochlorothiazide) are effective. Side effects such as hyperglycemia, hypokalemia, hypomagnesemia and hyperuricemia may develop, but are minimal with such low doses.

Selective beta blockers: Have been shown to reduce cardiovascular morbidity and mortality in people with diabetes. However, in these cases cardio-selective preparation in low doses are preferred and caution should be exercised, particularly in patients predisposed hypoglycemia.

Beta blockers may interfere with awareness of and recovery from hypoglycemia and cause worsening of peripheral vascular disease by causing vasospasm, their use may be associated with an adverse effect on lipid status and blood glucose control.

Angiotensin-converting enzymes (ACE) inhibitors: Have been shown to reduce microalbuminuria and delay the onset and progression of diabetic nephropathy. They have no adverse effects on lipid status or glucose levels, but may cause hyperkalemia in patient with renal impairment and in those taking potassium sparing drugs or potassium supplement. The ACE inhibitors are contraindicated in pregnancy and should therefore be used with caution in women of child bearing age. In people with renal artery stenosis ACE inhibitors may include impairment of renal function.

Alpha-receptor blockers: Have no adverse effects in lipid or glucose control, but may cause postural hypotension especially in people with autonomic neuropathy.

Calcium channel blockers: Can also be effectively used to low BP. They have no adverse effects on lipid and glucose metabolism.

Diabetic Neuropathy

Neuropathy is common in all patients with diabetes and may be detected soon after the onset of the disease. Neuropathy can affect the sensory, motor and autonomic nervous systems (ANS), and can be disabling the systems. At the initial visit, question asked regarding symptoms related to the sensory (numbness, anesthesia, incoordination, etc.) and ANS (gastrointestinal and bladder symptoms, sexual dysfunction, postural light-headedness). The above history and physical examination should be done at least annually during the follow-up visits. If the patient has neuropathy at the initial visit, its progress should be monitored.

Prevention and Management

Neuropathic involvement can be prevented or delayed by good glycemic control. If it persists in spite of good blood glucose control, during treatment may be indicated. Analgesics may be given, but if ineffective, tricyclic antidepressants such as amitriptyline may also be used for this purpose. Reassurance that pain will eventually decrease with time is needed.

Diabetic Foot

Severe foot lesions requiring amputation are one of the major complications of diabetes.

Prevention

The main approaches to prevention are:

- Identification of high-risk individuals
- Early detection of foot lesions, e.g. trauma infection or ulcers
- Intensified foot care should be ensured for patient at high-risk such as those with:
  - Poor foot hygiene
  - Symptoms and/or signs of neuropathic involvement
  - Evidence of peripheral vascular disease
  - Nephropathy or significant retinopathy
  - Foot deformities and chronic orthopedic or rheumatic disorders.
- Each person with diabetes should be educated on the rules of foot care.

Rules of foot care

1. Examine both feet carefully every day for injuries such as blisters, cuts, bruises or infection. Use a mirror to look at the bottom of the feet; do not apply henna coloring to easily visualized foot injuries or problems.
2. It is important to keep feet clean. Wash with soap and warm water (never use hot water), dry carefully especially between the toes.
3. If feet are too dry, apply mild cream/lotion such as Vaseline or olive oil except between the toes.
4. Do not walk barefoot even at home; protect feet when walking in sandy beaches or near swimming pools.
5. Do not smoke because it decreases the blood circulation. In diabetes, this may cause peripheral vascular disease, which may result in amputation of the feet.
6. Wear proper fitting socks, preferably cotton or well-fitting stocking.

7. Examine shoes every day for foreign objects (stones, pins), which may injure the feet and also for new lesions (redness ulcer).
8. Trim toe nails regularly straight across using an emery board, not too short and after washing when the nails are soft.
9. Do not cut or remove calluses by oneself, report to the physician.

MANAGEMENT OF PATIENT WITH BURNS

At the Scene

First Aid

The first priority is to remove the causality from further damage, e.g. extinguish burning cloths. Flames travel upwards and continue to burn the face, neck and scalp, if the casualty is upright. With the casualty horizontal on the ground, smoother the flames with a coat rug or similar heavy materials if the fire was in an enclosed space and there is smoke present. Remove the casualty to fresh air. If clothing is still smoldering, douse with water, clothes saturated with hot liquids act as a hot poultice. They should be removed quickly or cooled by drenching with cold water. With these exceptions, the active cooling of extensive thermal burns is of debatable value and should never be allowed to delay the removal of the casualty to hospital.

Corrosive burns: The removal of corrosive chemicals from the skin is just as urgent as extinguishing the flames of blazing clothing copious quantities of water should be used and particular attention must be paid to the eyes. Contaminated clothing should be removed irrigation of the affected parts should continue until the ambulance arrives and if possible be continued during the journey to the hospital. Any known information concerning nature of the chemical should accompany the casualty to hospital.

Admission to Hospital

First Things First

In accident and emergency department:

- Make sure there is a clear airway
- Indication for endotracheal intubation include deep burns of the face.

In addition to the burns, there may be other injuries that need to be taken into account in declining over all priorities.

Priorities

- Make sure there is a clear airway
- Brief history of accident
- Brief general examination
- Set up a reliable plasma drip
- Take blood samples

- Provide analgesia
- Catheterize the bladder
- Reassess the patients general condition
- Reassess the burn
- Check the priority
- Attend to the burn wound
- Look out for complications.

In the Accident and Casualty Department

Assessment of the Burn Wound

The cause of the injury and the time that it occurred should be ascertained and recorded. Even quite experienced staff can mistake the depth of a burn, at this stage it is sufficient to distinguish between erythema and actual skin damage, if the history is of a corrosive or chemical burn irrigation with water should be continued. A thermal burn should not be interfered with at this time. There is a need to make a quick estimate can be made mentally by using the rule of nines, which indicates in an easily remembered form. The percentage of total body surface area accounted for by various part of the body, 9% each for arms and head, 18% each for legs, front of trunk and back of trunk for part of the body that only small areas of burn. It is useful to remember that the palmar surface of the patients hand constitutes about 1% of the body surface area. Simple erythema is excluded from the estimate and if the total burn is more than 15–20% in an adult or 10–15% in child intravenous infusion is indicated with extensive burns 30% and more, it is both essential and urgent.

Setting up the Intravenous Drip

Unless both arms burned to the extent of deep charring, it will be possible to find a vein in one or other forearm or antecubital fossa. If the vein can be seen venipuncture is satisfactory, otherwise a cut down should be performed. In either case, the largest possible cannula should be inserted and secured firmly. A long narrow catheter is a bad choice.

Fluid and Electrolytes Imbalance

Evaporative water loss through the burn contributes to the client's diminished fluid volume and compromised hydration status. Evaporative loss are evidenced by a low BP, decreased urine output, dry mucous membranes and poor skin turgor:

- Urine output diminishes to less than 30 mL/h
- Elevated blood urea nitrogen (BUN) until the client adequately hydrated
- Absence of bowel sounds
- Nausea and vomiting and abdominal distention
- Approximately, 18–36 hours after burn injury, capillary membrane integrity begins to be restored.

Blood Samples

If a blood sample can be obtained from the cannula before the drip set is connected, it will save time and the need for a venipuncture a few minutes later.

Choice of Infusion Fluid

Fluid resuscitation is used to minimize the fluid shifts. The goal of fluid resuscitation is to maintain vital organ perfusion, while avoiding the complications related to either inadequate or excessive fluid administration. Several formula recommended by the American Burn Life Support (ABLS), e.g. consensus formula for fluid resuscitation. For adults, Ringer's lactate solution 2–4 mL × body weight × percentage burns.

$$\text{For example, } 2 \times 50 = \frac{100 \times 40}{4{,}000} = 4{,}000 \text{ mL}$$

If burned client is delayed 2 hours in reaching an emergency department those 2 hours must be considered in any calculation of needed fluid. However adjustment to the fluid infusion rate is based on client's physiological response, e.g. urine production, vital sings and lung sounds. The infusion rate is adjusted so that half of the estimated volume is administered in the first 8 hours postburn. The remaining half of the estimated resuscitation volume is administered over 16 hours. The expected plasma requirement for the period up to 4 hours postburn is between 0.5 and 0.65 mL/kg body weight/ percentage burn. Hence 73 kg patient with 55% burn is likely to needed between 2,000 and 2,600 mL of plasma in the first 4 hours postburn.

Airway and Breathing

Fires kill more people by asphyxia than by burns and as with any other accident. The first medical priority is the management of the airway and breathing, if the fire is in an enclosed space, carbon monoxide poisoning may occur, sometimes to the extent of producing unconsciouness. In this case, control of the upper airway will be important as well as providing 50% oxygen in air to breathe. The specific problems of smoke inhalation will be considered.

Upper Airway Obstruction

The main threat to the upper airway occurs when laryngeal edema develops following direct thermal injury caused by the inhalation of flame, hot gases or steam. Occasionally, aspiration of hot liquids during scalding of the face produces similar damage. Whenever there are burns or scalds of the face, consider the need for airway support, in general the more severe the thermal injury, the earlier will laryngeal obstruction become apparent in the most severe cases, obstruction is virtually inevitable within a few hours and may occur with little warning.

Pulmonary Damage

The inhalation of hot gases can produce burns down to the terminal bronchi, but only steam can carry sufficient heat into the lungs to produce thermal damage in the alveoli, an unusual injury with a very bad prognosis. Much commoner is smoke damage essentially a corrosive burns of the lungs, resulting from products of combustion.

Analgesia

The requirement for analgesia during the shock phase of burns is often small. With full thickness skin burns, there is seldom any complaint of pain because sensory end organs in the skin have also been destroyed. Even when the burns are partial thickness and the survival of sensory end organs can clearly bee demonstrated by pinprick, it is unusual for the patient to complain of continuing pain. However some patients will complain of pain and most will be affected by fear and discomfort and the provision of analgesia at an early stage is an important part of treatment. Injection morphine is the drug of choice.

Catheterization of the Bladder

Due to knowledge of the flow rate and composition of the urine provides vital information concerning both the effectiveness of resuscitation and functional status of the kidneys themselves an indwelling catheter should be inserted. The bladder is emptied, urine volume is measure thereafter:

1. **Prevent tetanus:** Burns even minor ones are susceptible of tetanus, tetanus toxoid should be administered.
2. **Prevent infection:** Controlling infection is a major components of burn management, standard precautions to be followed in caring for all client.

Wound Care

Dressing

The purpose of a burn dressing is to absorb the exudate from the wound and as for as possible, to prevent colonization of the wound by pathogenic bacteria, ideally, then it should be absorbent, on adherent (to facilitate dressing changes) and should act as a barrier to prevent outside bacteria penetrating to the wound surface. These properties are usually obtained by combination of bacterial ointment on the wound, covered by an absorbent pad held in place by bandages. For the treatment of extensive full thickness burns, it is important to prevent, delay or limit the colonization of the wound by gram-negative bacteria to this end, three agents have been shown to have useful:

- 0.5% silver nitrate soaks
- 1% silver sulfate cream
- Mafenide cream.

Changing the dressing

Changing a large burn dressing can be daunting experience and without careful planning, it will be exhausting for both patient and staff. Dressing on full thickness burns will need to be changes at least on alternate days and although it can be a painful procedure, sedation seldom necessary.

Nutritional Support

The calorie and protein intake should be provided by the enteral route if at all possible. parenteral feeding is necessary occasionally, whatever the source of the supplementary feed, its introduction to the patient must be gradual, if nausea are regurgitation occurs, the volume of feed is reduced for a day are two. Abnormalities of vitamine metabolism occur in burn cases and there is also an increased utilization of iron for erythropoietin. Consequently, iron and vitamin therapy should be routine from the end of the shock phase until healing is complete.

Nursing Management

Nursing Diagnosis

- Impaired gas exchange related to carbon monoxide poisoning
- Ineffective airway clearance related to smoke inhalation
- Fluid volume deficit related to evaporative loss
- Pain related to tissue and nerve injury
- Hypothermia related to loss of skin microcirculation and open wounds
- Anxiety related to fear and emotional impact of burn injury
- Acute respiratory failure, shock.

Nursing Intervention

- Provide oxygen
- Assess breath sounds, respiratory rate, rhythm and depth
- Prepare for intubation and mechanical ventilation, if required
- Maintain patient airway and position patient appropriately
- Suction as required
- Monitor intake and output
- Weight patient
- Monitor urine output
- Maintain IV lines and regulate IV fluids
- Observe and monitor laboratory report, and report to physician significantly
- Monitor central venous pressure, if patient is on CVP line
- Monitor vital signs

- Administer analgesics as prescribed observe for respiratory depression
- Assess pain scale
- Assess body temperature frequently
- Provide emotional support
- Assess patient and family coping skill
- Explain all procedures to the patient and family in simple terms
- Monitor pulse oximetry arterial blood gas values and report
- Report any deteriorating condition to physician
- Assess progressive edema as fluid shifts occur
- Elevate burn extremities
- Prepare and assist during wound debridement
- Perform dressing based on need of the patient
- Maintain nasogastric tube insertion, feeding and monitoring
- Auscultate for bowel sounds and abdominal distention
- Assess stool for occult blood
- Document all procedure and medication.

Chapter 8

Mechanical Ventilation

TERMINOLOGY

End-expiratory pressure: The pressure at the end of expiration.

Flow rate: The speed at which the tidal volume is delivered, the usual setting is 40–100 L/min.

Fraction of inspired oxygen (FiO_2): It is the fraction inspired of oxygen or simply percentage of oxygen in a gas mixture. For example, the atmospheric air has FiO_2 of 21%. If a patient needs mechanical ventilation, FiO_2 is usually in the 30–40% range.

Functional residual capacity: The volume of gas remaining in the lung after a normal expiration.

Inspiratory-expiratory ratio (I:E): The ratio between the inspiratory and expiratory phase. Normally the ratio is 1:2–1:1.5.

Peak airway pressure: Pressure required to administering the set amount of tidal volume.

Pressure limit: The amount of pressure, which the volume-cycled ventilator can generate to deliver the preset tidal volume. The usual setting is 10–20 cm H_2O.

Respiratory rate: The number of breaths that the venti͵ator will deliver to the patient over a specific time period. The respiratory rate parameters are set above and below this number, and an alarm will sound if the patient's actual rate is outside the desired range.

Tidal volume: The volume of gas that the ventilator will deliver to the patient with each breath. The usual setting is 5–15 cm^3/kg.

MECHANICAL VENTILATOR

A mechanical ventilator is a machine that generates a controlled flow of gas into the patient's airways. Oxygen and air are received from cylinders or wall outlets, the gas is pressure reduced and blended according to the prescribed inspired oxygen tension (FiO_2), accumulated in a receptacle within the machine and delivered to the patient using one of many available modes of ventilation. The pediatric ventilatir as shown in Figure 8.1.

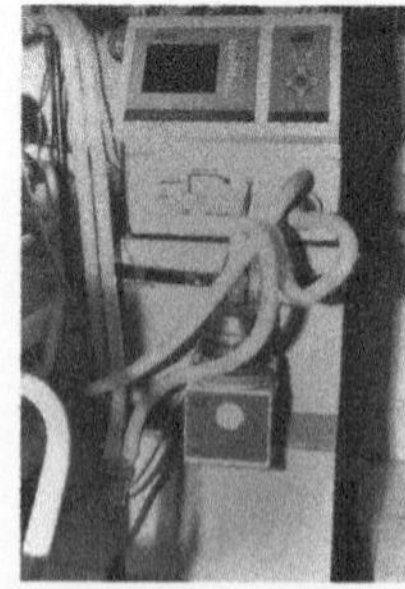

Fig. 8.1: Pediatric ventilator (*Courtesy:* Anil Baghi, Multispecialty Hospital, Ferozepur, Punjab)

METHOD OF MECHANICAL VENTILATION

Mechanical ventilation is the method in which FiO_2 moved in and out of the lungs. A vacuum is created and air flows in when ventilator is used. The positive pressure is necessary for gas exchange and keeps alveoli open. It is used supporting patient respiration until they recover to breathe independently. It can be continued until the decision is made to withdraw. The Roman physician Galen is the first to describe mechanical ventilation.

INDICATIONS

- Acute respiratory failure
- Inability to breathe
- To maintain adequate ventilation
- Hypoxia
- To maintain adequate oxygenation in diseased condition
- Cardiac or respiratory arrest
- Respiratory system injury.

CRITERIA/PREPARATIONS FOR USING VENTILATOR

Criteria for Starting Ventilatory Support

- Respiratory rate more than 35 breaths per minute
- Partial pressure of carbon dioxide (PCO_2) more than 60 mm Hg in a non-chronic obstructive pulmonary disease (COPD) case
- Partial pressure of oxygen (PO_2) less than 50 mm Hg in a non-cyanotic heart disease patient
- Signs of muscle fatigue
- Sweating
- Metabolic failure.

Complete Preparation for Rapid Sequence Intubation

- Ambu bag must be at hand
- Adequate size of face mask must be at hand
- One larger and one smaller than the predicted size of endotracheal tube (ETT)
- Adequate size laryngoscope blade
- Suction catheter must be at hand
- Magill forceps must be at hand
- Style for ETT must be at hand
- Preoxygenate for 3 minutes.

Set on Ventilator

Ventilator should be set on:

1. Continuous mandatory ventilation (CMV) for emergency ventilation and mode should be changed to synchronized intermittent mandatory ventilation (SIMV) + pressure support when emergency is over. Ventilator strategies are:
   - Minute volume: 100 mL/kg
   - Tidal volume: 10 mL/kg
   - Respiratory rate: 20 per minute initially and according to age and ventilator requirements
   - Maintain I:E ratio in the range of 1:2
   - Fraction of inspired oxygen should be 1.
2. Deep sedation/analgesics or induction agent may be used according to patient's requirements.
3. If nasogastric (NG) tube in place then suck out stomach content first.
4. Give muscle relaxant and ventilate the patient, while applying cricoids pressure.
5. Confirm appropriate position of ETT, fix it and connect to ventilator.
6. When possible, get arterial blood gases (ABGs) done 10 minutes before and 10 minutes after putting patient on ventilator and readjust the ventilator settings according to report otherwise treat clinically.
7. Drugs, which are already given must be continued during ventilatory support.
8. Cardiopulmonary resuscitation (CPR) trolley and resuscitation drugs must be at hand.
9. Get an X-ray of chest done as early as possible.

CLASSIFICATION

Types of Mechanical Ventilation

1. **Negative pressure ventilation:** Where air is essentially sucked into the lungs, creating negative pressure leads to expansion of the chest.
2. **Positive pressure ventilation:** Where air (or other gas mix) is pushed into the trachea. It works by increasing the patient's airway pressure through an endotracheal or tracheostomy tube.

Classification of Ventilators

- Volume controlled
- Pressure controlled
- Dual controlled.

Cycling

1. **Time cycled:** In pressure-controlled ventilation.
2. **Flow cycled:** Such as in pressure support.
3. **Volume cycled:** This occurs in volume-controlled ventilation.

Nurses are responsible for preparation setting, monitoring, observing, troubleshooting, assisting extubation and teach the family.

MODES OF VENTILATION

Modes means the way the client receives breaths from the ventilators (Table 8.1).

Table 8.1: Modes of ventilation

Sl No.	Volume modes	Characteristics
1.	Control ventilation (CV) or continuous mandatory ventilation (CMV)	In this mode, ventilator provides all minute ventilation to the patient, inspiratory time and positive end-expiratory pressure; conventional modes of CMV will deliver a preset volume of gas each time the client initiates a breath; if the client fails to initiate a breath within a preset amount of time, the ventilator will deliver a breath at a predetermined volume and rate.
2.	Assist control (AC) or assisted mandatory ventilation (AMV)	When patient initiates a spontaneous breath, a full volume breath is delivered. In this mode the ventilator provides a mechanical breath with either a preset tidal volume or peak pressure every time the patient initiates a breath.
3.	Intermittent mandatory ventilation (IMV) and synchronized intermittent mandatory ventilation (SIMV)	Patients can breathe spontaneously at their own rate. The ventilator synchronizes the mandatory breath with patient own inspiration. In this mode, the ventilator provides a preset mechanical breath (pressure or volume limited) every specified number of seconds. Within that cycle time, the ventilators senses the first patient breathing attempt within the cycle, it delivers the preset ventilator breath. If the patient fails to initiate a breath, the ventilator delivers a mechanical breath at the end of the breath cycle.
4.	Positive end-expiratory pressure (PEEP), continuous positive airway pressure (CPAP)	PEEP is applied positive airway pressure that keeps the alveoli open. CPAP is applied to a client with spontaneous respiration. PEEP has shown improvement in gas exchange and vital capacity.
5.	Pressure support ventilation (PSV)	For client with stable respiratory drive to overcome airway resistance from endotracheal tube. The patient must be able to initiate a breath in this modality. As the patient initiates a breath,

Contd...

Contd...

Sl No.	Volume modes	Characteristics
		the machine senses the spontaneous effort and supplies effort and supplies a rapid flow of gas at the initiation of the breath, throughout the breath.
6.	Auto mode	Designed to allow the ventilator to be interactive with the patient's needs by making breath by breath adjustments in both control and support modes.
7.	Pressure-regulated volume control	Assist control ventilation and the pressure control is titrated to the set tidal volume and is time cycled. Ventilator will give signal, if the tidal volume and maximum pressure limit setting incompatible.

SETTING OF MECHANICAL VENTILATION/MONITORING AND NURSING MANAGEMENT

Nurses are responsible for preparation, setting, monitoring, observing, troubleshooting, assisting extubation and teach the family (Tables 8.2 and 8.3).

Table 8.2: Nursing management

Sl No.	Parameter	Description
1.	Respiratory rate	Number of breaths the ventilator deliver; usual setting is 6–20 breaths per minute
2.	Oxygen concentration	Fraction of inspired oxygen delivered to the patient may be 21%
3.	Positive end-expiratory pressure (PEEP)	Usual setting is 3–5 cm H_2O
4.	Pressure support	Positive pressure used to augment patient inspiratory pressure as prescribed
5.	Inspiratory-expiratory (I:E) ratio	Duration of inspiration as prescribed
6.	Inspiratory flow rate and time	Speed with which the ventilator inspired (VI) is delivered
7.	Inspiratory flow rate	As prescribed
8.	Sensitivity	Determines the amount of effort that the patient must generate to initiate a ventilator breath
9.	High pressure limit	Regulate the maximal pressure

Complication

- Pneumothorax
- Airway injury
- Alveolar damage
- Ventilator-associated pneumonia

Table 8.3: Ventilator alarms

Alarm	Causes	Nursing intervention
High pressure alarm	Airway pressure meets or exceeds the pressure limit, ventilation is terminated when this alarm triggered caused by increased airway resistance Kink in endotracheal tube (ETT) Kink or water in ventilator tubing Caused by changes in lungs compliance pneumothorax	Assess ETT for kinks if orally placed, the patient is biting on this tube, reposition tube in oral cavity, place oral airway in patient to prevent biting Reposition tubing by emptying water from tubing or water trap A sudden increased peak airway pressure may indicate pneumothorax, assess for changes in breath sounds, drop in blood pressure (BP), increase in BP and worsening oxygenation, consult with physician on the need for chest X-ray and further therapeutic interventions
Low-exhaled volume	A leak or lose of tidal volume disconnection	Check all ventilator tubing connections and reconnect, if indicated
Apnea	Can be activated in IMV,* SIMV‡, CPAP†, PSV modes, alarm initiate breath within a preset period of time	Frequent apnea alarms may indicate the patient is not ready to wean and needs a more controlled mode of ventilation, patient may need assessment for sleep apnea or neurological impairment of the respiratory drive; may also indicate over sedation

*IMV, intermittent mandatory ventilation; †SIMV, synchronized intermittent mandatory ventilation; ‡CPAP, continuous positive airway pressure; §PSV, pressure support ventilation.

- Long-term disability due to inflammation
- Infection
- Barotraumas.

WEANING FROM MECHANICAL VENTILATOR

The process of reducing ventilator support and client resuming spontaneous ventilation is called weaning. Ventilation has to be weaned from the ventilator at some point of time, when extubation is done. Extubation refers to removal of the orotracheal or nasotracheal tubes from the patients.

Phases of Weaning

- Preweaning phase
- Weaning phase
- Outcome phase.

Indications for Weaning

1. Discuss with family members/significant others.
2. Before weaning the client who is under ventilator care, formal assessment is required and irrespective of weaning mode selected, all team members should be familiar with the weaning process and plan are as follows:
   - Client lungs should be reasonably clear on auscultation
   - Correction of underlying cause
   - Satisfy adequate oxygenation
   - Satisfy hemodynamic stability, fluid and electrolytes, acid-base balance
   - Tolerance of trial may lead to extubation
   - Client ability to initiate an inspiratory effort
   - Patient instructed to take deep breath and peek of inspiration, the cuff should be deflated
   - After removal, the patient should be encouraged to deep breath and cough, suctioned as needed, supplemental oxygen should be applied.

Triggering Mechanism

All breaths given to the client must be initiated or triggered. Triggering mechanism can be based on:

1. **Time triggered:** The ventilator will trigger a breath after a preset time, the client who cannot breath on their own.
2. **Pressure triggered:** The ventilator senses the patient's inspiratory effort by way of a decrease in the baseline pressure.
3. **Flow triggered:** When the client can initiate a breath, the ventilator completes the breath by sensing the flow of the air.
4. **Negative pressure inhalation:** As soon as the client initiates a breath, the ventilator is triggered to produce inhalation.

VENTILATOR CHECKLIST

Responsibility

Nurse in-charge of intensive care unit (ICU).

Checklist

1. Ventilator is placed bedside of the patients before patient arrives.
2. All gas connectors are secured into appropriate wall sockets.
3. Breathing circuit is attached to the ventilator for every patient; all filters are checked for proper functioning.
4. Ventilator is switched on and following functions are checked:

- Expired tidal volume is almost equal to the set inspired tidal volume showing there is no major leak in the circuit
- Respiratory rate is same as set on the ventilator
- Ventilator is able to give 100% oxygen
- All available modes, [synchronized intermittent mandatory ventilation (SIMV) and pressure support ventilation (PSV)] are checked for proper functioning
- Expiratory pressure is within normal limits, i.e. around 20 cm H_2O
- All alarm setting are reviewed and checked.

NUTRITIONAL SUPPORT OF PATIENT ON VENTILATOR

Responsibility

Nurse in-charge of ICU/dietitian.

Supportive Measures

1. Any patient who stays on ventilator for more than 24 hours will be given nutritional support.
2. Routes of nutritional support are:
   - Enteral
   - Parenteral.
3. Calculate caloric requirements by formula: 40 kcal/kg/24 h for adults and 100 kcal/kg/24 h for children below 10 kg by weight.
4. In the initial phase (non-catabolic state) 60–70% of the calculated calories are provided. However, after 3–4 days once the patient goes into catabolic state, 100% of the caloric requirements is fulfilled.
5. Nutrients include:
   - Carbohydrate 60–70% of the calculated calories
   - Fats 30–40% of the calculated calories
   - Proteins are not included, while calculating the calories requirements, proteins are given in a dose of 1–15 g/kg 24 h and if serum creatinine is more than 2 g then proteins should be given about 1 g/kg/24 h.
6. Vitamin C 500 mg shall be given to every patient, who needs nutritional support.
7. Multivitamins shall be given with macroelements and microelements.
8. Details of nutritional support provided during last 24 hours must be recorded on monitoring chart.
9. Nutritional support is calculated for next 24 hours on daily basis in the morning round.

CLEANING AND ASEPSIS OF VENTILATOR

Responsibility

Nurse in-charge of ICU.

Aseptic Measures

- Ventilator cleaning and asepsis will be carried out after every use
- Breathing circuit and humidifier filter must be changed after every use
- Only disposable breathing circuit must be used in ICU
- External case of ventilator will be cleaned with damp cloth soaked in detergent daily
- Change bacterial filter daily.

CHANGE OF BREATHING CIRCUIT OF VENTILATORS

Responsibility

Nurse in-charge of ICU.

Measures

- Breathing circuit will be changed for each patient
- No breathing circuit will be used without bacterial filter
- Always use disposable breathing circuit
- In extreme emergency and lack of disposable breathing circuit, a reusable type can be used
- Breathing circuit is dipped in Cidex (glutaraldehyde) solution for 2 hours then hanged till it is dry, afterwards it is autoclaved before reuse.

CHANGE OF CONDENSER HUMIDIFIER OF VENTILATOR

Responsibility

Nurse in-charge of ICU.

Measures

- Filter and water of condenser humidifier will be changed after every use
- Only distilled water will be used in humidifier
- Humidifier water level should be checked every 2 hours and level should be maintained.

NURSING INTERVENTION FOR PATIENT ON MECHANICAL VENTILATION

- The airway of a mechanically ventilated patient includes the ETT, tracheostomy or mask ventilator and tubing, frequently, assesses the mask and tube for leaks and the ventilator tubing for kinks and blockage
- Explain the procedure to the patient/significant others (informed consent as per institutional policy)
- Check all ventilator setting and alarm connection
- Assess both patient and ventilator for adequate breathing
- Check patient respiratory rate and work of breathing if the ventilator rate and respiratory rate differ, the ventilator may be disconnected or he/she may be taking spontaneous breaths
- Check ETT placement, ensure ETT is in secure and right position
- Check alarm function
- Monitor respiratory rate, tidal volume, oxygen flow rate, positive end-expiratory pressure (PEEP) and airway pressure
- Provide adequate humidity via the ventilator
- Administer sedatives and opioid analgesics as ordered
- Silence ventilator alarm during suctioning empty condenser water from water traps, monitor effects of ventilator changes on oxygenation
- Auscultate breath sounds, respiratory rate, lung compliance every hourly for 2 hours
- Observe obstructed airway
- Monitor ABGs and pulse oximetry
- Auscultate for presence of lungs sounds
- Monitor the effect of position changes on oxygenation
- Assist in frequent position changes/turn immobilized patient every 2 hour
- Perform suctioning to remove secretion
- Always use septic technique/wear personnel protective equipment
- Perform assisted range of motion exercise
- Use safety device for limbs
- Maintain skin integrity
- Keep an oropharyngeal airway ready
- Keep additional intubation equipment and Ambu bag ready
- Communicate with family member about the ventilator requirement
- Inform family about client's inability to verbalize and develop means of communication, provide pencil/paper/place a calling bell within reach of patients
- Encourage the patient to verbalize their feelings.

- Take precaution on pressure points
- Observe for any electrolyte imbalances
- Monitor nutritional status and administer feeding as prescribed
- Monitor bowel sounds
- Provide oral hygiene frequently
- Moisten lips with lubricant jelly
- Identify any complication and prompt report
- Make yourself visible
- Watch for dysrhythmia, tachycardia, bradycardia and feeble peripheral pulses
- Maintain and monitor all medications as prescribed
- Watch for signs of progress and deterioration.

Alert

- Check ventilator setting and alarm limits and connection at least every hour and after suctioning
- Use oral airway when required to prevent compression of ETT
- Monitor ABGs and arterial oximetry according to ICU protocol
- Monitor for signs of accidental extubation, in such cases inform concerned physician for reintubation, maintaining ventilation and oxygenation with face mask and Ambu bag
- Determine level of consciousness and check protective reflexes as required
- Check any leakage
- If water in expiratory limb of ventilator, remove water from tubing and check humidifier setting
- Check heater wire in humidifier
- If leakage in cuff, check cuff pressure
- Verify the feeding tube
- Special precaution to eyes to prevent corneal abrasion, lubricate the eye
- Carefully suction as necessary.

Goal

Maintaining patent airway is the main goal:

- Regular suctioning
- Oxygen saturation monitoring
- Proper positioning
- Periodical ABG
- Chest physiotherapy.

Chapter 9 Immediate Postoperative Care in Recovery Room or Postanesthesia Care Unit

The goal of the postoperative phase is the patient's returns, as quickly as possible, to an optimal level of functioning. Nursing has a very important role during the postoperative period in promoting a rapid, smooth and comfortable patient recovery from the traumatic effects of surgery. Wound healing should be promoted and postoperative complication should be prevented. The immediate postanesthetic period is critical. The patient must be observed very closely and must receive intensive physical and psychological support until the major effects of the anesthetic have worn off, and the overall condition of the client becomes stable. The nurse is largely responsible for the patient at this time.

The patient is accompanied to recovery room or postanesthesia care unit (PACU) by the anesthesiologist and another member of the operation team. The recovery room nurses assess the patient's status, obtain a report and begin recording the recovery room notes. Much of the nursing care in the immediate postanesthetic period depends on the surgical procedure performed and type of anesthesia given.

COMPETENCY FOR PACU NURSES

Postanesthesia care unit nurses should demonstrate competency in:

- Physical assessment (e.g. heart rate and lung sounds)
- Management or physiologic emergency (e.g. airway hemorrhage and cardiac arrest)
- Additional competency should include certification in cardiopulmonary resuscitation (CPR), both basic life support (BLS) and advanced cardiac life support (ACLS).

ADMISSION TO POSTANESTHESIA CARE UNIT

The circulator should call the PACU nurse before the patient leaves the operation room to give the estimated time of arrival in the PACU and to advice of a need to have any special life-support equipment on standby for immediate physiological and psychological status is reported to PACU nurse. Any necessary life-support equipment such as ventilator is connected. The PACU nurse connects electrocardiography electrodes, attaches a pulse oximetry lead and place a blood pressure (BP) cuff on the patient.

The PACU nurse is responsible for assessing the patient and assimilating the data. The flow of activity is as fast paced, but directed to the immediate physiologic needs of the patient.

POSTOPERATIVE REPORT AND GENERAL NURSING CARE FOR ALL PATIENTS IN RECOVERY ROOM

The postoperative report will vary according to the type of anesthesia and the surgical procedure, the anesthesiologist and surgeons' preference, and the policy and procedures. The main emphasis is placed on the needs of the patient in the immediate postoperative period. It continues until the patient is discharged from the PACU.

Management

- Pulmonary ventilation
- Circulation
- Fluid and electrolyte balance
- Prevent injury
- Promote comfort.

Assessment Parameters

Assess the parameters such as airway patency, vital signs, BP reading, level of consciousness, patient's position, tissue oxygenation, dressing or suture lines, fluid lines and tubes, etc. (Table 9.1).

Table 9.1: Postanesthetic assessment

Parameter	Assessment
Airway	Patency, presence/adequacy of artificial airway
Vital signs	Respiratory rate, depth, character, heart rate (pulse, pulse oximetry or cardiac monitor) and blood pressure (cuff or arterial line)
Pressure reading	Pulmonary artery wedge pressure, central venous pressure (CVP) and intracranial pressure
Level of consciousness	Ability to follow commands, sensation and ability to move extremities following regional anesthesia
Patient's position	Position to facilitate breathing to prevent pressure on body parts or invasive lines and to promote comfort
Tissue oxygenation	Skin color, temperature, moisture, nail beds color, capillary refilling lips, oral mucosa, pulse oximetry, peripheral pulse and presence of strength
Dressing/Suture lines	Dressing dry or minimal drainage, suture lines (if visible) color approximation of wound edges
Fluid lines/tubes	Intravenous fluid, rate amount in bottle/bags/infusion site Other lines (e.g. CVP line, arterial line), patency, connection, character and amount of drainage, Ryle's tube drainage, urine output, quality and color; note and record fluid coming out of dressing

Nursing Diagnosis

Possible nursing diagnosis for the anesthesia patients includes:

- Ineffective airway clearance related to effects of general anesthesia
- Impaired gas exchange related to anesthetic, narcotics incisional pain
- Fluid volume deficits, potential related to blood loss, food and fluid deprivation and vomiting
- Potential for hypothermia related to altered thermoregulatory ability and cool ability
- Alteration in sensory perception related to effects of medications and anesthesia
- Altered comfort, pain related to incision and tissue trauma
- Impaired skin integrity related to operative incision
- Potential for injury related to sensory deprivation as a result of preanesthetic medications and anesthesia.

Nursing Intervention

Maintaining Airway Ventilation

1. **Maintaining airway patency:** Airway obstruction is usually caused by falling back of the relaxed tongue against the pharynx, trachea or bronchial tree:
   - Positioning: Side lying or semiprone position with the head tilted back (if not contraindicated) and the jaw supported forward
   - Artificial airway: Allow metal, plastic or rubber airway to remain in place until the patient begins to wake up and trying to eject the airway. Some patients may return from the operation room with an endotracheal tube (ETT)
   - Removal of secretion: Oropharyngeal suctioning is usually done, tracheal suctioning may be indicated.
2. **Maintaining adequate ventilation:**
   - Oxygen therapy: Oxygen is administered by nasal cannula, disposable face mask, ETT or tracheostomy tube, if one is in place
   - Breathing exercise: Deep breathing exercises are started as soon as the patient is fully conscious and able to follow instruction.
3. **Maintaining circulation:** Vital signs, blood pressure, pulse and respiration rate are usually taken as follows:
   - Every 15 minutes until stable, continued for as long as the patient is in the recovery room and for at least 1 hour after leaving the recovery room (RR)
   - Every ½ hour for 2 hours
   - Every 4 hours, until ordered otherwise.

Note: More frequent monitoring may be required depending on patient's condition and the surgical procedures done. Hypotension and cardiac dysrhythmias are the most common cardiovascular complications in the immediate postanesthetic period, early detection and management of these complications depends on frequent assessment of the patient's vital signs.

Promoting Normal Temperature

- Monitor for signs of hypothermia such as persistent of low body temperature shivering and patient reporting of feeling cold
- Use of warming methods and warm blankets are usually applied when cold present.

Maintaining Fluid Balance

- Careful monitoring of intravenous (IV) fluids and urine output is important to ensure adequacy of fluid replacement and prevention of fluid overload
- Fluid deficit may result from inadequate replacement of body fluids loss during surgery or continued fluid loss as in bleeding and vomiting
- Fluid excess may occur from large volume of fluids replaced by IV fluids, when kidney function is inadequate as evidenced by oliguria.

Preventing Injury

To prevent falls, side rails on the structure or bed are raised until the patient is fully awake.

Relieving Pain

- Postoperative pain management in the RR is usually under the direction of the anesthesiologist
- Pethidine is usually given by intramuscular injection, as prescribed.

Promoting Psychological Comfort

1. Immediate postanesthetic period is often frightening to the patient, psychological support is very important for physical and emotional well-being. Good psychological support usually results in faster recovery from anesthesia, fever complications and less incisional pain.
2. Frequent orientation to place and reassurance of not being alone done, while patient is awakening from anesthesia.
3. Inform patient that operation is over and recovery from anesthesia is satisfactory.
4. Careful explanation of procedures has to be given to patient even if patient does not appear alert.

Observe

Following observations should be monitored:

- Breath sounds are clear
- Respiratory rate is 12–20 breaths per minute and regular
- Oxygen saturation levels are within normal limit
- Blood pressure and temperature return to normal limits
- Skin should warm and dry, pulse is regular, urinary output usually slightly less than fluid intake
- Pulmonary edema does not occur
- Sleep is quite and face is relaxed.

Discharge from Recovery Room

Criteria for discharging patients from RR are as follows:

- Vital signs should are stable and indicate normal respiratory and circulatory function
- Patient is awake or easily aroused and can call for assistance when in need
- Postsurgical complications have been thoroughly evaluated and are under control
- After regional anesthesia, motor and partial sensory functions have returned to normal.

POSTOPERATIVE NURSING

1. Transfer of the patient to the clinical unit/ward.
2. Two ward nurses usually accompany the patient from the operating room. A report is given by the recovery room nurse about the surgery and condition of the patient. The patient's chart is also handed over.
3. The patient's room is prepared to facilitate patient transfer and monitoring. Most surgeons discuss the result of the surgery with the family immediately after surgery and also visit the patient to describe the findings and to provide reassurance.

Preparing Room for the Patients Return from the Surgery

- Make an open surgical bed to facilitate easy transfer of patient
- Provide sufficient cover/blanket (patient may feel cold)
- Clear passage way to the bed
- Provide necessary equipment:
  - Intravenous stand
  - Stethoscope and BP apparatus
  - Thermometer

- Kidney/Emesis basin
- Suction apparatus
- Oxygen cylinder or centralized oxygen with nasal cannula or mask
- Any special equipment as required. For example, tracheostomy set for post-thyroidectomy patient.

Patient Assessment on Return to Ward from Recovery Room

Subjective Data

Patient is asked for symptoms of discomfort.

Objective Data

1. **Respiratory status:**
   - Patency of airways
   - Respiration-depth rate and characteristics.
2. **Circulatory status:**
   - Skin, color and temperature
   - Capillary refilling
   - Intravenous fluid, flow rate, amount in bag/bottle patency of tubing and IV cannula
   - Insertion site.
3. **Neurological status:**
   - Level of consciousness
   - Ability to move extremities.
4. **Dressing:** Presence of bleeding.
5. **Drainage tubes:**
   - Presence and patency of tubes, nasogastric tube, urinary catheter, chest tube, etc.
   - Amount character of drainage
   - Comfort
   - Presence of pain, nausea and vomiting.
6. **Comfort:**
   - Presence of pain, nausea and vomiting
   - Patient positioned for comfort and to facilitate ventilation/breathing.
7. **Safety:**
   - Necessity for side rails
   - Call bell within reach.

Postoperative Nursing Care

Maintain Aeration

- Encourage deep breathing and coughing exercise and yawn maneuvers for all persons following inhalant anesthesia
- Use additional ventilatory maneuvers such as incentive spirometer, for person at risk for pulmonary complications
- Encourage body position changes, at least every 2 hours for bedridden patients
- Encourage maximum activity within the prescribed limits
- Monitor breath sounds until the patient is ambulatory.

Maintain Circulation

- Provide elastic stockings for person at risk for thrombophlebitis
- Encourage bed exercise and ambulation within prescribed limits
- Instruct patient to elevate legs when sitting, unless contraindicated
- Avoid postoperative leg massage.

Maintain Fluid and Electrolyte Balance

- Monitor intake and output until patient is taking oral fluids equal to at least 1,200 mL output
- Monitor IV fluid flow to provide required fluids
- Assess patient for fluid overload, especially small-sized elderly patient's, monitor body weight
- Encourage oral fluids as soon as permitted
- When oral intake is permitted, encourage high-protein foods and fresh fruits to supply needed potassium.

Maintain Nutrition

- Teach the patient to select foods high in protein and vitamin C to enhance wound healing
- Encourage carbohydrate intake for energy supply
- Suggest more frequent smaller meals for the anorexic person.

Maintain Elimination

- Encourage micturition in the early postoperative period
- Encourage fluids and maximal activity within prescribed limits to prevent constipation
- Use measures to encourage defecation, if the patient has not had a bowel movement 2–3 days after peristalsis returns.

Promote Activity

- Encourage leg exercise for the bedridden patient and during the early postoperative period
- Encourage patient to carry out activities of daily living (ADL) and to turn self in bed within the limitations of pain and fatigue
- Encourage progressive ambulation, as soon as permitted.

Promote Comfort

- Teach pain reliving measures such as relaxation exercise and position changes
- Remove causes of pain other than incisional, such as loosening the tight bandages
- Encourage the use of transcutaneous electrical nerve stimulator
- For 48 hours following major surgery, offer prescribed analgesics as prescribed intervals before pain becomes severe
- Carry out usual comfort measures, if vomiting occurs
- Encourage ambulation and exercises, and consider use of rectal tube, if gas pains are present
- Give the patient opportunity to talk about concern related to surgery
- Teach the patient:
  - Care of self, according to specific surgery performed
  - Community resources available for assistance as needed
  - Dietary and activity restrictions, according to surgery performed
  - Gradual resumption of normal activity
  - Avoidance of heavy lifting, pushing or pulling for at least 6 weeks after major surgery
  - Importance of medical follow-up visits.

Advantages of Early Postoperative Ambulation

1. **Increase in rate and depth of breathing by:**
   - Prevention of atelectasis and from hypostatic pneumonia
   - Increased mental alertness from increased oxygenation to brain.
2. **Increase in circulation:**
   - Nutrients required for wound healing
   - Prevention of thrombophlebitis/deep vein thrombosis (DVT).
3. **Increase in kidney function by means of:**
   - Prevention of urinary retention
   - Increased micturition.
4. **Increase in metabolism:**
   - Restoration of nitrogen balance
   - Prevention of loss of muscle tone.

5. **Increase in peristalsis:**
   - Promotion of expulsion of flatus/gas
   - Prevention of abdominal distention
   - Prevention of constipation
   - Prevention of paralytic ileus.

Common Postoperative Discomfort

- Nausea and vomiting
- Thirst
- Constipation and gas cramps/abdominal distention
- Pain
- Hiccups
- Restlessness.

Postoperative Complications

- Shock
- Hemorrhage/Bleeding
- Deep vein thrombosis
- Pulmonary complications:
  - Atelectasis
  - Aspiration
  - Pneumonia
  - Pulmonary embolism.
- Urinary retention
- Intestinal obstruction
- Wound infection due to postoperative dehiscence/evisceration
- Postoperative psychological disturbances/depression.

Postoperative Nursing: Cardiac Surgical Patient

The postoperative nursing care of the cardiac patient starts from the preoperative assessment of the patient, which gets further tailored according to the kind of operation performed. With so many diversified cardiac operations along with their altered physiology and its associated hemodynamic changes, which ensure mandates that all the nurses involved in the care of these sick patients must understand what kind of illness they are dealing with. The results of cardiac surgery have a direct bearing on the precision of operative technique used, perfection and the adequacy of postoperative care. We must stick to the old adage 'a stitch in time saves nine' a good cardiac nurse should be precise, very observant of the changes and spontaneous in taking certain decision. A nurse must learn to anticipate the problems that could occur after any given cardiac operation.

After the patient is received in the cardiac recovery as a systematic approach should be extended, so as to nothing is missed:

1. Check all the records, if they have been received. Talk to the anesthetist and surgeons to find out, what kind of operation has been performed? Was there any complication during the operation, etc.
2. Go through the patient's details and history of illness once again.
3. Connect all the monitoring lines to the monitor.

Now, the main task begins to systematically analyze all the organ system of the body:

1. Examine all the peripheral pulses and record their volume frequently as per institutional policy.
2. Check the skin temperature proximally and the farthest point, i.e. finger and toes.
3. Manually check the BP by a mercury manometer.
4. Observe the electrocardiogram (ECG), very important to note the rate rhythm and the pattern, if there are any changes in the preoperative ECG, discuss with concerned doctor.
5. Now, check the invasive pressure, they give lot of information about the cardiac stability such as:
   - Arterial trace, systolic, diastolic and the mean
   - Central venous pressure
   - Pulmonary artery pressure, systolic, diastolic and the mean
   - Left atrial (LA) pressure, if there is a LA line is connected.
6. Cardiac output, cardiac index and single ventricle physiology (SVP) to be recorded.
7. Record the core and peripheral temperature and chart the gradient, if the gradient is high with core being low. Warming matters or blankets should be used.
8. Some patient may be connected to the intra-aortic balloon pump (IABP) or left heart support devices, so care is to be taken about these and how to manage.

Neurological Status

- Check level of consciousness
- Check for papillary reactions and record
- Check for limb movements
- Reflexes.

Respiration Status

Since most of the cardiac patients are intubated and artificially ventilated, must ask the concerned doctor, what is the ventilation plan for a given patient, as depending on the surgery performed it could range from few hours to few days. However, the following steps are important:

- Ensure the ETT is properly secure
- Check the mark where it is fixed and note it down
- Ensure the cuff is properly inflated and there is no tracheal air leak
- Do endotracheal suction to keep it patency
- Connect to the ventilator and check the settings, and confirm with doctor
- Check for the air entry and bronchospasm
- Check the arterial blood gas and ascertain adequacy of ventilation and oxygenation
- Connect the pulse oximetry
- Connect the end-tidal carbon dioxide ($ETCO_2$) monitor
- Institute chest physiotherapy as early as possible, so as to restore lung functions as early as possible.

Renal Status

Urinary output is a good indicator of adequate cardiac output. Normally, it is about ½–1 mL/kg/h. Therefore, an hourly check on urinary output is maintained. If it is less than ½ mL/kg/h, check for the cardiac output, CVP or cardiac filling pressure and systemic BP.

Gastrointestinal Status

Since after anesthesia, hemodilution, uses of cardiopulmonary bypass (CPB) or induced hypothermia could reduce the gastric motility and certain drugs can give rise to ulceration, one must check the intestinal motility on return and then every 4 hourly, if bowel sounds are reduced or less, then check with the doctor for further course.

Hematological Status

For cardiac operations, large doses of anticoagulants are administered. Preoperative bleeding increases, therefore to reduce the associated problems with this certain measure as required. It includes:

- Monitoring of hemoglobin
- Monitoring of platelets count
- Monitoring of activated clotting time, prothrombin time (PT), activated partial thromboplastin time (APTT), etc.
- Thromboelastography.

Back and Generalized Nursing Cares

Since cardiac operations are lengthy procedures, the pressure points in the body can suffer a barotrauma or neurotrauma, therefore physiotherapy should be started after return to the intensive care.

Biochemical and Other Hematological Investigation

To check for heart, brain, liver, kidney and hematological system, functioning with intelligent, timely and aggressive approach many lives can be saved with least morbidity and mortality.

DISCHARGE CRITERIA FROM CRITICAL CARE AREA

Objective Parameters Model

Vital Signs

- Pulse < 40 or >150 beats per minute
- Systolic arterial pressure < 80 mm Hg or 20 mm Hg below the patient's usual pressure
- Mean arterial pressure < 60 mm Hg
- Diastolic arterial pressure > 120 mm Hg
- Respiratory rate > 35 breaths per minute
- Temperature < 36°C and > 38°C.

Laboratory Values

- Serum sodium < 110 mEq/L or > 170 mEq/L
- Serum potassium < 2.0 mEq/L or > 7.0 mEq/L
- Arterial partial pressure of oxygen (PaO_2) < 50 mm Hg
- pH < 7.1 or > 7.7
- Serum glucose > 800 mg/dL
- Serum calcium > 15 mg/dL
- Toxic level of drug or other chemical substance is hemodynamically or neurologically compromised
- Radiography/Ultrasonography/Tomography.

Transfer Out Policy from Intensive Care Unit

Responsibility

Treating physician.

Subjective Parameters

Feeling of improvement in clinical condition, corroborated by objective findings.

Objective Parameters

- Vital parameters (pulse, BP and respiratory rate) stabilized within normal range
- Patient is not on invasive ventilatory support

- Patient is not on vasopressor agents
- Patient is not on invasive hemodynamic monitoring
- Patient is maintaining adequate oxygenation and ventilation.

Transfer to Another Hospital

Transfer in Intensive Care Unit

- All resuscitated 'blue code' patients
- Patient requiring continuous monitoring postprocedure
- Any patient:
  - Variation in vital parameters (pulse, BP and respiratory rate)
  - Patient requires invasive ventilatory support
  - Patient requires invasive hemodynamic monitoring
  - Patient is at risk of impending cardiorespiratory arrest.
- Poor general condition requiring extensive nursing care.

INFECTION CONTROL PROCEDURE IN INTENSIVE CARE UNIT

Waste Disposal Policy

Categorization of Waste

1. **Non-risk waste:**
   - General waste such as papers, unused tubing, packing of drugs, infusion bags, etc.
   - Cooked or food-related waste.
2. **Risk waste:**
   - Infected waste
   - Human blood and blood products
   - Collection from chest drains
   - Used empty syringes.

   Note: All syringes must be cut before disposal.
3. **Sharp:**
   - Used and unused hypodermic needles (all needles must be cut before disposal)
   - Style of peripheral cannula and central lines
   - Empty glass ampule.
4. **Chemical waste:**
   - Expired drugs
   - Disinfectant and germicides used for cleaning.

5. **Human biological waste:** Parts of human body amputated during surgery.
6. Radiological waste.

Separation and Disposal

Separate the waste according to following color coding system:

1. **Non-risk waste:** Throw it in black-colored bucket containing black-colored polythene bag. When filled-dispose off this black bag.
2. **Risk waste:** Throw it in yellow-colored bucket containing yellow-colored polythene bag. When filled, dispose off this yellow bag.
3. Sharps are kept in a puncture proof hard bag, which is of yellow color.
4. **Disposal points (DPs):** It should be in different areas from where waste is collected at least twice a day.
5. **Collection of waste:** Waste is collected from DPs at 10 hours and 18 hours.
6. **Disposal of collected waste:** All bags are collected from the whole hospitals twice in a day, they are carried to a place outs side the main hospital building.

Cleaning the Hospital

Cleaning the hospital is carried out at least twice a day unless required more frequently, e.g. in operation theater (OT) or intensive care unit (ICU). Sweepers are not allowed to use 'jharoo' or 'pucharas' anywhere in the hospital. Garbage is collected at the spot and then throwed away according to waste disposal policy. Floor is then disinfected with phenyl; floor polishes are not allowed, because it may cause injuries to the patients and relatives, and attracts dust.

Cleaning and Disinfection of Bathroom

Bathrooms are cleaned at least twice a day unless needed more frequently. Toilet bowls and wash basins are cleaned with detergent, and then disinfected with phenyl. More permanent stains cleaned with carbolic acid in strength of 1/20.

VISITOR POLICY IN CRITICAL CARE AREA

Visitor Policy

1. No attendants allowed stay with patient.
2. Only one visitor at a time can go and have a look at his/her patient.
3. Only two visitors per patients.

4. In ICU, every visitor:
   - Must change their shoes at the entrance provided by ICU staff
   - Must wear a gown over his/her cloths provided at the entrance
   - Must not touch anything/anybody in ICU
   - Must not touch his/her patient without permission
   - Must not bring any utensil/eatable item for his/her patient
   - Must not stay for > 3 minutes inside ICU
   - Rights of admission are reserved and are on the discretion of Manager on duty.
5. Special dress in more vulnerable areas. The whole staff, if ICU wears special dresses. Once changed to the specific dress nobody is allowed to leave the area without changing back to civil dresses.
6. Changes of shoes, caps and face masks in ICU: No individual is allowed to enter in ICU without changing shoes provided for the purpose. Visitors and doctors, who are supposed to go nearer to the patients in ICU, must also wear cap and face mask.

CHANGE OF PATIENTS' POSITION IN BED

Responsibility

Nurse in-charge of the case.

Changing Position

- Must be done 2 hourly unless specified otherwise.
- Should be done by nurse in-charge of patient.
- Always move whole body, i.e. neck with trunk in case of spine injury.
- One person will hold the endotracheal tube (ETT) (if patient on ventilator support) or neck of patient, while other two will move the trunk.
- During every change of position:
  - Sponge the patient with lukewarm water
  - Disinfectant with cloth soaked in chloroxylenol solution (Dettol)
  - Apply talcum powder
  - Perineal and urethral areas are cleaned with normal saline-soaked towels
  - Soft support (pillows) are given on one side and between legs
  - Massage legs and heals
  - Keep heals over soft things, e.g. gloves filled with water
  - Look for the pressure sores on pressure areas.

Section 2

Critical Care in Nephrology/Urology

Chapter 10

Genitourinary Disorders and Nursing Management

STRUCTURE OF THE KIDNEY

Urinary system consists of the following structures:

- Two kidneys
- Ureters
- Urinary bladder
- Urethra.

Gross Structure

Kidneys are bean-shaped organs, about 11 cm long, 6 cm wide, 3 cm thick and weight 150 g. Lies on the posterior abdominal wall, on one each side of vertebral column, behind the peritoneum and below the diaphragm, they extend from the level of 12th thoracic vertebra to the third lumbar vertebra, the right kidney is usually slightly lower than the left.

Microscopic Structure

The kidney is composed of about 1–2 million functional units, the nephron and a smaller number of collecting ducts. The collecting ducts are supported by a small amount of connective tissue, containing blood vessels, nerves and lymph vessels. The nephron consists of a tubule closed at one end, the other end opening into a collecting tubule. The closed or blind end is indented to form the cup-shaped glomerular capsule (Bowman's capsule), which almost completely encloses a network of tiny arterial capillaries, the glomerulus. These resemble a coiled tuft, the remainder of the nephron is about 3 cm long and is described as:

- Proximal convoluted tubule
- Medullary loop (loop of Henle)
- Distal convoluted tubule, leading into a collecting duct.

The kidneys receive about 20% of the cardiac output. After entering the kidney at the hilum, the renal artery divides into smaller arteries and arterioles. In the cortex an arteriole, the afferent arteriole, enters each glomerular capsule and then subdivides into a cluster of tiny arterial capillaries forming the glomerulus:

1. Renal capsule: Cavity within the kidney at the level of hilum is the renal sinus, it is lined by the renal capsule.
2. Renal cortex surrounded by fibrous capsule it consists of two parts. Renal column, these consist of cortical tissue, which extends from the

surface to the renal sinus. Other cortical arches, these arches are cortical matter present between the base of pyramid and surface of kidney.

3. Ureter is thick-walled tubes extending from the corresponding kidney to the urinary bladder. They are two in numbers and lie in relation to the posterior abdominal wall, which carry urine from the kidneys to the urinary bladder. They are about 25–30 cm long with a diameter of about 3 mm.
4. Nephron is the functional unit of the kidney. There are about 1.3 million nephrons in each kidney.
5. Production and secretion of renin, which controls blood pressure (BP).

MAIN FUNCTIONS OF THE KIDNEYS

1. Formation and secretion of urine, which regulates total body water, electrolyte and acid base balance and enables excretion of waste products, urine is stored in the bladder and excreted by the process of micturition.
2. Production and secretion of erythropoietin, the hormone that stimulates formation of red blood cells. The lifespan of erythrocytes is about 120 days.
3. Filtration takes place through the semipermeable walls of the glomerulus.
4. Regulation of extracellular fluid volume by controlling the water and electrolyte balance.
5. Control acid-base balance of the body.
6. Eliminate waste products such as ammonia, urea, uric acid, creatinine, etc.
7. Waste products of protein metabolism are excreted.
8. Electrolytes levels are controlled and pH (acid-base balance) is maintained by excretion of hydrogen ions.
9. The excess of sodium need will be excreted mainly in urine and sweat.
10. The minimum urinary output, i.e. the smallest volume required to excrete body waste products is about 500 mL/day.
11. The kidneys regulate blood pH by increasing or decreasing the excretion of hydrogen and bicarbonate ions as required.
12. Maintain buffering system.
13. Normal pH of urine varies from 4.5 to 8 depending on diet, time of the day and number of other factors.

RENAL SYSTEM: ESSENTIAL CONCEPTS

Development

1. Kidneys development begins during the first few weeks of gestation, but is not complete until the end of the 1st year after birth.
2. Infants are unable to excrete a water load at the same rate as older children and adults; glomerular filtration and absorption do not reach adult capabilities until age 1–2 years.

3. Newborns are more prone to develop severe acidosis.
4. Sodium excretion is also reduced during infancy and the kidneys are less adaptable to sodium deficiency or excess.

Psychosocial Implications

1. **Infants:** Comforting the infant following threatening procedures and acceptance by parents and family members in vital to the development of a positive body image.
2. **Children:** Problems of immobilization frustrate the children's drive for independence; allowing the children to participate in care as appropriate, maybe helpful.
3. **Preschoolers:** At this stage, body image awareness is heightened and the child's natural curiosity about the body may be stimulated by physical examinations. The child's active fantasy life can contribute to fear of the simplest procedures.
4. **School-age children:** Appearing different from peers is extremely anxiety producing, as are prohibitions on diet, sports and other activities that focus the child's differences from age-mates.
5. **Adolescents:** Because of an adolescent's increased need for independence, the enforced dependence imposed by rigorous therapeutic regiments can increase feelings of resentment and rebelliousness.

Normal Urine Values in Children

The normal values for different parameters of urine are indicated in Table 10.1.

Table 10.1: Normal urine values in children

Parameters	Normal ranges
Color	Pale yellow to dark amber
Clarity	Clear
Volume (mL/day) newborn	50–300
Child	500–1,000
Thereafter	800–2,000
Leukocytes	< 5
Erythrocytes	< 10
Fresh specimen	< 10,000
Leukocytes infant	0–1
Osmolarity (mOsm) premature	50–600
pH	5.0–7.0
Protein	Negative

Contd...

Contd...

Parameters	Normal ranges
Specific gravity (random)	1.00–1.020
	1.001–1.030
	> 1.025 after fluid restriction
	Negative
Sugar	0
Ketones	0

ASSESSMENT AND DIAGNOSTIC MEASURES

History Taking

- Physical assessment and psychosocial assessment
- History of urinary or urological problems
- Nurse determines previous health history: Assess any history of diabetes mellitus, hypertension, metabolic problems, skin or upper respiratory problems, urinary calculi.

  The alteration in the function (signs and symptoms) of urinary tract can be:
- Pain
- Changes in voiding
- Gastrointestinal (GI) symptoms.

  Elicit the previous history of the following.

Pain

The nurses assess the sites of pain, onset, location, duration, associated manifestations, episodes and current treatment:

1. **Renal pain:** A dull aching pain in the costovertebral angle, radiating to the umbilicus. Flank pain radiating to the lower abdomen or epigastrium.
2. **Urethral pain:** Back pain radiating to the abdomen, upper thigh, testis and labium.
3. **Bladder pain:** Lower abdominal pain or over the suprapubic area associated with urgency, tenesmus and terminal dysuria.
4. **Urethral meatus pain:** With irritation of the bladder neck or urethra it is due to infection, trauma or foreign body in the lower urinary tract.
5. **Scrotal pain:** Results from inflammation and edema of the epididymis or testicle or from torsion of the testicle, perineal and rectal fullness indicates acute prostatitis or prostatic abscess.
6. **Back and leg pain:** It is due to metastasis of cancer of the prostate to the pelvic bones.
7. **Penile shaft pain:** Originates from urethral problems.
8. **Pain in the glans penis:** It is due to prostatitis.
9. **Epididymal pain:** Results from acute infection.

Changes in Voiding

1. **Urinary frequency:**
   - Voiding that occurs more often than usual (normally from 5 to 6 times plus once occasionally at night)
   - Caused by infection, disease in the urinary tract, metabolic disease as in diabetes mellitus, hypertension and drugs such as diuretics.
2. **Urgency:** It is a strong desire to void caused by:
   - Inflammatory lesion in bladder, prostate or urethra
   - Acute bacterial infection
   - Chronic prostatitis in male
   - Chronic posturethrotrigonitis (inflammation of urethral end trigone of bladder).
3. **Burning on urination:** Caused by urethral irritation or bladder infection.
4. **Dysuria:** Painful or difficult voiding.
5. **Hesitancy:** Undue delay and difficulty in initiating voiding it is caused by:
   - Compression of urethra
   - Neurogenic bladder
   - Outlet obstruction.
6. **Nocturia:** An excessive urination at night caused by:
   - Decreased renal concentrating ability
   - Heart failure
   - Diabetes mellitus
   - Incomplete bladder emptying.
7. **Urinary incontinence:** Involuntary loss of urine caused by:
   - Injury of the external urinary sphincter
   - Acquired neurogenic disease
   - Severe urgency from infection.
8. **Stress incontinence:** Intermittent leakage of urine caused by:
   - Sudden strain
   - Weakness of sphincter mechanism.
9. **Enuresis:** Involuntary voiding during sleep caused by:
   - Physiological causes as in age < 3 years old
   - Functional as in obstructive disease of the lower urinary tract.
10. **Polyuria:** Large volume of urine voided in a given time, it is caused by:
    - Diabetes mellitus
    - Diabetes insipidus
    - Chronic renal failure
    - Diuretics
    - Excessive fluid intake.
11. **Oliguria:** A small volume of urine out between 100 and 500 mL/24 h.

12. **Anuria:** Absence of urine in the bladder, output is less than 100 mL/24 h, it is caused by renal dysfunctions due to:
    - Shock
    - Trauma
    - Incompatible blood transfusion
    - Drug toxicity.
13. **Urine retention:** The inability to urinate despite the patient's urge to do so.
14. **Hematuria:** The presence of red blood cells (RBCs) in the urine is caused by:
    - Cancer in the genitourinary tract
    - Acute glomerulonephritis
    - Renal tuberculosis
    - Blood dyscrasias (abnormal clotting)
    - Anticoagulant therapy
    - Neoplasm
    - Trauma
    - Extreme exercise.
15. **Proteinuria (albuminuria):** An abnormal amount of protein in the urine caused by acute and chronic renal diseases.

Gastrointestinal Symptoms

Because the GI tract and urinary tract have common autonomic and sensory enervation and because of renointestinal reflexes, nausea, diarrhea, abdominal discomfort, paralytic ileus, vomiting, GI hemorrhage and appendicitis may be accompanied by urinary symptoms.

Diagnostic Test of Urinary Dysfunction

Urinalysis

Urinalysis performed on a clean catch specimen, midstream specimen, first morning specimen, a specimen obtained with a catheter or 24-hour urine collection:

1. **Urine color and clarity:** Pale yellow or amber clear.
2. **Urine odor:** Aromatic (because of ammonia).
3. **Measurement of urinary acidity and specific gravity:** 1.003–1.030.
4. **pH:** 4.5–8.0 measures free hydrogen ion in urine.

Renal Function Test

- Specific gravity to assess the renal concentration ability
- Osmolarity of urine
- Creatinine clearance

- Serum creatinine test
- Serum urea nitrogen.

X-ray and Other Imaging Studies

- Kidney, ureter and bladder X-ray (KUB)
- Computed tomography (CT) provides information about kidney perfusion
- Magnetic resonance imaging (MRI)
- Drip infusion pyelography
- Excretory urography [intravenous (IV) urogram or IV pyelogram]
- Retrograde pyelography
- Cystogram or cystourethrogram
- Renal angiography
- Ultrasound.

Endourology

1. **Cystoscopy:** It is direct visualization of the urethra and bladder by using a cystoscopy.
2. **Renal and urethral brush biopsy:** Through a urethral catheter, the suspected lesion is brushed back and forth in order to obtain cells and surface tissue fragments for histological analysis.
3. **Renal endoscope:** Introduction of a fiberoptic scope into the pelvis of the kidney through an incision (pyelotomy) or percutaneous to view the interior of the renal pelvis, remove calculi, biopsy of small lesions and aid in the diagnosis of renal hematuria and renal tumors.
4. **Needle biopsy of the kidney:** It is useful in evaluating the course of renal disease and in obtaining specimens for electron and immunofluorescent microscopy. It can be done percutaneously or opened through a small flank incision.
5. **Radioisotope studies:** A radiopharmaceuticals are injected. IV studies are obtained with a scintillation camera placed posterior to the kidney with the patient in a supine, prone or sitting position. It provides information about kidney function.
6. **Urodynamic measurements:** They provide physiological and structural tests to evaluate bladder and urethral function by measuring:
   - Rate of urine flow (uroflowmetry)
   - Bladder pressure during voiding and at rest (cystometrogram)
   - Interior urethral resistance (urethral pressure profiles)
   - Bladder and detrusor pressures, sphincter activity, bladder innervation
   - Cystourethrogram—visualization of urethra and bladder.

URINARY TRACT INFECTION (TABLE 10.2)

Definition

It is the presence of pathogenic microorganisms in the urinary tract with or without signs and symptoms. Urinary tract infections occur equally in boys and girls. After the first year, more common in girls than boys infants and toddlers often present non-specific symptoms of unexplained fever, abdominal pain, diarrhea, irritability, etc.

Cystitis

Cystitis is an inflammation of the urinary bladder that is mostly caused by ascending infection from the urethra .it occurs more often in adolescence. Cystitis or inflammation of the bladder wall; caused by bacteria lead to decreased flow of the urine. This infection higher in women probably because the female urethra is shorter and lies closer to the anal, and vaginal openings. Usually occurs in hospitalized client due to improper catheter care.

Etiology

- Fecal contamination
- Cystoscopy
- Presence of catheter
- Close proximity of vagina and anus
- Unhygienic underwear
- Wearing wet garments
- Hospitalization.

Table 10.2: Urinary tract infection

Sites of infection	Name of the condition
Bladder	Cystitis
Urethra	Urethritis
Prostate	Prostatitis
Kidney	Pyelonephritis

Common Organism Causing Cystitis

- *Chlamydia trachomatis*
- *Trichomonas vaginalis*
- *Neisseria gonorrhoeae*
- *Escherichia coli*
- *Klebsiella.*

Signs and Symptoms

- Change in voiding pattern
- Urgency, frequency, burning, pain on urination, nocturia, pain or spasm in the region of the bladder and suprapubic area
- Pyuria (WBCs in the urine) bacteria and often RBCs (hematuria) are found on examination of urine and positive urine culture
- Burning and pain while urinating
- Incomplete emptying of the bladder

- Occasional hematuria
- Frequency of voiding
- Dysuria

Medical Management

Antibiotics therapy to promote comfort, based on culture and sensitivity report specific treatment should be started, advice plenty of oral fluids and adherence to complete antibiotics course as prescribed. Patient should consult healthcare provider still his/her culture result is negative. Most commonly used pharmacological agents include urinary antibiotics such as sulfonamides, trimethoprim, and sulfamethoxazole and ciprofloxacin/ Cipro/nitrofurantoin.

Nursing Management

Nursing diagnosis

Nursing diagnosis based on the assessment data may be:

- Pain and discomfort related to inflammation and infection of the urethra, bladder and other urinary tract structures
- Knowledge deficit regarding factors predisposing to infection and recurrence, and pharmacological therapy.

Goals

- Relief of pain and discomfort
- Increase knowledge of preventive measures and treatment modalities.

Nursing Intervention

Relieving pain and discomfort by

- Antimicrobial, antispasmodic as prescribed
- Children are treated in home prior to treatment with any drugs
- Heat to perineum
- Hot tub baths relieve urgency, discomfort and spasms
- Encourage patient to drink liberal amounts of fluids to promote renal blood flow and flush the bacteria
- Avoid irritating fluids such as coffee, tea, colas
- Frequent voiding 2–3 hours is encouraged to empty the bladder completely
- Advise children to drink more fluids
- A short acting sulfonamide or ampicillin prescribed is usually advised.

Patient Education

- Parents are informed of the factors that predispose children to urinary tract infection and methods they can use to prevent their occurrence

- Female children should taught to wipe front to back when performing perineal hygiene and to use clean tissue for each wipe
- Reduce pathogens by hygienic measures
- Shower rather than tub bath
- Clean around the perineum
- Drink liberal amount of fluids 2–3 liters of water every day
- Void every 2–3 hours
- Take the ordered medication after emptying the bladder and just before sleeping
- Monitor and test the urine for bacteria
- Modify the diet dietary changes needed to keep the urine acidic and to reduce bladder irritation avoid irritating fluids such as coffee, tea, colas, tomatoes, spicy foods.

Evaluation and Expected Out Come

Relief of the manifestations by following the health teaching given.

Urethritis

Inflammation of the ureter commonly associated with pyelonephritis.

Pyelonephritis

Inflammation of the interstitial tissues and pelvis of the kidney, it can be acute or chronic. Chronic pyelonephritis is repeated bouts of acute pyelonephritis. Acute pyelonephritis is an inflammation of the renal parenchyma. The common cause is bacterial infection. Bacteria found in the intestinal tract.

Clinical Manifestations

- Pyelonephritis usually infection of lower urinary tract via the ascending urethral route
- Reduced host resistance (e.g. calculi, malignancy, hydronephrosis)
- Vary from mild fatigue to the sudden onset of chills, fever, vomiting, malaise, flank pain
- Usually asymptomatic unless an acute exacerbation occurs
- Fatigue ,headache poor appetite, polyuria, excessive thirst, weight loss
- One of the risk factor is pregnancy.

Diagnostic Study

- History and physical examination
- Urine analysis
- Complete blood count

- Urine culture and sensitivity
- IVP or CT
- Ultrasonography

Types

Acute pyelonephritis

Usually occurs with introduction of instruments such as catheter or cystoscopy, assessment reveals high fever, chills, nausea, flank pain; patient experience several days, urine may be cloudy or bloody.

Chronic pyelonephritis

More likely to occur after chronic obstruction Persistent and recurring infection may produce progressive scarring of the kidney Associated factor is present like retrograde or backward movement of urine from lower to upper urinary tract.

Management

Medical management

Usually prescribed, IV, antibiotics, ampicillin, vancomycin, trimethoprim, sulfamethoxazole (Bactrim, Septran) check with urine culture and sensitivity, fluoroquinolones (ciprofloxacin, norfloxacin. As prescribed by the physician.

Nursing management

- History and physical examination, previous history of urinary tract infection, urinary frequency, hesitancy, urgency, pain, dysuria, nocturia
- Objective data such as Fever chills
- Laboratory data.

Nursing Diagnosis

1. Altered urinary elimination related to urinary tract infection.
   Goal: Patient will experience normal urinary elimination.
   Nursing intervention: As follows
   - Monitor urinary elimination
   - Obtain urinary culture and sensitivity report
   - Encourage liberal water 3–4 L/day
   - Assess pain
   - Administer prescribed medication (urinary analgesics)
   - Apply warm compressor to suprapubic area/flank area.
2. Ineffective therapeutic management.
   Goal: Client will manage effective therapeutic regimen.
   Nursing intervention: As follows:

- Administer medication as prescribed, urinary analgesics and antibiotics
- Encourage fluid intake 3–4 liter
- Assessment of laboratory data
- If fever present antipyretics administration
- Monitor urinary function
- Assess vital signs.

3. Pain related to inflammatory process.
   Goal: Client will report there is no pain.

NEPHROTIC SYNDROME

Characterized by severe Proteinuria leading to edema, hypoalbuminemia and hypercholesterolemia

Etiology

- Congenital nephritic syndrome is caused by an autosomal recessive gene
- Secondary nephritic syndrome occurs after glomerular damage of unknown or presumed etiology (e.g. acute or chronic glomerulonephritis)
- Nephritic syndrome occurs in 2 of 100,000 children per year
- It primarily affects preschoolers; with the most common age of ones between 1½ and 3 years.

Clinical Manifestations

Clinical manifestations include:

- Weight gain
- Per orbital edema, ascites, peripheral edema and edema in the labia or scrotum
- Respiratory difficulty secondary to pleural effusion
- Anorexia and diarrhea secondary to edema of the intestinal mucosa
- Dark, frothy urine
- Oliguria
- Pallor
- Irritability
- Fatigue, lethargy
- Increased susceptibility to infection.

Diagnostic Tests

- Massive proteinuria
- Proteinemia
- Elevated serum cholesterol.

Nursing Management

- Prednisone at a dose of 2 mg/kg/day to reduce proteinuria or as prescribed
- Cyclophosphamide for a child failing to respond to steroid therapy
- Monitoring for increased edema and taking daily measurements of abdominal girth, weight, intake and output, BP, and pulse.
- Providing good skin care.
- Improve nutritional status by providing a high protein, high-calorie diet
- Help the family by answering questions and providing information on diagnosis tests and treatments.

ACUTE POSTSTREPTOCOCCAL GLOMERULONEPHRITIS

An acute poststreptococcal glomerulonephritis (APSGN), self-limiting autoimmune disease that follows group A β-hemolytic streptococcal infection (e.g. pharyngitis, impetigo). The most common type of acute glomerulonephritis.

Etiology

- The precipitating streptococcal infection commonly occurs in the upper respiratory tract or skin
- Incidence varies with the particular environmental prevalence of primarily affects early school-age children
- Onset commonly occurs within 7–14 days after antecedent infection
- Immune complexes lodge in glomeruli, leading to inflammation and obstruction; subsequent decreased glomerular filtration and tissue injury results in excretion of RBCs and casts.
- Kidneys enlarge, and sodium and water are retained leading to edema, protein is excreted in urine.

Clinical Manifestations

Clinical manifestations include:

- Hematuria resembling tea or cola
- Oliguria
- Weight gain
- Periorbital and generalized edema
- Pallor
- Irritability
- Fatigue lethargy
- Mild to moderately elevated blood pressure
- Urinalysis indicates the presence of protein, RBCs, WBCs and casts with associated increase in urine specific gravity.

Nursing Management

- Assess fluid status by monitoring intake and output, taking and recording daily weights, and observing for edema
- Administer prescribed medications as ordered
- Stimulate the child by providing quiet, ambulatory play activities
- Maintain adequate caloric intake and good nutrition by planning meals around the child's dietary preferences and serving meals in a pleasant atmosphere
- Impose sodium, potassium or fluid restrictions, as ordered
- Support the child and parents by explaining and answering questions about diagnosis, treatment and home care
- Educate the parents on treatment, home care and follow-up.

WILMS' TUMOR

Wilms' tumor is a highly malignant neoplasm it may affect one or both the kidney, usually occurs at the age 1–3 years, mainly caused by congenital anomalies.

Clinical Manifestation

- Presence of abdominal mass
- Spread to urinary tract
- Hematuria
- Spread to other organs early (metastasize).

Diagnosis

- Abdominal X-ray
- IVP
- CT
- Renal arteriography
- Urine analysis
- Hematologic and coagulation studies.

Nursing Management

- Different type of therapy will be administered depending on stage of the tumor
- Preparing child for diagnostic procedure
- Emotional support for parents and child
- If patient selected for surgery preoperative and postoperative care, usually kidney surgery (nephrectomy will be performed. Preoperative teaching

should also include what the parents and child can expect during the postoperative care

- Postoperative radiation therapy will be explained to the parents
- Chemotherapy and radiation therapy will be started
- Educate the parents about chemotherapy and radiation therapy its side effect and its management
- Chemotherapy side effect includes alopecia, anorexia, constipation, diarrhea, fatigue ulceration, nausea. And suggested nursing management should be implemented.

Chapter 11 Urological Disorders and Nursing Management

URINARY TRACT INFECTION

Definition

Urinary tract infection is the presence of pathogenic microorganisms in the urinary tract with or without signs and symptoms (Table 11.1).

Cystitis

Cystitis is an inflammation of the urinary bladder that is mostly caused by ascending infection from urethra, which occurs more often in women. Cystitis or inflammation of the bladder wall, caused by bacteria leads to decreased flow of urine. This infection is higher in women, probably because the female urethra is shorter and lies closer to the anal and vaginal openings. Usually occurs in hospitalized client due to improper catheter care.

Etiology

- Feminine hygienic condition
- Fecal contamination
- Cystoscopy
- Presence of catheter
- Improper catheter care
- Close proximity of vagina and anus
- Sexual intercourse increase the risk of cystitis
- Unhygienic underwear
- Wearing wet garments
- Postmenopausal women have increased risk
- Hospitalization
- Diabetes mellitus
- Urinary calculus.

Table 11.1: Infection based on site of occurrence

Sites of infection	Name of the condition
Bladder	Cystitis
Urethra	Urethritis
Prostate	Prostatitis
Kidney	Pyelonephritis

Common Organism Causing Cystitis

- *Chlamydia trachomatis*
- *Trichomonas vaginalis*
- *Neisseria gonorrhoeae*

- *Escherichia coli*
- *Klebsiella.*

Signs and Symptoms

- Change in voiding pattern
- Urgency, frequency, burning, pain on urination, nocturia, pain or spasm in the region of the bladder and suprapubic area, pyuria (white blood cells in the urine) bacteria and often red blood cells (hematuria) are found on examination of urine and positive urine culture
- Burning and pain, while urinating
- Incomplete emptying of the bladder
- Occasional hematuria
- Frequency of voiding
- Dysuria.

Medical Management

Antibiotics therapy to promote comfort, based on culture and sensitivity report specific treatment should be started, advice plenty of oral fluids and adherence to complete antibiotics course as prescribed. Patient should consult healthcare provider, still his/her culture result is negative. Most commonly used pharmacological agents include urinary antibiotics such as sulfonamides, trimethoprim, sulfamethoxazole and ciprofloxacin/cipro and nitrofurantoin.

Nursing Management

Nursing diagnosis based on the assessment data, may be:

- Pain and discomfort related to inflammation and infection of the urethra, bladder and other urinary tract structures
- Knowledge deficit regarding factors predisposing to infection and recurrence and pharmacological therapy.

Goals

- Relief of pain and discomfort
- Increase knowledge of preventive measures and treatment modalities.

Nursing intervention

1. **Relieving pain and discomfort by:**
   - Antimicrobial, antispasmodic as prescribed
   - Heat to perineum
   - Hot tub baths relieve urgency, discomfort and spasm
   - Encourage patient to drink liberal amounts of fluids to promote renal blood flow and flush the bacteria
   - Avoid irritating fluids such as coffee, tea and colas
   - Frequent voiding 2–3 hours is encouraged to empty the bladder completely.

2. **Patient education:**
   - Reduce pathogens by hygienic measures
   - Shower rather than tub bath
   - Clean around the perineum
   - Drink liberal amount of fluids 2–3 L of water everyday
   - Void every 2–3 hours
   - Take the ordered medication after emptying the bladder and just before sleeping
   - Monitor and test the urine for bacteria
   - Modify the dietary changes needed to keep the urine acidic and to reduce bladder irritation avoid irritating fluids such as coffee, tea, colas, tomatoes and spicy foods.

Evaluation—expected outcome

Relief of the manifestations by following the patient education given above.

Urethritis

Inflammation of the ureter commonly associated with pyelonephritis.

Pyelonephritis

Inflammation of the interstitial tissues and pelvis of the kidney and it can be acute or chronic. Chronic pyelonephritis is repeated bouts of acute pyelonephritis. Acute pyelonephritis is an inflammation of the renal parenchyma. The common cause is bacterial infection. Bacteria found in the intestinal tract.

Clinical Manifestations

- Pyelonephritis usually infection of lower urinary tract via the ascending urethral route
- Reduced host resistance (e.g. calculi, malignancy and hydronephrosis)
- Vary from mild fatigue to the sudden onset of chills, fever, vomiting, malaise and flank pain
- Usually asymptomatic unless an acute exacerbation occurs
- Fatigue, headache, poor appetite, polyuria, excessive thirst and weight loss
- One of the risk factor is pregnancy.

Diagnostic Study

- History and physical examination
- Urine analysis
- Complete blood count
- Urine culture and sensitivity

- Intravenous pyelogram (IVP) or computed tomography (CT) scan
- Ultrasonography.

Types

Acute pyelonephritis: Usually occurs with introduction of instruments such as catheter or cystoscopy, assessment reveals high fever, chills, nausea, flank pain; patient experience for several days, urine may be cloudy or bloody.

Chronic pyelonephritis: More likely to occur after chronic obstruction. Persistent and recurring infection may produce progressive scarring of the kidney. Associated factor is present as retrograde or backward movement of urine from lower to upper urinary tract or benign prostate hyperplasia (BPH).

Medical Management

- Usually prescribed as intravenous (IV)
- Antibiotics: Ampicillin, vancomycin, trimethoprim and sulfamethoxazole (Bactrim, Septra)
- Check with urine culture and sensitivity
- Fluoroquinolones (ciprofloxacin, norfloxacin as prescribed by the physician).

Nursing Management

1. History and physical examination: Previous history of urinary tract infection, urinary frequency, hesitancy, urgency, pain, dysuria and nocturia.
2. Objective data, e.g. fever and chills.
3. Laboratory data.

Nursing diagnosis I

Altered urinary elimination related to urinary tract infection.

Goal

Patient will experience normal urinary elimination.

Nursing intervention

- Monitor urinary elimination
- Obtain urinary culture and sensitivity report
- Encourage to drink liberal water 3–4 L/day
- Assess pain
- Administer prescribed medication (urinary analgesics)
- Apply warm compressor to suprapubic area/flank area.

Nursing diagnosis II

Ineffective therapeutic management.

Goal

Client will manage effective therapeutic regimen.

Intervention

- Involve patient and family members in care
- Explain medications required
- Advised to adhere medication prescribed
- Report to healthcare provider any adverse signs and any symptoms appears
- Advised to adhere fluid intake.

Nursing diagnosis III

Pain related to inflammatory process.

Goal

Client will report there is no pain.

Nursing intervention

- Administer medication such as urinary analgesics and antibiotics as prescribed
- Encourage fluid intake 3–4 L
- Assessment of laboratory data
- If fever present, antipyretics administration
- Monitor urinary function
- Assess vital signs.

NEPHROTIC SYNDROME

Nephrotic syndrome is a symptom complex commonly accompanying glomerular disease and characterized by severe proteinuria leading to edema, hypoalbuminemia and hypercholesterolemia.

Etiology and Incidence

1. Congenital nephritic syndrome is caused by an autosomal recessive gene. The disorder does not respond to usual therapy and the infant usually dies within the 1–2 years after birth.
2. Secondary nephritic syndrome occurs after glomerular damage of unknown or presumed etiology (e.g. acute or chronic glomerulonephritis).
3. Minimal change disease, so named because the histological changes seen by electron microscopy are limited to effacement of epithelial foot processes, accounts for 80% cases of nephritic syndrome in children aged 2–5 years. Onset often is preceded by a non-specific viral illness occurring 4–8 days before onset.
4. Nephritic syndrome occurs in two out of 100,000 children per year.
5. It primarily affects preschoolers; with the most common age of onset between 1½ and 3 years.
6. Incidences in boys is double than in girls.

Pathophysiology

1. Disturbance in the glomerular basement membrane leads to increased permeability to protein.
2. Protein leak through glomerular membrane resulting in:
   - Protein, especially albumin in urine (hyperalbuminuria or proteinuria)
   - Decreased serum albumin level (hypoalbuminemia).
3. Decreased colloidal osmotic pressure in capillaries leads to fluid shifting, causing fluid to accumulate in interstitial spaces and body cavities, particularly in the abdomen (ascites).
4. Massive fluid shift leads to hypovolemia, which stimulates the renin-angiotensin system to increase secretion of antidiuretic hormone (ADH) and aldosterone, leading to sodium and water reabsorption and further increased edema.
5. Hyperlipidemia occurs for as yet poorly understood reasons.

Assessment Findings

1. **Common clinical manifestations include:**
   - Weight gain
   - Periorbital edema, ascites, peripheral edema and edema in the labia or scrotum
   - Respiratory difficulty secondary to pleural effusion
   - Anorexia and diarrhea secondary to edema of the intestinal mucosa
   - Signs of malnourishment (may be masked by edema)
   - Dark and frothy urine
   - Oliguria
   - Pallor
   - Irritability
   - Fatigue and lethargy
   - Increased susceptibility to infection.
2. **Laboratory studies and diagnostic tests may reveal:**
   - Massive proteinuria
   - Proteinemia
   - Elevated serum cholesterol
   - Effacement of epithelial cell foot processes seen in electron microscopy.

Nursing Diagnoses

- Activity intolerance
- Body image disturbance
- Altered family processes

- High risk for fluid volume deficit
- Altered growth and development
- High risk for infection
- Knowledge deficit
- Altered nutrition; less than body requirements
- Impaired tissue integrity.

Planning and Implementation

1. Administer prescribed medications as ordered, which may include:
   - Prednisone at a dose of 2 mg/kg/day to reduce proteinuria
   - Immunosuppressant therapy (usually cyclophosphamide) for a child failing to respond to steroid therapy
   - Spironolactone in combination with hydrochlorothiazide to treat severe edema
   - A broad-spectrum antimicrobial agent to reduce the risk of infection.
2. Assess for fluid volume deficit by monitoring for increased edema and taking daily measurements of abdominal girth, weight, intake and output, BP and pulse.
3. Prevent skin breakdown by checking areas of edema for skin breakdown, ensuring frequent position changes, using scrotal supports in boys and providing good skin care.
4. Maintain or improve nutritional status by providing a high-protein and high-calorie diet. Offer small frequent meals of preferred foods in a pleasant atmosphere.
5. Monitor for signs of infection and take precaution to prevent infection [the child is susceptible to secondary infections because of the loss of immunoglobulin (a protein) in urine].
6. Conserve the childs energy by enforcing bedrest and encouraging quiet activities.
7. Help to improve the child's self-concept by providing positive feedback, emphasizing strengths and encouraging social interaction and pursuit of interests.
8. Support the family by answering their questions and providing information on diagnosis tests and treatments.
9. Provide patient and family teaching, covering:
   - Signs and symptoms of relapse to watch for and report
   - Urine testing for albumin
   - Medication dosage schedule, administration techniques and side effects
   - Special dietary instructions
   - Infection prevention measures
   - Skin care.

Evaluation

1. The child exhibits reduced edema and ascites, absence of skin breakdown and infection, and urine output within acceptable range.
2. Parents verbalize knowledge of the disorder, treatments, medications, home monitoring, diet instructions and follow-up care.
3. The child resumes or maintains age-appropriate development and participates in age-appropriate activities as tolerated.

ACUTE POSTSTREPTOCOCCAL GLOMERULONEPHRITIS

Acute poststreptococcal glomerulonephritis (APSGN) is an acute, self-limiting autoimmune disease that follows group A β-hemolytic streptococcal infection (e.g. pharyngitis and impetigo); the most common type of acute glomerulonephritis.

Etiology and Incidence

- The precipitating streptococcal infection commonly occurs in the upper respiratory tract or skin
- Incidence varies with the particular environmental prevalence
- The APSGN primarily affects early school-age children
- Incidence in boys is double that in girls.

Pathophysiology

- Onset commonly occurs within 7–14 days after antecedent infection
- Some theorized that streptococcal infection is followed by release of a membrane such as substance from the specific organism, which is antigenic in nature
- Antibody is formed in response and an immune-complex reaction occurs
- Immune complexes lodge in glomeruli, leading to inflammation and obstruction; subsequent decreased glomerular filtration and tissue injury result in excretion of red blood cells (RBCs) and casts
- Kidney enlargement, sodium and water are retained leading to edema, protein is excreted in urine
- Most children with APSGN recover completely, but some develop chronic disease
- Although rare, complications are associated with APSGN the most serious include hypertensive encephalopathy, pulmonary edema and acute renal failure.

Assessment Findings

1. Common clinical manifestations include:
   - Hematuria resembling tea or cola
   - Oliguria
   - Weight gain
   - Periorbital and generalized edema
   - Pallor
   - Irritability
   - Fatigue lethargy
   - Mild to moderately elevated BP.
2. Onset of complications can lead to serious sequelae, if not detected and treated early, signs and symptoms of complications include:
   - Markedly elevated BP, headache, dizziness, abdominal discomfort and vomiting and altered level of consciousness possibly progressing to seizures (hypertensive encephalopathy)
   - Coughing, restlessness, paroxysmal nocturnal dyspnea (pulmonary edema).
3. Urinalysis indicates the presence of protein, RBCs, white blood cells and casts with associated increase in urine specific gravity.
4. Other laboratory study data may reveal:
   - Mild anemia and leukocytosis
   - Positive antistreptolysin O (ASO) titers indicating a recent streptococcal infection
   - Elevated erythrocyte sedimentation rate
   - Elevated blood urea nitrogen (BUN) and creatinine levels.
5. Renal biopsy, if done, shows an increased number of cells in each glomerulus.

Nursing Diagnoses

- Diversional activity deficit
- Altered family processes
- Fluid volume deficit
- Fluid volume excess
- High risk for infection
- Knowledge deficit
- Altered nutrition: Less than body requirements.

Planning and Implementation

1. Ensure early detection of complications by closely monitoring BP and respiratory rate.

2. Assess fluid status by monitoring intake and output, recording daily weights and observing for edema.
3. Administer prescribed medications as ordered, which may include:
   - Intravenously diazoxide and furosemide to treat severe hypertension
   - Methyldopa or hydralazine, usually in conjunction with reserpine or furosemide, to treat mild hypertension
   - Digitalis to combat circulatory overload
   - Antibiotics to treat existing streptococcal infection
   - Diuretic therapy, such as hydrochlorothiazide or furosemide or severe edema.
4. Stimulate the child by providing quiet, ambulatory play activities.
5. Maintain adequate calorie intake and good nutrition by planning meals around the child's dietary preferences and serving meals in a pleasant atmosphere.
6. Impose sodium, potassium or fluid restrictions as ordered.
7. Support the child and parents by explaining and answering questions about diagnosis, treatment and home care.
8. Refer the child and family to a community health nurse for home visits, as needed, to help them for adjusting to home managements.
9. Provide patient and family teaching, covering:
   - The need for medical evaluation and culture of all sore throats
   - Home care measures, including urinary testing, BP monitoring activity, diet instructions, infection—prevention measures, and signs and symptoms of potential complications to watch for, and report (the child will require monitoring of urinalysis and BP, for 6 month and then every 3–6 month until he/she has been symptom free for 1 year)
   - Medication dosage schedule, administration techniques and side effects
   - The possible need for peritoneal dialysis or hemodialysis, if renal failure occurs.

Evaluation

1. The child demonstrates improved urine output, maintains weight, adheres to diet restrictions and is free from life-threatening complications.
2. Parents verbalize knowledge of treatment, home care and follow-up.

CRYPTORCHIDISM (UNDESCENDED TESTICLE)

Failure of one or both testes to descend through the inguinal canal to the normal position in the scrotum.

Etiology/Incidence

- Possibly caused by delayed descent, prevention of descent by mechanical lesion or endocrine disorder
- More common in premature infants.

Nursing Diagnoses

- Body image disturbance
- Risk for infection
- Risk for fluid volume deficit
- Pain
- Knowledge deficit.

Planning and Implementation

1. Administration of human chorionic gonadotropin (HCG) has produced descent of the tests in some children. Testes may have descended spontaneously in many of these cases.
2. Orchiopexy surgery to achieve permanent fixation of the testis in the scrotum. Surgery should be performed between the age 1 and 3 to prevent damage to the tissues and to lessen emotional concerns related to body image.

Postoperative Nursing Management

- Prevent contamination of the suture line, a suture is placed in the lower portion of the scrotum
- Administer antibiotics as prescribed to prevent infection
- Administer wound care by using aseptic technique, inspect incision for drainage or signs of infection
- Providing emotional support regarding body image
- Continue reassurance about appearance of genitalia
- Maintain discussions regarding reactions
- Focus on activities that child can perform and accomplish
- Measure and record accurate intake and output
- Administer analgesics as ordered and according to assessment of complaints on pain restlessness, crying or withdrawal.

Evaluation

1. Child and family verbalizing to understanding of surgery.
2. Child and family verbalizing relief that defects can be surgically repaired and reconstructed.
3. Incision without drainage or signs of infection.
4. Vital signs stable urine output adequate.

HYPOSPADIAS

Malposition of the urethral opening.

Etiology and Incidence

- It is frequently associated with other urogenital tract anomalies
- Although rare, it is the most common disorder involving the penis
- Possibly due to decreased testosterone production in early gestation
- Increased chance for incidence with future male siblings
- Rare in girls.

Pathophysiology

- The urethra opens on the ventral aspect for the penis
- In severe forms, interfere with the inability to procreate
- Inability to void with the penis in the normal elevated position
- In female, the urethra opens into vagina.

Diagnostic Tests

- Usually not difficult to diagnose due to visual anomaly
- Chromosomal and hormonal studies in severe cases of genotypic/phenotypic (sex determination)
- Renal ultrasound, IVP voiding cystourethrography to determine associated defects.

Nursing Diagnoses

- Anxiety
- Pain
- Body image disturbance
- Knowledge deficit
- Impaired physical mobility
- High risk for impaired skin integrity
- Constipation.

Planning and Implementation

Preoperative nursing management

Prior to surgical repair, the family is given an explanation of the elements of the procedure and its goals.

Postoperative nursing management

1. Mobility is severely limited for the first 48–72 hours following surgery and moderate restrictions are maintained for 7–10 days until the suprapubic tube and dressings are removed.
2. During the first 2–3 postoperative days, child is confined to the bed and required to remains in a supine position.
3. Prepare the parents for this period of limited mobility and encourage them to obtain multiple diversionary activities that the child may engage in, such as story books, toys that can be manipulated, while the child is supine.
4. Administer analgesic as ordered.
5. Pillows or other supports are used to afford maximal mobility.
6. Maintain adequate hydration:
   - Measure urine
   - Encourage fluids as needed.
7. Provide adequate fiber-rich foods.
8. After Foley catheter is removed, chart when the child voids through the meatus, report to the doctor:
   - Character of flow, presence of spray, dribbling and leaking pain
   - Expect pain on the first voids, should decrease subsequently.

Evaluation

- The parents verbalize their relief that defects can be repaired
- The child interacts with other children, despite immobility during the postoperative period.

RENAL CALCULUS

An abnormal stone formed in body tissues by an accumulation of minerals. (calcium oxalate, calcium phosphate and uric acid). Stone may be found any where from the kidney to the bladder and vary in size from minute granular deposits, small sand size to big size as small apple.

Etiology

- High-serum calcium
- High-urine calcium
- Infection
- Urinary stasis for longer time
- Hyperparathyroidism
- Excessive intake of vitamin D.

Assessment

1. Pain, discomfort, severity, location, radiation, associated symptoms, relieving factors and aggravating factors.
2. Signs and symptoms of urinary tract infection, chills, fever, dysuria, frequency, hesitancy.
3. Obstruction: Frequent urination with small amounts of oliguria or anuria.
4. Urine hematuria, stones and gravel.
5. History factors, which predispose the patient to urinary tract stones as family history of stones, bone marrow disorders, use of chemotherapeutic agents, inflammatory bowel disease, high calcium or purines diet, dehydration, prolonged immobilization and infection.
6. Patient knowledge about renal stones and measures to prevent their occurrence or reoccurrence.
7. Associated manifestations as nausea, vomiting, diarrhea and abdominal distention.

Diagnosis Findings

- Kidney, ureter and bladder (KUB) X-ray
- Ultrasonography
- Blood chemistry, serum calcium, uric acid, creatinine sodium and pH
- Dietary, medication history and family history.

Medical/Nursing Management

- Control the pain
- Antibiotics as prescribed
- Hot baths or moist heat to the flanks area
- Increase the fluids
- If stone is not removed, use extracorporeal shock wave lithotripsy or surgically remove the stone
- Monitor the patient pain closely.

Nursing Diagnosis

- Pain and discomfort related to inflammation, obstruction of urinary tract
- High risk for infection and obstruction related to blockage of the urinary tract by a stone or edema
- Knowledge deficit regarding prevention of occurrence of renal stones.

Patient Education and Home Care

- Encourage the patient to follow a regimen to avoid further stone formation
- Maintain a high fluid intake

- Avoid sudden increase in environmental temperature
- Increase fluid after excessive sweating
- Increase fluid in the evening to prevent urine concentration at night
- Perform urine culture every 1-2 months of the 1st year and periodically thereafter
- Increase mobility whenever possible
- Avoid excessive ingestion of vitamin especially, vitamin D
- Instruct the patient about signs and symptoms of complications
- Instruct the patient about the importance of following up assessment of kidney function
- Explain to the patient about the medications, their actions and importance.
- Instruct the patient to monitor his/her urine pH
- Direct the patient to report to the hospital promptly.

RENAL FAILURE

When the kidneys are unable to remove the body metabolic wastes or perform their regulatory functions result in accumulation of toxic wastes, increased serum urea and creatinine level. Reduced kidney function, it is of two types:

- Acute renal failure
- Chronic renal failure.

Acute Renal Failure

Sudden loss of kidney functions to clear waste products and regulate fluid and electrolyte balance and accumulation metabolic waste products.

Causes

1. **Prerenal:**
    - Hypovolemia (hemorrhage and dehydration)
    - Extensive surgery in the elderly
    - Septicemia (septic shock).
2. **Intrarenal:**
    - Damage to the glomerular or kidney
    - Prolonged renal ischemia
    - Hemoglobinuria (transfusion reaction, hemolytic anemia, crush injury, burns and massive tissue injury)
    - Exposure to nephrotoxic agents
    - Acute glomerulonephritis
    - Acute pyelonephritis.

3. **Postrenal:**
   - Urinary tract obstruction, calculi tumors, prostatic hypertrophy and strictures
   - Due to obstruction distal to the kidney as pressure rises, decreased glomerular filtration rate (GFR).

Clinical Manifestations

- The patient appears critically ill is lethargic
- Persistent nausea, vomiting and diarrhea
- Dry skin and mucous membranes
- The breath may have the odor of urine
- Drowsiness, headache, muscle twitching and convulsion
- Scanty urinary output may be with blood, urine with low specific gravity
- Daily rise in the serum creatinine value
- Severe hyperkalemia, which may leads to dysrhythmias and cardiac arrest
- Decrease in serum calcium levels
- Anemia due to uremic gastrointestinal lesions reduced RBCs lifespan and reduced erythropoietin production.

Management

Goals: To restore normal chemical balance and prevent complications. The treatment modalities include the following:

1. **Dialysis:** Hemodialysis, peritoneal.
2. **Reduce potassium levels:**
   - Monitoring serum electrolyte levels and electrocardiography (ECG)
   - Reduce patient catabolic chemical status
   - Administering ion exchange (sodium sulfate) orals or by retention enema and eliminate sources of potassium.
3. **Management of fluid balance:**
   - Record daily body weight
   - Measurement of central venous pressure (CVP), serum and urine concentrations, fluid losses, BP and clinical status of the patients intake and output recording, edema distention of jugular veins and retention of fluid excess
   - Dietary proteins are limited to approximately 1 g/kg during oliguric phase and then high-protein diet after the diuretic phase
   - High carbohydrates: Restrict foods and fluids containing potassium and phosphorus such as banana, citric juice and coffee
   - Monitor the patient for complications

- Inform patient's family about patient condition.
- Bedrest to reduce patient's metabolic rate.
- Prevent and/or treat fever and infection.
- Maintain asepsis with invasion lines and catheter.
- Skin care to avoid dryness, breakdown, excoriation and itching. Massage bony prominences, turn the patient frequently and bath with cool water frequently.

Chronic Renal Failure (Uremia)

Chronic renal failure is a progressive irreversible deterioration in renal and function the body ability to maintain metabolic, fluid and electrolyte balance fails. The end result is uremia, a syndrome resulting from an excess urea in the blood.

Causes

- Chronic glomerulonephritis
- Pyelonephritis
- Uncontrolled hypertension
- Hereditary lesion as polycystic kidney disease
- Vascular disorders
- Obstruction of the urinary tract
- Renal disease secondary to systemic disease
- Infection
- Drugs
- Toxic agent
- Environmental and occupational agents.

Clinical Manifestation

- Flank pain
- Azotemia
- Edema of the extremities, sacral area and abdomen
- Hypernatremia (excessive sodium in the blood) and hypertension
- Hyperkalemia (excessive amount of potassium)
- Disturbances in acid-base balance
- Begins with fatigue and lethargy
- Headache, general weakness
- Decreased urinary output
- Fatigue anorexia, nausea, vomiting and diarrhea
- Bleeding tendencies
- Mental confusion

- Decrease in salivary flow, thirst and metallic taste in mouth
- Loss of smell and taste
- Parotitis and/or stomatitis
- Fluid volume overload
- Electrolyte imbalances
- Elevated BUN, creatinine.

Without treatment, these symptoms become more marked and metabolic abnormalities of uremia affect every body system:

- The patient becomes more and more drowsy
- The respirations becomes Kussmaul
- Deep coma develops often with convulsions (myoclonic jerks)
- A white powdery substance (uremic frost) appears on the skin
- Death soon follows, if there is no treatment.

Medical Management

Goals: As follows:

- Retain kidney function
- Maintain homeostasis for as long as possible.

Treatment: Based on symptoms with restricted diet and fluid intake, and medication:

- Treat the reversible causes
- Dialysis
- Kidney transplantation.

Nursing Management

Nursing diagnosis I

Excess fluid volume related to inability of the kidney to excrete water.

Nursing intervention

- Monitor intake, output and daily weight
- Monitor vital signs, report any significant findings
- Monitor laboratory values as prescribed
- Allow fluid as prescribed usually 500–1,000 mL as condition permits
- Provide personal hygiene specially skin care.

Nursing diagnosis II

Altered nutrition less than body requirements.

Nursing intervention

- Monitor body weight daily
- Advise food as decided by dietitian and physician
- Monitor bowel function

- Monitor GI symptoms
- Offer frequent and small meals/snacks.

Nursing diagnosis III

Risk for infection related to impaired immune system.

Nursing intervention

- Observe for any signs and symptoms of infection
- Maintain aseptic precaution
- Allow the fruit as advised by physician
- Advise the patient to avoid contact with infected person
- Reduce visitors.

Chapter

12

Dialysis

The process of separating colloids and crystalline substances in solution by the differences in their rate of diffusion through a semipermeable membrane or dialysis is a technique in which substances move from the blood through a semipermeable membrane into a dialysis solution (dialyzate).

PRINCIPLES OF DIALYSIS

Dialysis involves diffusion of particles from an area of high to lower concentration:

- To remove poison and excessive amounts of drugs
- To correct serious electrolytes and acid-base imbalance
- To remove nitrogenous waste product such as urea, uric acid and creatinine in patient with chronic end-stage renal disease.

The principles of diffusion, osmosis and ultrafiltration are involved in dialysis.

Diffusion

Diffusion is the process in which solid particles or matter in a fluid moves from an area of higher concentration to an area of lower concentration resulting in an even distribution of the particles in the fluid.

Osmosis

Osmosis is the movement of a pure solvent such as water, through a semipermeable membrane from a solution that has a lower solute concentration to one that has a higher solute concentration. The membrane is impermeable to the solute, but is permeable to the solvent. The rate of osmosis depends on the concentration of solute. Osmosis is the movement of fluid from an area of lesser to an area of greater concentration of solute. Glucose is added to the dialyzate and creates an osmotic gradient across the membrane, pulling excess fluid from the blood.

Ultrafiltration

A type of filtration sometimes conducted under pressure through filters with very minute pores, as used by an artificial kidney ultrafiltration can separate large molecules from smaller molecules in body fluids. The excess fluid is removed by creating a pressure differential between the blood and dialyzate solution with a combination of positive pressure in the blood compartment or negative pressure in the dialyzate compartment.

INDICATION FOR DIALYSIS

- Dialysis removes excess water and nitrogenous waste
- Reducing the manifestation of renal failure
- Useful in acute renal failure or as a permanent life-sustaining treatment
- Control uremia
- Physically prepare the client to receive transplanted kidney.

Hemodialysis involves the use of artificial kidney to remove waste products and excess water from the patient blood. Main object is to remove excess water by artificial kidney called dialyzer, used artificial semipermeable membrane. In hemodialysis, the blood contain toxin and nitrogenous wastes is diverted from the patient to a machine, a dialyzer, where toxin are filtered out and removed, and the blood is returned to the patient.

VASCULAR ACCESS

Vascular right of entry must be established to allow blood to be removed, cleansed and returned to the patient's vascular access.

Arteriovenous Fistula

For hemodialysis, permanent vascular access is created surgically (usually in the forearm) by joining (anastomosing) an artery to a vein, either side-to-side or end-to-side, it needs 2–3 months to mature. Then it will accommodate large quantity of blood flow.

Arteriovenous Graft

A biological and semibiological or synthetic graft material between artery and vein for patient, who is not candidate for arteriovenous fistula (AVF) can be created subcutaneously.

Patient Education

Nurse who takes care of the patient should be cautious and advise, but not to use harsh tone:

- Discuss why hemodialysis is necessary
- Explain problems, complication and their management during hemodialysis
- Advise dietary and fluid restriction as per physician's prescription
- Show how to take care of AV fistula
- Inform to observe and report side effects such as skin allergy, signs and symptoms of infection
- Advise to take precaution, while traveling, exercising, working or during family activity

- Identify learning need of patient
- Report any painful muscle cramps
- Report signs and symptoms of headache, nausea, vomiting, restlessness and drowsiness
- Follow prescribed dietary protein, sodium, potassium and fluid requirements
- Fluids are restricted to an amount equal to the daily urine output plus 500 mL/day
- Recording daily weight
- Allow the patient and relatives to express their feelings
- Take medication as prescribed.

PREDIALYSIS ASSESSMENT OF HEMODIALYSIS PATIENT

Definition

An assessment of condition of the patient prior to commencing hemodialysis treatment is required. The assessment includes physical, social and psychological aspects to detect and manage any immediate identifiable problems for further action and to enable the planning of an individualized treatment in line with their dialysis prescription.

Purposes

- To ensure safe and effective treatment planned according to the patient's dialysis prescription
- To identify any issues that require further action and follow-up to ensure that the patient receives individualized therapy and thus, maintain optimum quality of care.

Conditions

- The procedure (Table 12.1) should be carried out by an experienced dialysis nurse
- Applies to all registered nursing personnel working in the dialysis centers
- This procedure can be undertaken by an inexperienced dialysis nurse undertaking a specific educational training program, provided they are closely supervised by an experienced dialysis nurse at all time
- A strict aseptic technique should be maintained throughout the procedure in accordance with the policy and procedures of aseptic technique
- Hand hygiene should be performed according to policy and procedures on handwashing.

Equipment

- Stethoscope
- Blood pressure apparatus
- Weighing scale
- Thermometer
- Patient's file.

Table 12.1: Procedure for predialysis assessment

Nursing actions	Rationales
1. *Impression of general condition*	
• General enquiry to the patient about health and well-being since last dialysis treatment and situation on the day of treatment • Objective assessment of the visual picture of the patient's walking (easily, general), demeanor or any other signs of potential complications, e.g. dyspnea and muscle weakness	• Vital information about the patient can be learned as soon as he/she arrives for treatment • More extensive assessment is required before the patient is commenced on dialysis therapy • Any patient's complaint may require immediate action before dialysis therapy can be commenced
2. *Weight*	
• Weigh patient ensuring that he/she is in the same clothes, etc. as per previous dialysis treatments; an appropriate person should check the weight of the patient • Observe general condition, observing for complications such as hypotension • Document findings and interpret information obtained • If any abnormalities detected, inform the physician for further action	• It is necessary to compare predialysis weight with that at the end of the previous dialysis to assess the weight gained and to be able to plan dialysis treatment in the light of expected dry weight and the information gained from the patient as per step one • Further action may be necessary if there are abnormalities detected, which may result in a change in analysis prescription
3. *Check and record vital signs*	
• Blood pressure • Pulse rate, rhythm and fullness • Temperature • Volume status: – Presence and absence of edema – Neck vein distention – Skin turgor	• Vital signs and fluid status of the patient should be in the normal range, if there is deviation from the normal range, the physician should be informed and further action taken, which may include revision of dialysis of prescription
4. *Review*	
• Review laboratory reports for treatment of biochemical and hematological data, interpret data and note findings for further action	• It is essential that all data is reviewed to ensure that patient safety is maintained; it is essential to maintain accurate and complete

Contd...

Contd...

Nursing actions	Rationales
• Review previous dialysis treatment records for notes, remarks and action to be taken • General review of all findings to ensure that dialysis treatment can be planned according to the individual requirements	records of data obtained to allow monitoring of treatment responses and the detection and management of any complications • If any abnormalities are detected, an appropriate member of the team should take appropriate action; required patient education should be noted for further planning
5. *Assessment of vascular access*	
• Question the patient about the fistula/ vascular access since last dialysis treatment • Observe overall appearance of limb/site for signs of swelling, etc. • Carefully observe the fistula/site for signs of infection, evidence of fistula/ site for bruit, thrill, volume and any signs of pain or oozing, etc.	• It is essential that potential complications will be eliminated before dialysis treatment is commenced • It is important to maintain accurate and complete records of data obtained to allow monitoring of treatment responses, detection and the management of any complications
6. *Documentation of findings*	
• The results of the assessment and the treatment goals should be recorded and signed by the nurse undertaking the assessment • Any notes or instructions for this or a subsequent dialysis treatment must be clearly identified	• There has to be accountability for the delivery of dialysis treatment and evidence of the therapy management to achieve the goals of the dialysis prescription • It is necessary to ensure that there is continuity of care from one dialysis treatment to the next to maintain patient safety and well-being

PRIMING OF HEMODIALYSIS BLOODLINES AND DIALYZER

Definition

Priming is a process in which normal saline is rinsed and filled into the dialyzer and bloodlines to expel air and sterilant to expand the membranes to achieve effective surface area.

Purpose

To demonstrate a safe and skilled method of priming hemodialysis bloodlines and dialyzer.

Conditions

- Applies to all registered nursing personnel working in dialysis centers
- This procedure (Table 12.2) can be undertaken by an inexperienced dialysis nurse undertaking a specific educational training program, provided they are closely supervised by an experienced dialysis nurse at all times
- Practice universal precautions and aseptic technique according to policy and procedures on infection control
- The machine should be fully functional and alarm testing has been completed.

Equipment

- Dialyzer
- Arterial and venous bloodlines
- Intravenous set with Luer lock
- One 20 mL syringe
- Blood-lined clamp as required
- Three 500 mL sodium chloride (NaCl) 0.9% (two for priming and one for washback at the end of dialyzer).

Table 12.2: Procedure for priming hemodialysis bloodlines and dialyzer

Sl No.	Nursing actions	Rationales
1.	Wash and dry hands as per policy and procedures on handwashing	To prevent cross infection
2.	Place dialyzer in holder with arterial side down **Alert:** Please note specific requirements of the machine	To expel air from extracorporeal circuit
3.	Place one bottle of normal saline (500 mL) on the intravenous (IV) stand with primed drip set	IV normal saline should be attached and available throughout the procedure
4.	**Arterial line:** Apply clamp to patient's end of the arterial line with attached spike saline, which is on stand	The saline will run through the line, if not clamped
5.	Place arterial line on the machine	To expel air
6.	Prime heparin line by opening the line to air and reapply screw	
7.	Connect arterial line to the dialyzer 'A' port	

Contd...

Contd...

Sl No.	Nursing actions	Rationales
8.	Connect pressure transducer as required	To monitor measure where facility is available
9.	Release clamp and prime with saline by gravity until pump segment is full of saline and reapply the clamp as before	To expel all air from lines
10.	**Venous line:** Place venous chamber in air detector	To ensure there is continuous monitoring of air
11.	Connect venous line to dialyzer 'V' port	
12.	Place patient end of the venous line into sterile drainage bag and ensure venous end clamp is opened	
13.	Connect pressure transducer	
14.	Priming hollow fiber dialyzer	To facilitate normal saline to flow
15.	For first 500 mL bottle, switch on the blood pump 100–150 mL/min	To wash and remove air bubbles
16.	Make sure that extracorporeal circuit, if filled with saline	To prevent air embolism
17.	Tap gently over the dialyzer to facilitate air removal	To facilitate air removal and prevent clotting
18.	Raise fluid levels in 'A' and 'V' chamber as necessary (as per the specifications of the machine)	To ensure chambers remain full and prevent air entry into extracorporeal circuit
19.	Turn off blood pump after finishing first bottle of saline; return dialyzer to upright position	To prime dialyzate compartment
20.	• Ensure conductivity is at correct level then connect dialyzate line to the dialyzer • Ensure that dialyzate flow is in opposite direction to the blood flow	To create counter current flow and maximize dialyzer efficiency
21.	Prime the dialyzate compartment, remove air from it and place it; place dialyzer arterial end down	
22.	Connect second 500 mL of normal saline to arterial line and complete priming with 200 mL blood pump speed	To remove minute bubbles and through washing of sterilant
23.	Switch off blood pump	
24.	Clamp 'A' and venous bloodlines	

Contd...

Contd...

Sl No.	Nursing actions	Rationales
25.	Join 'A' and 'V' bloodlines together with connector, prepare for recirculation (if these facilities are available)	To facilitate recirculation
26.	Release both 'A' and 'V' clamps	
27.	Connect IV saline to 'A' port, open the clamp in IV drip set and arterial port	To replace ultrafiltrates saline
28.	Switch on blood flow 10–100 mL/min in order to recirculate and save the sterile drain bag/container	To use as a receiver when bleeding during connection
29.	Just before connecting to the patient clamp arterial line, open venous line and drain 100 mL of saline to the sterile container	To take out all ethylene oxide, which is remaining inside the blood tube and dialyzer
30.	Clamp arterial venous and recirculation line and commence hemodialysis	
31.	**Alert:** For priming of the flat dialyzer, it is necessary to prime the dialyzate side first prior to the blood compartment in order to open up the dialyzate compartment; the dialysis pressure set of 200 mm Hg	
32.	Ensure the conductivity is at correct level	
33.	Connect dialyzate lines to the dialyzer; prime the dialyzate compartment and make sure all air is expelled	
34.	Pressure test dialyzer: Check that upper alarm unit on the venous pressure gauge is set at 300 mm Hg clamp venous line	

HEMODIALYSIS

Using Anticoagulant

Definition

Heparin is an anticoagulant used to prevent platelets aggregation in order to maintain the extracorporeal circuit. It inhibits the generation and activity of thrombin (factor XIa).

Purpose

Heparin is used routinely to anticoagulate the blood during hemodialysis.

Conditions

- Applies to all registered nursing personnel working in the dialysis centers
- These procedures (Table 12.3) can be performed by a nurse undertaking nephrology/hemodialysis training provided he/she is closely supervised by experienced dialysis nurse at all times
- A strict technique should be maintained throughout the procedure in accordance with the policy and procedure of aseptic technique
- Hand hygiene should be performed according to policy and procedure on handwashing.

Equipment

- Heparin pump (as per the hemodialysis machine)
- Syringe
- Heparin.

Heparin-free Dialysis

Alert

Heparin-free dialysis is not a routine dialysis, follow-up the treating physician's order. The total volume to be given has to be calculated for inclusion in weight loss during hemodialysis (Table 12.4).

Table 12.3: Procedure for hemodialysis using anticoagulant

Sl No.	Nursing actions	Rationales
1.	• After preparing the access site for dialysis, administer the initial bolus dose of heparin as prescribed • Loading dose: Calculation of heparin is to be done as per prescribed dose	To initiate the desired action of heparin during the 1st hour of hemodialysis
2.	Start regular heparin infusion prescribed	To reinforce the desired action of heparin bolus
3.	Monitor heparin pump hourly	To serve as a guide in adjusting appropriate dose of heparin
4.	Stop the heparin infusion 1 hour before the end of hemodialysis (patient having AVF*) and 2 hour (patient with AVG†) according to patients clotting time see annex about clotting time continue to give heparin until the end of hemodialysis (patients having temporary access)	To prevent prolonged bleeding on the access site after the removal of needles and to maintain the lumens patency

*AVF, arteriovenous fistula; †AVG, arteriovenous graft.

Table 12.4: Procedure for heparin-free dialysis

Sl No.	Nursing actions	Rationales
1.	See physician order for use of heparin in priming procedure	To perform the right procedure
2.	At the last bottle of saline for priming, rinse the extracorporeal circuit with saline containing 3,000, i.e. of heparin	To reduce the propensity for extracorporeal circuit clotting
3.	Rinse the dialyzer every 30 min (during dialysis) rapidly with 100 mL saline, while occluding the blood interline	To reduce the propensity for extracorporeal circuit clotting
4.	Use of ultrafiltration (UF) controller to adjust the transmembrane pressure (TMP)	To achieve body weight

Indications

- Pericarditis
- Recent surgery after, which bleeding would be dangerous
- Coagulopathy
- Thrombocytopenia
- Intracerebral hemorrhage
- Any active bleeding.

CONNECTING A PATIENT WITH ARTERIOVENOUS FISTULA TO HEMODIALYSIS MACHINE

Definition

Connecting a patient with AVF to the hemodialysis machine (Fig. 12.1).

Purposes

- To demonstrate safe and skilled use of dialysis equipment
- To demonstrate safe and skilled venipuncture technique
- To prevent complications and hazards that can occur when cannulating AVF and when commencing dialysis
- To safely prepare and administer prescribed dialysis treatment.

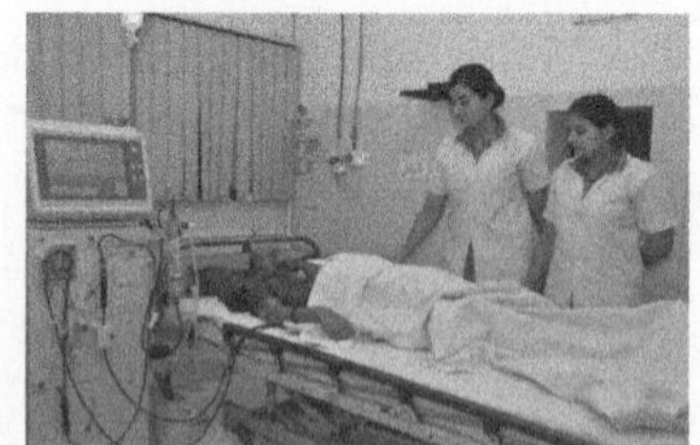

Fig. 12.1: Patient in dialysis (*Courtesy:* Anil Baghi, Multispecialty Hospital, Ferozepur, Punjab)

Conditions

1. Apply to all registered nursing personnel working in the dialysis centers.
2. This procedure (Table 12.5) can be performed by a nurse undertaking

nephrology/hemodialysis training program and provided he/she is closely supervised by experienced dialysis nurse at all times.

3. A strict aseptic technique should be maintained throughout the procedure in accordance with the policy and procedure of aseptic technique.
4. Hand hygiene should be performed according to policy and procedure on handwashing.
5. Rotating fistula needle must be used where possible.

Equipment

- Hemodialysis chart
- On/Off pack
- Skin disinfectant
- Sterile gloves
- Two fistula needles
- Syringes: 20 cc × 1, 10 cc × 2, 1 cc × 1
- Injection: Heparin, lidocaine (1%)
- Laboratory specimen, tubes and specimen bags
- Laboratory requisition forms.

Table 12.5: Procedure for connecting a patient with arteriovenous fistula to the hemodialysis machine

Sl No.	Nursing actions	Rationales
1.	Ensure that the patient had finished meal at least 1 hour before commencing hemodialysis	Eating during dialysis can result in vomiting and hypotension during dialysis
2.	Patient should change from outdoor clothes into clothes worn specifically during treatment	To prevent infection
3.	Supervise the patient in washing the fistula arm with HiBiSCRUB	To prevent infection
4.	Check predialysis instructions and ensure that the machine is set up as per dialysis prescription and following predialysis assessment	To make sure that the patient is receiving appropriate treatment
5.	Clean the table as per policy and procedures on infection control	To prevent infection
6.	Wash and dry hands as per policy and procedure on handwashing	To prevent cross infection
7.	Open out on/off pack and layout sterile field	

Contd...

Contd...

Sl No.	Nursing actions	Rationales
8.	Place all necessary accessories in the sterile field	
9.	Wash and dry hands as per policy and procedure on infection control	To prevent cross infection
10.	• Assesses fistula to identify sites for insertion of needle; assessment of fistula is carried out when patient is in a comfortable position • Refer predialysis policy for general fistula preparation and assessment	Assessment is carried out to ensure needle are inserted in the correct position to achieve maximum blood flow
11.	Clean the patient fistula with disinfectant (use thumb forceps for cleaning the limb) and put the limb on a sterile towel	
12.	Don gloves and prepare fistula, heparinized needle, if no blood sample is required	Heparinized saline may interfere with the effectiveness of sample
13.	Apply manual or mechanical tourniquet above insertion site to select sites for distal needle and local anesthesia, if required	The need to assess the fistula prior to insertion of fistula needles
14.	Give local anesthetic subcutaneously to sites according to the preference of the patient	To minimize pain for the patient
15.	Apply manual or mechanical tourniquet above insertion	To examine fistula patency and strength, and to make vessels prominent for needling
16.	**Insertion of arterial needle:** Insert the needle at least 5 cm away from the site of arteriovenous anastomosis insertion (the site should be changed)	To avoid puncturing of anastomosis and to prevent fistula complications
17.	Release pressure	
18.	Secure the needle in position by tape, check the flow by aspirating the blood using 10 mL syringe; take any samples required and then flush with heparinized saline	To ensure the correct placement of needle, to ensure needle remains patent
19.	Second nurse to flush dialyzer with 100 mL normal saline whilst the first nurse inserts fistula needles	To remove any air pockets and flush out ethylene oxide

Contd...

Contd...

Sl No.	Nursing actions	Rationales
20.	Clamp the needle tubing and recap	To avoid spillage of blood, to prevent infection and maintain safety
21.	**Insertion of venous needle:** Insert venous needle in a suitable position site away from arterial needle; secure the needle in position with tape, check blood flow and administer heparin-loading dose	To minimize recirculation
22.	Clamp the needle tubing and recap	To avoid spillage of blood, to prevent infection and maintain safety
23.	Attach 'A' line to 'A' needle, 'V' line into sterile plastic bag	
24.	Turn on blood pump slowly to 100 mL/min	To prevent a rapid reduction in plasma volume and therefore prevent its consequences
25.	It is necessary to perform a straight connection for some patients (no bleeding out)	Some patients cannot tolerate bleeding out on single or recurring circumstances
26.	When the blood reaches the bubble trap, turn off blood pump and clamp the venous line	To minimize blood loss
27.	When bleeding out, observe patient for any deterioration in his/her condition	To prevent complications
28.	Connect venous bloodline to venous needle	To maintain the patient safety
29.	Unclamp venous bloodline to venous needle	
30.	Secure the bloodlines	
31.	Restart blood pump and increase the speed gradually to the prescribed pump speed	To ensure and maintain countercurrent
32.	Turn the dialyzer with 'A' blood port uppermost	
33.	Make sure that the machine is in dialysis mode	
34.	Set up the machine with the dialysis prescription	

Contd...

Contd...

Sl No.	Nursing actions	Rationales
35.	Place on/off pack on top of the machine for postdialysis use	
36.	Wash and dry hands as per policy and procedure on handwashing	To prevent cross infection
37.	*Check and record:* • General condition • Blood pressure/Pulse • Pump speed • Venous pressure • Transmembrane pressure • Ultrafiltration rate (UFR) • Hourly weight reduction • Heparin dose	
38.	Obtain and record observation hourly or more frequently depending on the condition of the patient	To maintain safety of the patient
39.	Ensure that the patient is comfortable	
40.	Clean and tidy the area	

DISCONNECTING A PATIENT WITH ARTERIOVENOUS FISTULA FROM HEMODIALYSIS MACHINE

Definition

Disconnecting patient with AVF from the hemodialysis machine.

Purposes

- To disconnect the patient AVF from hemodialysis machine on completion of treatment
- To investigate malfunction in the system or patient tolerance.

Alert

An air washback should not be performed under any circumstances. Any reported occurrences, results in disciplinary action.

Conditions

1. Applies to all registered nursing personal working in dialysis center.
2. Closed methods (Table 12.6) should be carried out by an experienced dialysis nurses.
3. Open method (Table 12.7) should be carried out by two experienced dialysis nurses.

4. Contraindications to carry out the closed method:
   - If the needle is facing fistula
   - If there is high residual pressure within the fistulae, brachial fistula, graft
   - If there is any evidence of clotting in the dialysis lines.

Table 12.6: Closed procedure

Sl No.	Nursing actions	Rationales
1.	Check time treatment elapsed	To establish treatment completed
2.	Collect all equipment and bring the trolley to patient bedside	To prevent cross infection promote efficient use resources
3.	Explain the procedure to be undertaken to the patient; make a preliminary evaluation of the patient's condition before disconnecting hemodialysis, reports any abnormalities	To ensure that the patient has completed the treatment
4.	Wash and dry hands as per policy and procedure on handwashing	To prevent cross infection
5.	Collect any required blood samples from 'A' port in 'A' bloodline	To provide accurate laboratory data to enable continuity of procedure
6.	Switch off transmembrane pressure (TMP) or ultrafiltration (UF) mode, adjust all alarm limits to minimum	To prevent further fluid loss, to improve washback, to minimize disruption during discontinuation procedure
7.	Connect 0.9% saline to the infusion port on 'A' line	To maintain continuity of extracorporeal circuit
8.	Stop blood pump, clamp 'A' lumen and line open saline to infusion port; give intravenous (IV) erythropoietin (EPO) when prescribed	To maintain safety
9.	Start blood pump speed and increase to 100–150 mL/min	To use saline efficiently during washback
10.	Apply a light pressure only on the 'V' line with fingers in order to facilitate the washback release blood stuck to lines	To facilitate an efficient washback observe venous pressure (VP) and venous site for signs of 'blown' fistula
11.	As the venous line clears, stop the blood pump taking in consideration the condition of the patient, e.g. blood pressure	To ensure that the washback reflects the need of the patient's condition
12.	Stop blood pump and clamp saline	
13.	Clamp the 'V' line and fistula needle	
14.	Unclamp arterial line and fistula needle, unclamp saline; apply gentle pressure by clamping the line	Air detector is not utilized, so additional caution is required during this part of the procedure

Contd...

Contd...

Sl No.	Nursing actions	Rationales
15.	Wash and dry hands as per policy and procedure on infection control	To prevent cross infection and to maintain aseptic technique
16.	Prepare medication, if required open on/off hemodialysis pack	
17.	Wash and dry hands as per policy and procedure on handwashing, don sterile gloves	To prevent cross infection, to maintain aseptic technique
18.	Disconnect the bloodlines from the fistula needles; connect both lines to the dual connector	To prevent blood spillage, to prevent cross infection
19.	Give any IV injections and flush with saline	As per prescription requirements
20.	Prepare gauze into pad, hold over 'V' needle site, withdraw the needle slowly and apply pressure immediately (avoid applying too much pressure while withdrawing needle)	To minimize pain, to ensure effective pressure applied to actual needle site and to minimize trauma to fistula
21.	Remove 'A' needle with same manner	To minimize pain, to ensure effective pressure applied to actual needle site, to minimize trauma to fistula
22.	Once homeostasis is achieved, apply small dressing to each site and observe for oozing	To ensure that the patient is safe to leave the dialysis unit
23.	Discard fistula needles as per policy and procedure on handwashing	To prevent cross infection
24.	Discard gloves	
25.	Wash and dry hands as per policy and procedure on handwashing	To prevent cross infection
26.	Refer to postdialysis evaluation of patient procedure for further management of the patient	
27.	Using unsterile gloves, prepare machine for sterilization, remove dialysis lines and dispose as per policy and procedures on infection control; clean machine and clamps as per policy and procedures on infection control	To maintain standards of infection control and prevent cross infection

5. This policy does not apply in the following circumstances:
    - Severe blood leak
    - Air embolism
    - Clotting of bloodlines

- Hemolysis of blood in extracorporeal circuit
- Extensive recirculation time.

Table 12.7: Open procedure

Sl No.	Nursing actions	Rationales
1.	Check time of treatment elapsed	To establish treatment time completed
2.	Collect all equipment and bring the trolley to patient bedside	To prevent cross infection, to promote efficient use of resources
3.	Explain the procedure to be undertaken to patient; make a preliminary evaluation of the patient's condition before disconnecting hemodialysis; reports any abnormalities	To ensure that the patient is fit to complete the treatment
4.	Both nurses wash and dry hands as per policy and procedure on handwashing	To prevent cross infection
5.	*First nurse (with machine):* Don unsterile gloves *Second nurse (assisting nurse):* Don sterile gloves	To maintain aseptic technique
6.	*First nurse:* Prepare any medication required and open on/off pack and required equipment	
7.	Second nurse (assisting nurse): Withdraw 5 mL saline for flushing arterial needle	
8.	*First nurse:* Switch off transmembrane pressure (TMP)/ ultrafiltration (UF) mode and adjust alarm limits	To prevent further fluid loss, to improve washback and to minimize disruption during discontinuation procedure
9.	*First nurse:* Disconnect saline from intravenous (IV) line and recap it; connect the IV set to dual connector; turn off blood pump	
10.	*First nurse:* Clamp 'A' line and 'A' fistula needle	
11.	*Second nurse (assisting nurse):* Disconnect 'A' line from fistula needle, take samples and flush arterial needle	To determine accurate postdialysis results and to minimize red cell loss
12.	*First nurse:* Connect 'A' line to dual connector, turn on blood pump to 100–150 mL/min; apply intermittent light pressure to facilitate a good washback	To determine accurate postdialysis results and to minimize red cell loss

Contd...

Contd...

Sl No.	Nursing actions	Rationales
13.	As venous line clears *First nurse:* Stop the blood pump taking in consideration the condition of the patient, clamp 'V' line and 'V' fistula needle	To quantify of saline given in the washback should reflect the clinical status of the patient
14.	*Second nurse (assisting nurse):* Disconnect 'V' line from needle and hand over to first nurse for disposal	
15.	*First nurse:* Check and record vital signs; report abnormalities	
16.	Prepare gauze into a pad, hold over first needle site, withdraw the needle slowly, apply pressure immediately (avoid applying too much pressure, while withdrawing needle)	To minimize pain, to ensure effective pressure is applied to actual needle site and to minimize trauma to fistula
17.	Remove second needle in the same manner	
18.	Once homeostasis is achieved, apply small dressing to each site and observe for oozing	To ensure that the patient is safe to leave the dialysis unit
19.	Discard fistula needles as per policy and procedures on infection control	To maintain safety and prevent cross infection
20.	Discard gloves	
21.	Wash and dry hands as per policy and procedure for further management of the patient	
22.	Refer to postdialysis evaluation of patient procedure for further management of the patient	
23.	Using unsterile gloves, prepare machine for sterilization, remove dialysis lines and dispose as per policy and procedures on infection control; clean machine and clamps as per policy and procedures on infection control	To maintain standards of infection control and prevent cross infection

Please refer institutional policy for discontinuation of hemodialysis in these emergencies. General remarks are given in Table 12.8.

Table 12.8: General remarks

Sl No.	Nursing actions	Rationales
1.	Heparin should be switched off 1 hour before disconnection on all fistula patients except otherwise indicated	To minimize bleeding posthemodialysis
2.	If hemodialysis is performed on a patient, who has temporary vascular access, e.g. subclavian vein catheter (SVC), jugular vein catheter (JVC) and permcath, then heparin infusion should be maintained until the end of dialysis	To prevent clotting of the catheter
3.	When applying pressure to the needle site do not use fistula clamps if the intravenous (IV) fistula is new	To prevent trauma
4.	While performing washback, do not apply forced pressure on the bloodlines if there is already clot present in 'V' chamber or dialyzer	Patient is oriented to time and place and is safe to leave the treatment center
5.	Remove fistula dressing 8–12 hour posthemodialysis	To prevent infection and bleeding
6.	Educate the patient to watch for bleeding or oozing from needle site, if so reapply the pressure	

Equipment

- Trolley cleaned according to policy and procedures on infection control
- On/Off hemodialysis pack
- Fistula clamps: Optional
- Saline (0.9%) 500 mL
- Intravenous infusion set
- One pair of sterile gloves
- One pair of unsterile gloves
- Micropore tape
- Sterile syringe 5 mL (open method only)
- Specimen containers (if required)
- Postdialysis medications
- Blood pressure (BP) apparatus and stethoscope.

POSTDIALYSIS ASSESSMENT OF HEMODIALYSIS PATIENT

Definition

Assessment of the patient's condition in hemodialysis treatment to evaluate the effectiveness of the treatment and whether the treatment goals were achieved. Additionally, undertake further action if any problems remain unsolved.

Purposes

- To ensure that a safe and effective treatment was given and that the patient is fit to be discharged from the treatment center
- To identify any issues that require further action and follow-up to ensure that the patient receives individualized therapy and thus, maintains optimum quality of care.

Conditions

1. The procedure (Table 12.9) should be carried out by an experienced dialysis nurse.
2. This procedure can be undertaken by inexperienced dialysis nurse undertaking a specific educational training program, provided that are closely supervised by an experienced dialysis nurse at all times.

Table 12.9: Procedure for postdialysis assessment

Nursing actions	Rationales
1. *Check and record vital signs*	
Blood pressure, pulse rate, rhythm and fullness, temperature	Vital signs should be in the normal range, if there is deviation from the normal range, the physician should be informed and further action is taken
2. *Evaluation of fistula and vascular access*	
Bleeding stopped and site is clean then dry dressing applied and secured, patient is educated about dressing management	To ensure that there is no excess bleeding and no hematomas, and that the patient is safe to leave the treatment center
3. *Weight*	
• Following assessment of blood pressure (BP) weighing patient, ensure that he/she is in the same clothes, etc. as for predialysis weight • Observe general condition; observing for complications, e.g. hypotension • Document findings and interpret information obtained • If any abnormalities detected, inform the physician for further action	• It is necessary to compare predialysis and postdialysis weight to evaluate whether the treatment goal has been achieved • Further action may be necessary if there are abnormalities detected, which may result in a change in dialysis presentation
4. *Mental status*	
The patient is questioned to ensure that he/she is aware of his/her situation and they are fit to return home as an outpatient	Patient is oriented to time and place, and is safe to leave the treatment center

Contd...

Contd...

Nursing actions	Rationales
5. *Administration of medications*	
• Ensure that prescribed medication are given • Administration of additional medications are required in the light of findings from the postdialysis evaluation • Document and sign for medication given or not; give and mention the reasons (if not) for not giving the medications	• It is essential that all medication to be given as prescribed, as this is an integral part of the dialysis treatment • It is essential to maintain
6. *General evaluations for other conditions and complications*	
General discussion with the patient to evaluate general well-being following dialysis with some general advice for subsequent home care	Further action may be necessary if there are abnormalities detected, which may affect the discharge treatment or result in a change to the dialysis prescription for a subsequent dialysis
7. *Documentation*	
Overall evaluation of the patient's conditions to be recorded and signed by the nurse undertaking the evaluation, any notes or instruction for subsequent dialysis treatment must be clearly identified and documented by the nurse carrying out the evaluation	There has to be accountability for the delivery of dialysis treatment and evidence of therapy management to achieve the goals of the dialysis prescription, it is necessary to ensure that there is continuity of care from one dialysis treatment to the next to maintain patient's safety and well-being

CONTINUOUS AMBULATORY PERITONEAL DIALYSIS WITH TEMPORARY ACCESS TO HEMODIALYSIS MACHINE

Procedure should be used for the patient with a permcath.

Definition

Temporary vascular access is used for the patient, who has no functioning permanent AV access. This includes acute and chronic patients requiring hemodialysis or other renal replacement therapy for subclavian vein catheter (SVC), jugular vein catheter (JVC), femoral vein catheter (FVC) and permcath.

Purpose

Provide temporary access to the venous circulation for the purpose of understanding hemodialysis and/or other form of extracorporeal renal replacement therapy or treatment.

Conditions

1. Two nurses of whom one should be an experienced hemodialysis nurse, should carry out this procedure (Table 12.10).
2. A strict aseptic technique should be maintained throughout the procedure in accordance with the policy and procedure on aseptic technique.
3. Hand hygiene should be performed according to policy and procedure on handwashing.
4. The catheter dressing must be changed at every dialysis session.

Table 12.10: Procedure for temporary access to hemodialysis machine

Sl No.	Nursing actions	Rationales
1.	Check the dialysis prescription	To obtain specific instructions for the management of the patient
2.	Identify the patient; ensure that patient is wearing identification bracelet with correct information (if patient is admitted in the hospital)	To fulfill requirements and hospital policy
3.	Explain the procedure to the patient and allow him/her to ask questions	To allay fears and gain patients confidence and cooperation and to promote patient education
4.	Ensure privacy	To avoid unnecessary embarrassment to the patient during the procedure
5.	Complete prehemodialysis assessment (refer to policy and procedure on predialysis assessment)	To ensure patient is fit for hemodialysis
6.	Wash and dry hands	To prevent cross infection
7.	Prepare on/off pack with all accessories	
8.	Remove dressing and tapes from the catheter 'do not use scissors'	To avoid damage to the catheter
9.	Inspect exit site for signs of infection; take swab for culture and sensitivity if indicated	To detect early signs of infection
10.	Wash hands with disinfectant (preferably HiBiSCRUB or Betadine); dry hands	To prevent infection
11.	Wear sterile gloves	To prevent infection
12.	Place sterile field under catheter; take gauze soaked with Betadine and place around 'A' and 'V' caps and extensions with gentle scrubbing clean for 3 min	To prevent cross infection

Contd...

Contd...

Sl No.	Nursing actions	Rationales
13.	Clean exit site with cotton balls soaked in Betadine, then cover with sterile gauze until treatment is completed	To clean and sterilize exit site
14.	Ensure that the extensions are clamped before removing the Luer-lock caps	To prevent air entry and blood leak
15.	Attach syringe to 'A' side open clamp aspirate 2 mL, clamp the 'A' side again and flush the contents on a piece of gauze	To remove priming heparin and check for blood clots
16.	If there is significant clotting, then remove 3–5 mL more blood and check for more clots	To ensure adequate blood flow for hemodialysis; if not seek medical advice
17.	Assess blood flow in 'A' by using 10 mL syringe filled with normal saline (2–3 mL)	
18.	Flush lumen with normal saline (take blood samples prior to this process, when required)	
19.	Repeat the step 14–17 for venous side	
20.	Administer the loading dose of heparin via the venous lumen	To heparinize the blood
21.	Initiate dialysis, as usual secure catheter and dialysis lines to ensure there is no traction on the catheter from hanging bloodlines	To avoid accidental pulling out of catheter

5. The catheter should be filled with heparin, when not in use. The concentration is 5,000 IU/mL, volume (capacity) and the amount used in according to the catheter volume (capacity) as per manufacturer's instruction.
6. Micropore tape:1.
7. Betadine antiseptic solution.

DISCONNECTING A PATIENT WITH TEMPORARY ACCESS FROM HEMODIALYSIS MACHINE

Definition

Disconnecting patient with temporary access from the hemodialysis machine.

Purposes

- Disconnect the patient with temporary access from hemodialysis machine on completion of treatment
- To investigate malfunction in the system or patient intolerance.

Alert

An air washback should not be performed under any circumstances; any reported occurrence results in disciplinary action.

Conditions

1. This procedure can be performed by a nurse undertaking nephrology/dialysis training program provided and he/she is closely supervised by an experienced dialysis nurse at all time.
2. Two nurses of whom one should be an experienced nurse should carry out the procedure.
3. A strict aseptic technique should be maintained throughout the procedure in accordance with the policy and procedure on aseptic technique.
4. Hand hygiene should be performed according to policy and procedure on handwashing.

Equipment

- Trolley cleaned according to policy and procedures on infection control policy
- On/Off hemodialysis pack
- Ampules (0.9%) × 2.10 mL
- Saline (0.9%) 500 mL
- Intravenous infusion set
- One pair of sterile gloves
- One pair of unsterile gloves
- Micropore tape
- Heparin 5,000 IU/mL
- Syringe 10 mL × 2 for flushing with normal saline
- Syringe 2 mL × 2 for heparin lock (volume to be infused as per manufacturer's instructions)
- Luer-lock caps: 2
- Mepore dressing: 2
- Antiseptic solution
- Antiseptic ointment
- Specimen container (if required)
- Postdialysis medications.

Procedures

Procedures are of two types:

- Closed procedure (Table 12.11)
- Open procedure (Table 12.12).

The general remarks regarding these procedures are given in Table 12.13.

Table 12.11: Closed procedure of disconnecting a patient with temporary access from hemodialysis machine

Sl No.	Nursing actions	Rationales
1.	Check time of treatment elapsed	To establish treatment time completed
2.	Collect all equipment and bring the trolley to patient bedside	To prevent cross infection and to promote efficient use of resources
3.	Explain the procedure to be undertaken to the patient; make a preliminary evaluation of the patient's condition before disconnecting hemodialysis and reports any abnormalities	To ensure that the patient is fit to complete the treatment
4.	Wash and dry hands as per policy and procedure on handwashing	To prevent cross infection
5.	Collect any required blood samples from 'A' port	To provide accurate laboratory data to enable continuity of procedure
6.	Switch off transmembrane pressure (TMP) or ultrafiltration (UF) mode, adjust all alarm limits to minimum	To prevent further fluid loss to improve washback to minimize disruption during discontinuation procedure
7.	Connect 0. 9% saline to the infusion port on 'A' line	To maintain continuity of extracorporeal circuit
8.	Stop blood pump clamp 'A' lumen and line open saline to infusion port; give intravenous (IV), EPO when prescribed	To maintain safety
9.	Start blood pump speed and increase to 100–150 mL/min	To use saline efficiently during washback
10.	Apply a light pressure only on the 'V' line with fingers in order to facilitate the washback release blood stuck to lines	To facilitate an efficient washback to minimize red cell loss
11.	As the 'V' line become pinkish, stop the blood pump taking in consideration the condition of the patient, e.g. blood pressure	To ensure that the washback and reflects the need of the patient condition
12.	Stop blood pump and clamp saline	
13.	Clamp the 'V' line and 'V' lumen	

Contd...

Contd...

Sl No.	Nursing actions	Rationales
14.	Unclamp 'A' line and 'A' lumen of temporary access	Air detector is not utilized, so additional caution is required during this part of the procedure
15.	Flush until line is pinkish; apply gentle pressure by clamping the line; clamp 'A' line and 'A' lumen of temporary access	To minimize saline infused to minimize red cell loss to prevent air embolism
16.	Wash and dry hands as per policy and procedure on infection control	To prevent cross infection
17.	Prepare medication if required; open on/off hemodialysis pack and assisting nurse comes to assist	To ensure aseptic technique can be undertaken
18.	Both nurses wash and dry hands as per policy and procedure on handwashing *First nurse:* Don sterile gloves *Assisting nurse:* Don unsterile gloves and removes gauze dressing *First nurse:* Place sterile fields under temporary access; take gauze soaked with Betadine and rub gently on the extensions for 2–3 min	To prevent cross infection and to maintain aseptic technique
19.	*First nurse:* Disconnect the bloodlines from the temporary access using gauze *Assisting nurse:* Connect both lines to the dual connector	To prevent blood spillage To prevent cross infection
20.	*First nurse:* Flush each lumen of the catheter with 10 mL 0.9% normal saline using separate syringes	To flush and clear blood cells
21.	*First nurse:* Push in one-go heparin 5,000 IU/mL into each lumen (volume as per manufacturer's instructions), clamp immediately *Note:* The clamp should not be opened once the catheter has been heparinized	To prevent clotting back flow
22.	*First nurse:* Apply sterile lock cap to each lumen *Assisting nurse:* Tape them with bridging tape *First nurse:* Wrap the lumen with sterile gauze *Assisting nurse:* Tape them	To maintain aseptic technique

Contd...

Contd...

Sl No.	Nursing actions	Rationales
23.	*First nurse:* Clean the skin at the catheter exit site with antiseptic solution and apply antiseptic ointment to the exit site	To prevent exit site infections
24.	*First nurse:* Make a sandwich dressing using Mepore (or other suitable alternative)	To provide occlusive dressing
25.	Both nurses discard glove, wash and dry hands	To prevent cross infection
26.	Refer to postdialysis evaluation of patient procedure for further management of the patient	To ensure patient treatment and condition is fully evaluated
27.	Using unsterile gloves, prepare machine for sterilization, remove dialysis line and dispose as per policy and procedure on infection control; clean machine and clamps as per policy and procedure on infection control	To maintain standards of infection control and prevent cross infection

Table 12.12: Open procedure for disconnecting a patient with temporary access from hemodialysis machine

Sl No.	Nursing actions	Rationales
1.	Check time of treatment elapsed	To establish treatment time completed
2.	Collect all equipment and bring the trolley to patient bedside	To prevent cross infection and to promote efficient use of resources
3.	Explain the procedure to be undertaken to patient; make a preliminary evaluation of the patient's condition before disconnecting hemodialysis and reports any abnormalities	To ensure that the patient is fit to complete the treatment
4.	Both nurses wash and dry hands as per policy and procedure on handwashing	To prevent cross infection
5.	Assisting nurse with machine prepare any medication required; open on/off pack and required equipment	To maintain aseptic technique
6.	Both nurses don gloves; first nurse sterile gloves; assisting nurse unsterile gloves	To maintain aseptic technique

Contd...

Contd...

Sl No.	Nursing actions	Rationales
7.	*Assisting nurse:* Remove gauze dressing at the same time *First nurse:* Place sterile field under catheter	Maintain aseptic technique
8.	*First nurse:* Withdraw 5 mL saline for flushing 'A' lumen	To prevent clotting of lumen
9.	*Assisting nurse:* Switch off transmembrane pressure/ ultrafiltration (TMP/UF) mode and adjust alarm limits	To prevent further fluid loss to improve washback to minimize and disruption during discontinuation procedure
10.	*Assisting nurse:* Disconnect saline from intravenous infusion port and connect to dual connector; turn off blood pump	
11.	*Assisting nurse:* Clamp 'A' line *First nurse:* Clamp 'A' lumen of catheter	
12.	*First nurse:* Disconnect 'A' line from temporary access lumen using sterile gauze, take sample when necessary and flush 'A' lumen clamp immediately	To determine accurate postdialysis results, to minimize red cell loss and maintain patency and to prevent air embolism
13.	*Assisting nurse:* Connect 'A' line to dual connector, turn on blood pump to 100–150 mL/min and apply intermittent light pressure to facilitate a good washback	To determine accurate postdialysis results, to minimize red cell loss
14.	As venous line clears and becomes pinkish *Assisting nurse:* Stop the blood pump taking in consideration the condition of the patient *First nurse:* Clamp 'V' lumen *Assisting nurse:* Clamp 'V' line	The quantity of saline given in the washback should reflect the clinical status of the patient
15.	*First nurse:* Disconnect 'V' line from 'V' lumen using sterile gauze and hand over to the assisting nurse	To prevent air embolism
16.	*Assisting nurse:* Connect both lines to the dual connector	To prevent blood spillage and cross infection
17.	*First nurse:* Flush lumen of the catheter with 10 mL normal saline 0.9% using separate syringe	To flush and clear blood cell

Contd...

Contd...

Sl No.	Nursing actions	Rationales
18.	*First nurse:* Push in one—go heparin 5,000 IU/mL into each lumen (volume as per manufacturer's instructions)	To prevent clotting and back flow
19.	*First nurse:* Apply sterile Luer-lock cap to each lumen *Assisting nurse:* Tape the lumens with sterile gauze *Assisting nurse:* Tape them	To maintain aseptic technique
20.	*First nurse:* Clean the skin at the catheter exit site with antiseptic solution and apply antiseptic ointment to the exit site, make a sandwich dressing using Mepore (or other suitable alternative)	To prevent exit site infection and to provide occlusive dressing
21.	*Both nurses:* Discard gloves; wash and dry hands	To prevent cross infection
22.	Refer to postdialysis evaluation of patient procedure for further management of the patient	To ensure patient's treatment and condition is fully evaluated
23.	Using unsterile gloves, prepare machine for sterilization, remove dialysis lines and dispose as per policy and procedures on infection control; clean machine and clamps as per policy and procedures on infection control	To maintain standards of infection control and prevent cross infection
24.	Discard gloves	

Table 12.13: General remarks

Sl No.	Nursing actions	Rationales
1.	If hemodialysis is performed on a patient who has temporary vascular access, e.g. subclavian vein catheter (SVC), jugular vein catheter (JVC) and permcath, then heparin infusing should be maintained until the end of dialysis	To prevent clotting of the catheter
2.	While performing washback, do not apply forced pressure on the bloodlines if there is already cloth present in 'V' chamber or dialyzer	To prevent cloth dislodging and entering the circulation

PREOPERATIVE AND POSTOPERATIVE CARE OF ARTERIOVENOUS FISTULA

Purposes

- To maintain patency of fistula
- To prevent the occurrence of complications.

Policies

- The procedure is explained to the patient by the physician and consent is obtained
- The operation performed under brachial block or general anesthesia
- Vessels in the arm intended for AVF should not be punctured for any reason except for life-saving procedures
- In case of venography, puncturing should be performed in the veins of the dorsum of the hand and not on the inner aspect of the arm
- Nil by mouth is maintained for 6–8 hours prior to surgery
- All blood investigations should be available prior to surgery.

Procedures

1. **Preoperative care:**
   - Perform skin preparation of the arm from the shoulder to the wrist including the armpit
   - Have premedication available, if required.
2. **Postoperative care:**
   - Check for the thrill and listen for bruit to ascertain the patency of the fistula
   - Report immediately when the thrill or bruit is absent
   - Report if any cyanosis, pallor and/or numbness of fingers
   - Note an edema of operated arm
   - If bleeding occurs, inform the physician immediately and change dressing, observe wound site for further bleeding
   - Inspects wound on 3rd postoperative day; remove dressing and apply opposite dressing (transparent and quick drying, self-adhesive polyurethane film use over the wound site)
   - Instruct patient not to use tight watch, tight clothes, jewelry (rings or bracelet) in the operated hand especially the first 48–72 hours.
3. **Hand exercise:** Give soft cotton ball (size of tennis ball) rolled in gauze to the patient, instruct patient how to place the ball in the palm of the fistula arm and grip it lightly for 5 seconds (count 1-5) and release. Patient has to do this exercise immediately after recovery—three times a day for the vein to become prominent.

4. **Cleaning:** Both internal (Table 12.14) and external (Table 12.15) part of machine has to be cleaned. Purpose of external cleaning:

Table 12.14: Cleaning internal parts of machine

Sl No.	Nursing actions	Rationales
1.	Prepare the machine for cleaning (drain or rinse for removal of used fluid)	To remove contaminants, microorganism, organic origin such as proteins and glucose deposited in the fluid pathway
2.	Prepare the solution (sodium hypochlorite) refer to the machine manufacturer before performing this procedure	
3.	Put the designated tube to the solution and put the machine on cleaning mode	To fill machine with solution
4.	After filling finish, the machine must go for a mandatory rinse and this procedure will take 40–45 min	To flush out the cleaning solution

Table 12.15: Cleaning external parts of machine

Sl No.	Nursing actions	Rationales
1.	Prepare the machine for cleaning remove items such as disposable, extracorporeal line, forceps, etc.	To be able to clean the machine properly
2.	***Prepare the solution:*** • Use soap and water for ordinary cleaning • Dilute (milton 1%) into 5%, when there is blood spillage • Refer to the machine manufacturer before performing this procedure	
3.	Wipe the whole machine including dialyzate line with 'J' cloth	
4.	Soak the 'J' cloth with the solution and remove the excessive water	
5.	Soak again the machine with 'J' cloth	To remove soap solution

- To clean the external parts of the machine from blood and fluid spills
- This procedure is to be performed by medical orderly and supervised by nursing staff.

5. **Decalcification:** Purpose is to remove the participate from the machine (Table 12.16).
6. **Maintenance (service and performance):** This is detailed in Table 12.17.

Table 12.16: Decalcification

Sl No.	Nursing actions	Rationales
1.	Prepare the machine for decalcification (drain or rinse the machine)	To remove used dialyzate fluid from the machine
2.	Prepare the citric acid 20% solution refer to the machine manufacturer before performing this procedure	
3.	Put the designated tubes in the citric acid solution, rinse the machine	
4.	Drain and rinse the machine	To flush out the solution

Table 12.17: Maintenance (service and performance)

Sl No.	Nursing actions	Rationales
1.	The machine should be serviced every 2,000 hour and refer to the machine manufacturer before performing this procedure	To maintain the machine trouble free and during treatment to overall check the machine
2.	*Electronic calibration:* Check voltage and calibration	
3.	Change the old or discolored part, which needs replacement	
4.	• Check each part of the machine with the test equipment • Performance test should be performed every 2 month	Check and test main functions of the machine, e.g. conductivity, temperature, pressure and calibration
5.	Clean internal and external filters	Some filters may clog with organic participate needs cleaning
6.	Check overall performance of the machine	To ascertain that the machine is working properly

Possible Complications

- Edema of the arm
- Hemorrhage
- Infection
- Ischemia of hand
- Endocarditic to the bacterial infection
- Congestive heart failure (CHF)
- Thrombosis due to slow circulation or failure technique of anastomosis
- Pseudoaneurysm due to early use of the fistula before thickening of the walls of the veins
- Embolism.

Advice the Patient

- Avoid pressure on the fistula arm
- Avoid wearing tight watch, jewelry or cloths on the fistula arm
- Avoid the habit of using the fistula arm as armrest, while sleeping
- Continue hand exercise till further instructions from nurses
- Avoid carrying heavy items by the fistula arm
- Avoid excessive shaking of fistula arm
- Keep the area clean and hygienic
- If any bleeding occurs, apply pressure and report to the nearest medical center immediately.

MANAGEMENT OF HYPOTENSION DURING HEMODIALYSIS

Definition

A decrease in blood volume will result in decreased cardiac filling, which in turn will cause reduced cardiac output and ultimately hypotension.

Most Common Causes

- Excess decrease in blood volume
- Too low body weight
- High ultrafiltration (UF) and transmembrane pressure (TMP)
- Low conductivity [low-sodium (Na) dialysis solution]
- Antihypertensive drug therapy
- Hot dialysis fluid
- Due to cardiac failure and inability to increase cardiac rate
- Due to hemorrhage.

Conditions

The procedure of management of hypotension during hemodialysis (Table 12.18) can be undertaken by nursing staff, who is undertaking a specific educational training program provided and they are closely supervised by an experienced dialysis nurse at all time.

PREVENTION AND MANAGEMENT OF AIR EMBOLISM

Definition

Air embolism is the entry of air bubbles into the central venous system, (rarely arterial system) by direct or indirect access into the bloodstream through a central or peripheral route. The symptoms reflect and the end organ is affected.

Table 12.18: Procedure of hypotension management during hemodialysis

Sl No.	Nursing actions	Rationales
1.	Keep the patient in supine position with feet slightly elevated	To ensure sufficient blood supply to vital organs of the patient
2.	Minimize ultrafiltration (UF)	To prevent further hypotension
3.	Reduce blood pump	To prevent further hypotension
4.	Check blood pressure (BP) and pulse	To assess the degree of hypotension
5.	Initiate fluid replacement as prescribed, e.g. normal saline	
6.	Monitor BP and pulse	To monitor the patient's condition and assess whether hypotension has been corrected or not
7.	Start hypertonic solutions if needed, e.g. dextrose and albumin	To increase oncotic pressure and to attract fluid from extracellular space
8.	If the patient vomits, turn him/her to the side, clean the vomiting and elevate slightly the patient's head	To maintain patient comfort
9.	Communicate with the patient and reassure him/her	
10.	Monitor the condition of the patient and report progress to the treating physician	To prevent further hypotension
11.	Educate the patient about his/her condition and prevention of hypotension; avoid taking hypertensive drugs on the day of dialysis	To prevent further hypotension
12.	Document patient condition, medication given and response to treatment	

Entry of Air in the Heart

In seated patients, infused air will tend to migrate into the cerebral venous system without entering the heart causing obstruction to cerebral venous return with loss of consciousness, convulsion and even death. In recumbent patient, the air tends to enter the heart, generate foam in the right ventricle and pass on into lungs. At this point, dyspnea, cough and chest tightness can be expected. Further passage of air across the capillary bed into the left ventricle can result in air embolism to the arteries of the brain and heart, with acute neurologic and cardiac dysfunction.

Preventions

- Ensure all lines are secured
- Ensure all alarm systems are fully functioning
- Continual observation of all dialysis circuit
- Remove all empty containers attached to the dialysis circuit.

Purposes

- To ensure that a safe and hazard-free dialysis treatment is delivered.
- To identify any issues that require further action and follow-up to ensure that the patient receives safe individualized therapy and thus, maintain optimum quality of care.

Condition

The procedure of prevention and management of air embolism (Table 12.19) can be undertaken by a nursing staff, provided they are closely supervised by an experienced dialysis nurse at all times.

Table 12.19: Procedure for prevention and management of air embolism

Sl No.	Nursing actions	Rationales
1.	If hemodialysis 'on', clamp the venous line and stop the pump, if open access to central venous catheter (CVC), immediately clamp ports of CVC	If open access to CVC, immediately clamp ports of central catheter; prevent further air entry into the circulation
2.	Place the patient in a recumbent position on the left side with the head and chest tilted downward until the embolism is ruled out	To prevent the entry of air into the circulation and thereby into the cerebral blood vessels with the right ventricle acting as a bubble trap
3.	Administer 100% oxygen	To reduce cerebral hypoxia
4.	Seek medical assistance	This is a medical emergency that require further intervention
5.	Give prescribed intravenous (IV) therapy; IV infusion of low-molecular-weight dextrin or dextrose	To improve capillary perfusion of brain tissues
6.	Maintain observation and document events as they happen with administered medications; note effects of medications and condition of patient and response to management	Documentation of such events is essential for monitoring and follow-up the patient's condition

Contd...

Contd...

Sl No.	Nursing actions	Rationales
7.	Keep the patient for a minimum of 4–6 hour for close observation; transfer to intensive care unit for further management, if necessary	
8.	If the condition of the patient deteriorates, additional intensive support may be necessary	

HEMODIALYSIS HAZARDS

Power Failure During Hemodialysis

Purposes

- To be aware of the complications and hazards that can occur when power fails during hemodialysis
- To demonstrate safe and skilled technique (Table 12.20) in using dialysis equipment
- To complete the required hours of dialysis
- To prevent blood loss during power failure (hemodialysis and blood clot).

Table 12.20: Procedure for management of power failure during hemodialysis

Sl No.	Nursing actions	Rationales
1.	If the power is accidentally disconnected for individual patient, press the mute alarm, keep upon power return, eliminate all alarms and press dialysis start key	
2.	During power failure, call for help from all staff	
3.	Explain the procedure to the patient and reassure him/her	To allay fears and gain patient's confidence and cooperation
4.	Release venous air detector clamp; clamp the venous and arterial pressure monitor lines	
5.	Rotate the blood pump manually *Alert:* All nurses need to be very vigilant, because there are no machine alarms	
6.	Inform the electrical department if the generator has not been taken over	

Contd...

Contd...

Sl No.	Nursing actions	Rationales
7.	Continue rotating the pump for 15–20 min	To prevent clotting
8.	If the power failure last for > 20 min, reinfuse the blood manually as per the policy and procedure	To prevent distraction of red blood cells (RBCs)
9.	Heparinized the access and keep it patent	To prevent clotting
10.	If the power returns within 20 min fix the blood pump handle in place and reset all alarms	To commence safe dialysis
11.	Check all dialysis parameters	
12.	Press dialysis 'start' and commence dialysis	
13.	Take record of vital signs	To monitor the condition of the patient
14.	Document the incident including the time when the blood leak started, nursing intervention, the patient condition and the amount of blood lost (if any)	

Conditions

- All renal nurses must be aware of how to operate the blood pump manually
- All renal nurses must be aware of the complications of hazards that may occur due to power failure during hemodialysis, e.g. air embolism and blunt fistulae
- Hemodialysis machine should be always plugged to emergency sockets, if available.

Management of Blood Leak During Hemodialysis

Definition

The principal reasons for a true blood leak are defective dialyzer membrane, excessive TMP and rarely hemodialysis (Daugirdas and Ing, 1990). A blood leak is classified as minor (Table 12.21), when microscopic blood is detected by the monitor and confirmed by Labstix, if available. No visual blood is seen. A major blood leak (Table 12.22) results in a microscope loss of blood into the waste dialysis line.

A false blood leak results when the detector incorrectly identifies a blood leak. This can result from debris in the area of the detector or in the dialysis fluid or excessive air in the waste dialyzate line. The management is to ensure that there is no blood present and to call for technical assistance, if it cannot be cleared immediately. The machine must be withdrawn from service for maintenance.

Purposes

The principal reasons for a true blood leak are defective dialyzer membranes:

- To prevent blood leak during hemodialysis through attention to following manufacturer's instructions for the testing of hemodialysis machines before commencing hemodialysis
- To prevent complications related to blood leak, e.g. hemodialysis septicemia
- To ensure staffs are educated about actual and false blood leaks and their management.

Conditions

- Applies to all registered nursing personnel working in dialysis centers
- This procedure can be undertaken by dialysis nurse, who has undertaken a specific educational training program, provided they are closely supervised by an experienced dialysis nurse at all times.

Alert

- All renal unit nurses must be aware of the complications of hazards that may occur due to blood leak during dialysis

Table 12.21: Minor blood leak

Sl No.	Nursing actions	Rationales
1.	When blood leak alarm occurs, check for faulty blood leak detector and if so call for the technician assistance	To avoid confusion and save time
2.	Explain the procedure to the patient; allow him/her to ask questions	To gain confidence and cooperation
3.	Check the dialyzate lines for discoloration	To ensure whether it is a real blood leak or just a machine error or faulty alarm
4.	Collect 10 mL of dialyzate in a test tube and visually check for blood; check with Labstix, if available	To decide whether it is minor or major blood leak
5.	Return the blood leak is verified	To prevent massive blood loss
6.	Return the dialysis line in the lock; the alarm should stop when the line are clear (no blood)	

Contd...

Contd...

Sl No.	Nursing actions	Rationales
7.	Put the machine on rinse program	To clear blood from the dialysis lines
8.	Reassess the patient and decide whether to recommend dialysis	To ensure delivery of prescribed treatment
9.	Document the incident including the time, when the blood leak started, nursing intervention, the patient condition and the amount of blood lost (if any)	

Table 12.22: Major blood leak

Sl No.	Nursing actions	Rationales
1.	If blood leak is massive and the blood cannot be reinfused send a blood sample to check for hemodialysis and inform the physician on call *Nursing alert:* When a blood leak occurs, there is a risk of blood contamination from unsterile dialysis entering the compartment of the dialyzer	To identify the blood loss and check hemodialysis
2.	Put the machine on rinse program	To clear blood from the dialyzate lines
3.	Take and record vital signs	To monitor the condition of the patient
4.	Reassess the patient	To allay fears and gain patient's confidence and cooperation
5.	Document the incident including the time, when the blood leak started, nursing intervention, the patient condition and the amount of blood lost (if any)	
6.	Document the lot number of kidney and serial number	To report to the company

- All renal unit nurses must be able to differentiate a true blood leak from a false one
- A functional test must be completed on all machines prior to commencing hemodialysis to ensure patient's safety and well-being
- All the circuit must be checked to ensure connections are secure (repeated if there are changes made to the circuit during hemodialysis to ensure patient's safety and well-being)
- The blood leak sensitivity control knob must be kept at maximum, e.g. 10 at all time (Gambro machine)

- A spare machine must be kept ready for the use in case of emergency, e.g. faulty blood leak down detector
- Ensure that the patient is aware of the hazard and reassure him/her to allay fears and gain his/her confidence and cooperation.

Machine Breakdown During Hemodialysis

Purposes

- To provide guidelines regarding exchanging machine during dialysis
- To complete dialysis session without any complication
- To demonstrate safe and skilled technique of handling dialysis.

Conditions

- Two experienced nurses should carry out this procedure (Table 12.23)
- A spare machine should be kept ready at all times for use in case of emergency available
- All nurses working in renal unit must be aware of nursing responsibility in case of machine breakdown during dialysis
- The functional test in the machine must be completed prior to start each dialysis session
- This procedure should be carried out within 15–20 minutes to prevent complications.

Table 12.23: Management of machine breakdown during hemodialysis

Sl No.	Nursing actions	Rationales
1.	As soon as the machine breakdown, the nurse should call for help from another nurse	
2.	Switch off the machine and rotate the blood pump manually (after writing down the parameters on the machine)	
3.	Explain the procedure to the patient and reassure him/her	To allay fears and gain patient's confidence and cooperation
4.	Bring the spare machine to bedside and switch on	
5.	• Disconnect water inflow and drain connection from other machine and connect to spare machine; put concentrate stock in the dialyzate fluid and start functional test • Switch on the venous air detector by pass • If no spare machine, return blood as per policy and procedure	
6.	Once the spare machine is ready, clamp the arterial and venous pressure monitors, patient lines and heparin line	

Contd...

Contd...

Sl No.	Nursing actions	Rationales
7.	Release venous air detector clamp	
8.	Disconnect dialyzate lines from the dialysis and replace them in lock	
9.	With the assistance of the other nurse, remove gently the dialyzer and tubing from the faulty machine and connect to the spare machine *Alert:* Ensure that the catheter/fistula needles are in the site and the tubing are not pulled, while transferring	To recommence safe dialysis
10.	Attach dialyzate lines to the dialyzer	
11.	Fix arterial and venous lines and release all clamps	
12.	Reset all alarms *Alert:* Always check the system for air/blood clot	
13.	Check all dialysis parameters	
14.	Start hemodialysis and adjust the remaining dialysis time	To complete the required hour of dialysis
15.	Take and record vital signs	To monitor the condition of patient
16.	Document the incident including the time when the machine breaks down, time taken when transferring, time restarted, and presence/absence of blood clot in the system	

DISINFECTION, CLEANING, DECALCIFICATION AND MAINTENANCE OF HEMODIALYSIS MACHINE

Purposes

- To maintain dialysis machines clean, sterile and trouble free during the treatment
- To maintain the fluid and fluid pathway sterile and free from contaminates
- To remove precipitate due to the low solubility of calcium carbonate
- To remove blood spills and other solutions from the machine.

Conditions

- This procedure (except external cleaning) should be performed by renal dialysis technician)
- The machine should be serviced every 2,000 hours (mechanical servicing)
- Strict safety measures should be taken during the procedure
- Heat disinfection should be performed after each dialysis.

Alert

- Chemical disinfection should be performed weekly if the machine undergoes heat disinfection, otherwise two times a week
- Decalcification should be performed weekly
- For positive patient, chemical disinfection should be done for the machine after each dialysis
- The machine should be disinfected if not used more than 24 hours.

Equipment

- Disinfectant and cleaning solutions
- Tools for maintenance
- Test equipment
- Charts for service and performance.

Procedure

Heat Disinfection

Some machines can be put directly to heat disinfection (Table 12.24), step 1 and step 2 will be done automatically.

Table 12.24: Heat disinfection

Steps	Nursing actions	Rationales
1.	After dialysis, drain or rinse the machine	To remove used dialyzate from the inside of the machine
2.	Put the machine on heat disinfection, this procedure will take 40–45 min	To sterilize the machine

Chemical Disinfection

Sodium chlorite can be used as disinfectant and cleaning solution as it kills microorganisms and removes contaminants organic origin such as proteins and glucose deposited in the fluid pathway. Chemical disinfection is given in Table 12.25.

Table 12.25: Chemical disinfection

Sl No.	Nursing actions	Rationales
1.	Prepare the machine for chemical disinfection (drain or rinse the machine)	To remove used dialyzate from the inside of the machine
2.	*Prepare the solution:* • Sodium hypochlorite (5.25% diluted to 5% for some machine) are used to disinfectant recommended by the manufacturer • Refer to the machine manufacturer before performing this procedure	

Contd...

Contd...

Sl No.	Nursing actions	Rationales
3.	Put the pickup tube designated from chemical intake (disinfecting pot) into the solution	For filling the machine with chemical
4.	Press the chemical disinfecting button	To activate the functions
5.	When disinfection finishes the light will flash, then the machine has to go for a mandatory rinse program, this procedure will take 45–60 min	To flush out chemicals from the machine

Note: Citrosteril, Puristeril and Dialox are disinfectant, but they do not remove organic origin.

BLOOD TRANSFUSION DURING HEMODIALYSIS

Purposes

- To restore the blood volume
- To raise the hemoglobin level
- To raise deficiency of plasma proteins
- To replace the blood with hemolytic agents with fresh blood (exchange transfusion)
- To raise leukocytes count.

Definition

Blood transfusion is the transfusion of whole blood or its components such as blood cells and plasma from one person (donor) to other (recipient). This involves two procedures, the collection of blood from the donor and the administration of blood to the recipient (Tables 12.26 and 12.27).

Equipment

- Blood transfusion tubing (blood Y set within line filter)
- Packed cell or whole blood as ordered
- Blood warmer
- Flow sheet for recording
- Non-sterile gloves
- Materials for IV start.

Purpose

Increase client's hemoglobin and hematocrit for improved circulation and oxygen distribution.

Table 12.26: Procedure for blood transfusion during hemodialysis

Sl No.	Nursing actions	Rationales
1.	Determine if client knows for transfusion, ask if the client has had a transfusion or transfusion reaction in the past	Direct teaching prior to beginning transfusion
2.	Explain procedure to client, check for signed consent for transfusion, advice to report any chill, itching, rash or unusual symptoms	Provides reassurance facilitates and for professional safeguard cooperation prompt reporting of any reaction to transfusion necessitates
3.	Wash hands	Handwashing deter the spread of microorganisms
4.	Hang container of 0.9% normal saline with blood administration set to initiate intravenous (IV) infusion and follow administration of blood	Dextrose may lead to clumping of red blood cells (RBCs) and hemolysis, filter in blood administration set removes particulate materials formed during storage of blood
5.	Start IV, open by starting flow of normal saline	Not to cause damage to RBC
6.	Obtain blood product, where it was stored (with maintained temperature)	Unit at carefully controlled temperature (4–6°C)
7.	Complete identification and check as required by hospital policy	Some agency required two-registered nurse to verify information
8.	Identification number	Verify that unit number match
9.	Blood group and type	Verify that ABO group and Rhesus (Rh) type are the same
10.	Expiry Date	Safe storage of blood is limited to 35 day before blood cell begins to deteriorate
11.	Client's name	Never administer a blood to client without a name band
12.	Inspect blood for clots	If clots are present, blood should be returned to blood bank
13.	Take baseline set of vital signs prior to beginning transfusion	Any change in vital signs during transfusion may indicate a reaction
14.	Start infusion of the blood product in line filter with blood	Necessary if blood is to flow properly
15.	Start administration slowly	Transfusion reaction typically occur during this period and a slow rate will minimize the volume of RBC infused; if there had been no adverse effects during this time, the infusion rate is increased

Contd...

Contd...

Sl No.	Nursing actions	Rationales
16.	Check vital signs every 5 min for 5–15 min	If complication occurs, they can be observed and the blood can be stopped immediately
17.	Observe client for flushing dyspnea, itching, hives or rash, etc.	May be early indications of transfusion reaction
18.	Maintain the prescribed flow rate and assess frequently for transfusion reaction; stop blood transfusion and allow saline to flow, if you suspect a reaction, notify physician and blood bank officer	Rate may carefully be controlled and clients reaction must be monitored on a frequent basis; saline prevents hemolysis of RBC and clears reminder of blood in IV line
19.	Record administration of blood and client reaction; return bag to blood bank according to hospital policy	Provide for accurate documentation of clients response to blood transfusion

Table 12.27: Transfusion reaction and nursing activity

Sl No.	Transfusion reactions	Signs and symptoms	Nursing activities
1.	Allergic reaction allergy to transfused blood	Hives, itching and anaphylaxis	Stop transfusion immediately and keep vein open (KVO) with normal saline notify physician and administer medication as per instruction
2.	Febrile reaction, fever develops during infusion	Fever, chills, headache and malaise	Stop transfusion immediately and KVO with normal saline, notify physician and treat symptoms
3.	Hemolytic transfusion reaction, incompatibility of blood product	Immediate on set of facial flushing, fever, chills, headache, low back pain and shock	Stop transfusion immediately and KVO with normal saline notify physician, obtain blood sample from site and obtain first-voided urine if test shock present, send unit and filter tubes to blood bank
4.	Circulatory overload (too much blood administered)	Dyspnea, dry cough and pulmonary edema	Slow or stop infusion, monitor vital signs and notify physician
5.	Bacteria present in the blood	Fever, hypertension, dry flushed skin and abdomen pain	Stop infusion immediately, monitor vital signs and administer antibiotics as prescribed

Assessment

Assessment should focus on the following:

- Baseline vital signs, circulatory and respiratory status
- Doctor's prescription
- History of blood transfusions and reaction, if any
- Compatibility of client to blood (blood group and matching)
- Some agencies require that two registered nurses perform blood test of client, identification check, refer to agency policy
- Clients with a history of previous transfusion must be watched carefully for a transfusion reaction
- The maximum transfusion time for packed cells or whole blood is 4 hours
- The transfusion must be started within half-an-hour after getting the blood from the blood bank, otherwise the blood cannot be reissued
- Keep emergency medication on bedside.

HEMODIALYSIS SHUNT GRAFT AND FISTULA CARE

Equipment

- Non-sterile gloves
- Two pairs of sterile gloves
- Antiseptic cleansing agents or antiseptic swabs
- Topical antiseptic, if ordered
- Sterile 4" × 4" gauze pads
- Cannula clamps.

Purposes

- Maintain patency of access for dialysis.
- Detect complications of hemodialysis access site related to infection, occlusion or cannula separation.

Assessment

Assessment should focus on the following:

- Status of fistula, graft or cannula site and dressing
- Location of shunt, fistula or graft
- Vital signs
- Pulses distal to shunt, fistula or graft
- Color and temperature or extremity in which access is located, presence of pain
- Time and date when last dressing changed.

Note: Potential complications related to the presence of the shunt is cannula separation, hemorrhage can occur if the shunt is not clamped off until a new cannula is inserted, therefore a pair of clamps should be kept at the client's bedside at all times. Procedure is detailed in Table 12.28.

Table 12.28: Procedure for care of hemodialysis shunt graft and fistula

Sl No.	Nursing actions	Rationales
1.	Wash hands	Reduce microorganism transfer
2.	Explain procedure to the patient	Decreases anxiety
3.	Open antiseptic solution or antiseptic swabs and position for easy access; keep one package of gauze 4" x 4" dry	Decrease anxiety, facilitates cleaning process, provides gauze to cover shunt
4.	Don clean gloves	Reduce nurses exposure to body secretions
5.	Remove old dressing if present and check access site	Expose access site
6.	Discard dressing and gloves	Removes contaminated items
7.	Wash hands and don sterile gloves	Avoids site contamination
8.	Cleanse access area with antiseptic agents, for shunt care, begins at exit areas and work outward; discarding antiseptic swab or folded gauze pad after each wipe	Reduce contamination
9.	Lightly place two or three fingertips over access site and assess for presence of thrill (a palpable vibration should be present) assess site for extreme warmth or coolness	Test for adequate blood flow through shunt
10.	Apply topical ointment, if ordered	Prevent infection
11.	Place dry sterile gauze pads over access site	Reduces site contamination
12.	For shunt, cover with gauze pads and around extremity (wrap firmly that dressing is secure, but not too tight as to occlude blood flow) and tape securely; leave small piece of shunt tubing visible	Prevent accidental dislodgment of cannula
13.	Discard equipment and gloves then wash hands	Reduces spread of infection
14.	Place call light within reach	Enables client to communicate
15.	Assess status of dressing access site and pulse in affected extremity every 2 hour	

Contd...

Contd...

Sl No.	Nursing actions	Rationales
16.	During immediate postoperative period inform client family and staff of the following care instructions:	Prevents rupture and pain
	• Keep extremity elevated on pillow until instructed otherwise • Do not apply pressure or lift heavy objects with extremity • Do not allow access area to get wet during showering, bathing or swimming	
17.	Inform client's family and staff of the following care instructions: • Never perform following procedures on the affected extremity • Blood pressure assessment or any procedure that might occlude blood flow • Vein puncture or any procedure involving a needle stick; place signs over bedside prohibiting use of affected extremity for these procedures • Avoid restricting blood flow in affected extremity with tight fitting cloths, watches, name bands, knee high stockings, antiembolytic, restraints and so forth • Notify nurse immediately if bleeding or cannula disconnections are noted • Apply cannula clamps if disconnection is noted	• Facilitates cooperation with care of site, reduces fear and prevent undue injury • Present occlusion of blood flow • Prevent injury, clotting and infection • Prevents restriction of blood flow and injury to graft/shunt/fistula area • Prevent excessive bleeding • Prevent hemorrhage
18.	Documentation of the following should be noted: • Location of access site • Status of site and dressing • Vital signs • Status of pulse distal to access area • Color and temperature of extremity, presence of pain or numbness in extremity in which access is located	

Chapter 13 Peritoneal Dialysis

In peritoneal dialysis (PD), peritoneum is used as diffusible membrane, it involves repeated cycles of instilling dialysate into the peritoneal cavity allowing time for substance exchange and then removing the dialysate.

Peritoneal dialysis procedure performed to correct an imbalance of fluid or of electrolytes in the blood or to remove toxins, drugs or other waste normally excreted by the kidney. It is contraindicated in patient with extensive intra-abdominal adhesions, localized peritoneal infection or gangrenous or perforated bowels.

CONTINUOUS AMBULATORY PERITONEAL DIALYSIS

Preparation of Peritoneal Dialysis Machine

Purposes

- To prepare accurately the PD machine in accordance with the dialysis prescription
- To prevent cross infection.

Policy

- The physician order must be obtained
- All nursing staff working in the renal unit should be trained in the preparation of PD machine
- A strict aseptic technique should be maintained throughout the procedure in accordance with the policy and procedure of aseptic technique
- Hand hygiene should be performed according to policy and procedure on handwashing.

Equipment

- Trolley cleaned and wiped with 70% spirit
- Peritoneal dialysis lines and set
- Peritoneal dialysis on and off pack
- Sterile gloves
- Betadine skin cleanser in spirit
- Surgical mask: 2
- Injection heparin 1,000 IU/mL
- Peritoneal dialysis fluid of correct strength as ordered
- Micropore tape

- Additive drugs
- Drip stand
- Sterile hand towel
- Syringe 10 mL: 3
- Scissors
- Sterile gauze
- Specimen containers: 2
- Laboratory investigation form: 2.

Procedure

- Both nurses wash and dry their hands
- Clean bedside table with spirit
- Wear mask
- Open sterile drapes over the work surface touching only the covers
- Using non-touch technique, open lines and tip, and place them on the sterile area
- Open the on and off pack, and keep on the sterile area
- Pour Betadine into the container
- Wear sterile gloves
- Ensure that all screw, spikes and clamps closed
- Apply Betadine-soaked gauze swabs to the part of the line, which will be connected to the patient's catheter
- The second nurse (assisting nurse) set up the machine with desired volume dwelling and draining time
- Switch off power button and wait for few seconds to stop the alarm (alarm stops automatically once the machine is ready for priming)
- Wash and dry hands
- Pass the lines to the second nurse (assisting nurse) to attach to the machine taking great care to keep the spikes and the patient's end sterile
- The second nurse (assisting nurse) opens the cover of all bags one by one, which are hanging on the drip stand
- Clamp and connect the bags on all the spikes one after one
- Withdraw heparin injection as prescribed
- Add heparin to the peritoneal fluid
- Inject any additive drugs along with the heparin in separate syringe
- Ask the second nurse (assisting nurse) to open all clamps and press start button, the machine will automatically prime at the end of priming and the start button will be illuminated again
- Secure and cover sterile surface and patient connector with a sterile drape unit ready to commence PD
- Dispose of used equipment appropriately
- Wash and dry hands.

Peritoneal Dialysis

Equipment

- Dialysate fluid(s) ordered
- Medication additives ordered
- Syringes for adding additives
- Dialysis flow sheet
- Dialysate tubing
- Intravenous (IV) pole
- Sterile saline
- Antiseptic solution as per agency policy
- Clean gown
- Sterile gloves
- Gauze dressing pads (2" × 2" and 4" × 4" tape).

Purposes

Instill solutions into peritoneal cavity to remove metabolic end products, toxins and excess fluid from body when a kidney function is totally or partially ineffective.

Requirements

- Instruct each person in room to don appropriate protective masks for all persons in room, sterile gloves for nurse and assistant handling fluid bags
- All nursing staff working in the renal unit should be trained in connecting a patient to PD machine
- A strict aseptic technique should be maintained throughout the procedure in accordance with the policy and procedure of aseptic technique
- Handwashing should be performed according to policy and procedure on handwashing.

Procedure

The procedure for PD is detailed in Table 13.1.

Connecting a Patient to Peritoneal Dialysis Machine

Purposes

- To aid in the removal of toxic substances and metabolic wastes
- To assist in regulation body fluid and electrolyte balance
- To control blood pressure
- To remove excessive body fluid.

Table 13.1: Procedure for peritoneal dialysis

Sl No.	Action	Rationale
1.	Wash hands	Reduces microorganisms transfer
2.	Explain procedure to the patient	Decreases anxiety
3.	Check weigh of client for each dialysis session	Provides data needed to determine appropriate concentration of fluids clearance
4.	Place dialysate fluid in room temperature	Prevents abdominal cramps
5.	Don mask	Reduces spread of airborne microorganism
6.	Prepare dialysate with medication additives as ordered, label on bags	Avoids error that could affect end results of dialysis
7.	Insert dialysate infusion tubing spike into insertion port on dialysate fluid bag/battle and prime tubing, place fluid bag/bottle and prime tubing, place fluid bag on intravenous (IV) bag *Note:* Some tubing spikes are designed like a screw cap with a spike in the center of the cap	Eliminates air that may contribute to client discomfort
8.	Adjust position of bed, so that fluid hangs higher than the clients abdomen and drainage bag is lower than abdomen	Enhances gravitational flow, as fluid infuses and drains
9.	Provide privacy	Reduces embarrassment
10.	Don sterile gloves	Reduce contamination
11.	Remove old peritoneal catheter dressing and examine catheter site for catheter dislodgement or signs of infection, if leakage or abdominal drainage is noted	Assesses catheter intactness, facilitates identification of infection agent
12.	Discard dressing, gloves and wash hands	Reduces microorganisms transfer
13.	Cleanse at catheter site, cleanse site with a circular motion outward using peroxide or sterile saline on gauze or swab and allow to dry, apply antiseptic agents recommended; discard each swab or gauze after each wipe when cleansing site	Decrease microorganisms at catheter insertion site, reduces risk of peritonitis
14.	Using sterile technique apply dressing and secure tape	Protects site from microorganisms

Contd...

Contd...

Sl No.	Action	Rationale
15.	Don sterile gloves	Reduces microorganism
16.	Connect end of dialysate tubing to abdominal catheter	Connects tubing to begin dialysate infusion
17.	Clamp tubing from abdominal catheter to drainage bag	Prevents dialysate from leaking
18.	Check clients position (abdominal lower than height of fluids, which allows gravity to facilitate flow) check tubing for kinks or bends	Removes obstruction that could affect infusion rate
19.	Open dialysate infusion tubing clamps and allow fluid to drain into peritoneal cavity for 10–15 min; observe respiratory status infuses and remains in the abdomen (dwell time)	Infuses dialysate for fluid and electrolytes exchange in peritoneal cavity
20.	Allow fluid to dwell in abdomen for 20 minutes (or amount of time specified by doctor)	Allows time for proper exchange of fluid and electrolytes
21.	Open clamp leading to drain bag and allow fluid to drain for specified amount of time or until drainage has decreased to a slow drip (if all the fluid does not return reposition client and recheck tubing leading to drainage bag) For continuous ambulatory peritoneal dialysis (CAPD) client may fold dialysis bag and secure bag and tubing to abdomen or clothing, and allow fluid to dwell, while performing daily activities; to drain dialysate client would unfold and lower bag and allow fluid to drain from abdominal cavity; a new bag is then hung and infusion dwelling drainage cycle is repeated continuously	Allows end products of dialysis to drain
22.	Record amount of fluid infused and amount drained after each exchange, add balance of fluid infused and drained on appropriate flow sheet (if net output is greater than amount infused by a large margin 200 mL or more notify doctor)	Provides accurate record of fluids exchange for determining fluid balance

Contd...

Contd...

Sl No.	Action	Rationale
23.	Reassess the following client data every 30–60 min thereafter through exchanges vital signs, output, respiratory status, mental status, appearance of dialysate return, abdominal dressing (should be kept dry) and signs of lethal electrolytes imbalance	Alerts nurse to impending complications or need to change fluid and additive concentrations
24.	Check weight of client at end of appropriate number of fluids exchange	Provides data regarding efficiency of exchanges in removing excess fluid
25.	Obtain laboratory data as ordered and as needed	Provides data about clearance of metabolic wastes as well as electrolytes status
26.	When the total series of exchanges is completed empty drainage bag into graduated container; discard bag; tubing and cap peritoneal catheter	Removes fluid waste so that other fluid may drain
27.	Discard or restore equipment appropriately	Promotes clean environment
28.	Wash hands	Reduces microorganism
29.	Note the fluid balance, vital signs, weight, presence or absence of edema abdominal girth, status of catheter site, changes of laboratory data (blood gases, potassium, blood urea nitrogen, creatinine, hemoglobin, hematocrit) type and amount of dialysate and infused medication additives in dialysate	

Requirements

- All nursing staff working in the renal unit should be trained in connecting a patient to PD machine
- A strict aseptic technique should be maintained throughout the procedure in accordance with the policy and procedure of aseptic technique
- Handwashing should be performed according to policy and procedure on handwashing.

Equipment

- Trolley cleaned and wiped with 70% spirit
- Peritoneal dialysis on and off pack

- Sterile drape: 2
- Syringe 10 mL: 2
- Specimen container: 2
- Specimen bags: 2
- Sterile gloves
- Surgical mask
- Micropore tape
- Laboratory investigation form: 2
- Sterile cotton buds
- Betadine skin cleanser in spirit
- Sterile gauze
- Kidney basin
- Disposable apron
- Peritoneal dialysis flowchart
- Blood pressure (BP) apparatus.

Procedure

- Clean the trolley as appropriate
- Check the physician order and previous dialysis records
- Explain the procedure to the patient and provide privacy
- Place the patient in a comfortable position
- Take and record vital signs and weight
- Both nurses wear surgical mask
- Both nurses wash and dry their hands and wear gloves
- Place a sterile drape on the trolley
- Once nurse opens the PD on and off, pack 10 mL syringe and hands them over the nurse performing the procedure
- Arrange the instruments on the sterile field
- Pour Betadine solution into the gallipots using non-touch technique and remove the dressing from the peritoneal catheter
- Inspect the site for any unwanted leakage or infection and take swab, if appropriate
- Clean the PD catheter's site and surrounding area with Betadine solution then apply sterile dressing
- Wrap the catheter with a piece of gauze soaked with Betadine solution and then apply sterile dressing
- Change gloves.
- Using a 10 mL syringe aspirate the heparinized solution from a peritoneal catheter and discard it
- Use another 10 mL syringe to obtain PD fluid for routine microbiology tests

- Unclamp the catheter and PD catheters lines
- Secure the lines and catheter with plaster and press the start button on the machine (note the time and ensure that the dialysis button is illuminated and the fluid from the top bag is freely flowing into the peritoneal cavity)
- Leave the patient in a comfortable position
- Check BP and pulse at this point and maintain hourly or more frequent checks depends in patient conditions
- Maintain peritoneal flowchart
- Document in the nurses notes and report any abnormalities to the nurse in charge and the physician.

Connecting a Patient to the Dialysate

Purposes

- To aid removal of toxic substances and metabolic wastes
- To assist in regulating the fluid and electrolyte balance of the body
- To control BP
- To control severe intractable heart failure when diuretics no longer promote elimination of water and sodium.

Policy

- The procedure should be ordered by physician
- The procedure should be performed in the hospital by a physician or a continuous ambulatory peritoneal dialysis (CAPD) trained nurse
- The procedure is performed:
  - On patient who cannot tolerate hemodialysis
  - When all the vascular access procedures failed
  - In very old patient with cardiac diseases.
- A strict aseptic technique should be maintained throughout the procedure in accordance with the policy and procedure of aseptic technique
- The catheter insertion site should be checked for signs of infection, swab culture and sensitivity sent if any sign is present
- Handwashing should be performed according to the policy and procedure on handwashing.

Equipment

- Trolley wash with soap and water with 70% spirit
- Continuous ambulatory PD fluid
- Betadine antiseptic
- HiBiSCRUB
- Transfer set with adaptor

- Sterile gauze packs
- Mepore dressing (9 × 15 cm)
- Surgical mask
- Clean sheet/tray
- Surgical mask
- Sterile dressing set
- Sterile gloves
- Drugs/sterile syringe with needle (if required)
- Unsterile receiver for soiled dressing
- Drip stand with de block clamp
- Sterile sheet/Kinidrape
- Spirit swab
- Weighing scale (hanging).

Procedure

- Explain the procedure to the patient to gain cooperation
- Clean top trolley with a piece of gauze soaked with spirit then push to bedside
- Screen the bed to provide privacy
- Wear surgical mask
- Wash and dry hands
- Check CAPD fluid bag for:
  - Leakage
  - Correct type
  - Amount
  - Expiry date
  - Clarity
  - Color and place it near the edge of the trolley on the top shelf.
- Open the transfer set pack gently using aseptic technique (with clear side of the pack facing downwards) and place on the top shelf
- Open the outer pack of the CAPD fluid bag and place bag on the trolley with the connecting site hanging
- Disinfect hand
- Remove cap of the CAPD fluid bag and spray all around the exposed part of the connecting site
- Disinfect hand again
- Pick up gently on end of the transfer set and remove the cap
- With the left hand thumb and forefinger, hold the exposed connecting site of the CAPD fluid bag and quickly connect the transfer set to the site of the CAPD fluid bag (non-touch technique where the rest of the fingers are not facing the connecting site)

- Break the cone in the CAPD bag and then hang the bag on the drip stand
- Prime the transfer and clamp it, leaving the other end of the transfer set in the opened pack
- Open dressing pack and side the tray gently on the top shelf using aseptic technique
- Open adaptor pack sterile pack, Mepore sterile gloves, sterile gauze pack and slide them into the dressing set
- Pour in some Betadine antiseptic
- Prepare the patient
- Observe the exit site of the catheter for any signs of infection of ever granulation of tissue, if infected, take a swab culture and sensitivity and inform the physician; over granulation of tissue, is cauterized with silver nitrate
- Disinfect hand
- Clean exit site and area around with Betadine antiseptic
- Clean the Tenckhoff catheter with Betadine from bottom to top
- Place gauze soaked with Betadine antiseptic around the exit site and all around the Tenckhoff catheter for at least 3 minutes
- After 3 minutes, hold the catheter end with left and remove the gauze piece and discard them
- Place the sterile sheet around the catheter site and place the catheter on the sterile sheet
- Remove gloves, disinfect hands properly
- Clean and dry the catheter with dry sterile gauze
- Fix signal to noise ratio (S/N) adaptor
- Hold the S/N adaptor between the third and fourth finger of the left hand and hold the free end of the transfer set between the thumbs and forefinger of the left hand
- Remove the cap of the S/N adaptor and spray all around the exposed area for avoiding the lumen with Freka-DERM
- Quickly remove the cap of the transfer set and connect it to the S/N adaptor and tighten it well
- Place the connected site on the sterile sheet and release both clamps
- Allow the fluid to flow in
- Watch for any leakage at the connecting site, if present; tighten the S/N adaptor with the provided spanner, remove the sterile sheet
- Watch for oozing from the exit site of the catheter
- Disinfect hands; apply sterile Mepore as dressing at the exit site
- When fluid has gone in completely, fold and coil the tubing around the folded bag and secure it around the patient's abdomen or place it in the pocket
- Make patient as comfortable as possible

- Remove the trolley and discard soiled swabs, wash hands
- Dispatch specimen it taken to the laboratory
- Document the procedure in the CAPD chart.

Changing Transfer Set

Purpose

To prevent infection.

Policy

- The procedure should be performed in the hospital by a physician or a CAPD trained nurse
- A strict aseptic technique should be maintained
- The set should be changed every 6 months or whenever it contaminated
- Handwashing should be performed in accordance with the policy and procedure on handwashing.

Equipment

- Trolley washed with soap, water and 70% spirit
- Spirit
- Non-sterile gauze pieces
- New drainage bag
- New transfer set
- Sterile sheet/Kinidrape
- Clean sheet/Tray
- Surgical mask
- Small dustbin.

Procedure

- Explain the procedure to the patient to gain cooperation
- Bring the prepared trolley beside the patient
- Screen the patient to provide privacy
- Wear surgical mask
- Wash and dry hands
- Clean top shelf of trolley with gauze soaked in spirit
- Open the transfer set pack gently using aseptic technique and place the opened pack with the tubing inside on a corner of top shelf (place clear side of pack downwards)
- Open the new drainage bag, pack and place the bag besides the transfer set pack with the connecting site hanging freely not touching the edge of the trolley

- Open sterile sheet and leave the sheet lying within the pack on the top shelf of the trolley
- Place freak aspect and Freka-DERM on the top shelf at one corner
- Place clean tray below the level of the patient
- Place the dustbin beside the patient
- Disinfect hands properly with Freka-SEPT (turn aside, away from the trolley)
- Remove the cap of the new drainage bag and spray all around the exposed connecting site with FrekaDERM (avoid the lumen)
- Disinfect hand with properly with Freka-SEPT
- Take one end of the transfer set, remove cap and quickly connect it to the drainage bag and clamp the transfer set
- Disinfect hands with Freka-SEPT
- Place sterile sheet underneath the Tenckhoff catheter and let the connecting site lie on the sheet
- Spray all around the connecting site of the Tenckhoff catheter and old transfer set with Freka-SEPT
- Disinfect hands with Freka-SEPT
- Disconnect the old transfer set from the Tenckhoff catheter and discard it into the dustbin
- Hold the Tenckhoff catheter end in between third and fourth finger of left hand, and spray all around the exposed connecting site avoiding the lumen
- Pick up the other end of the new transfer set; hold it with the left thumb and forefinger
- Remove the cap of the new transfer set and quickly connect it to the Tenckhoff catheter
- Place the connected site on a dry area of the sterile sheet
- Place the drainage bag on the clean tray below the level of the patient
- Release clamps of the Tenckhoff catheter and transfer set, allow about 100 mL of fluid to drain into bag (count 1–10), this is to flush out any bacteria present in the cube
- Clamp both tubes
- If due for exchange of fluid, patient can continue with his/her exchange otherwise fold the bag with tubing coiled around the bag and secure it to patients abdomen
- Document the procedure in the patient file.

Dialysate Bag Exchange

Purposes

- The procedure should be performed by a physician or a CAPD trained nurse

- A strict aseptic technique should be maintained throughout the procedure in accordance with the policy and procedure of maintained technique
- Number of exchange to be done daily should be ordered by the physician
- The type of the CAPD fluid and drugs to be given should be prescribed by the physician
- Wash and dry hand should be performed according to the policy and procedure on handwashing
- Weight and BP of the patient should be taken and recorded in the CAPD chart
- The exit dressing should be changed every morning after taking bath.

Equipment

- Trolley washed with soap, water and wiped with 70% spirit
- Continuous ambulatory PD fluid (type as required)
- Freka-SEPT or HiBiSCRUB
- Freka-DERM
- Betadine antiseptic
- Spirit/Spirit swab
- Sterile gauze packs
- Mepore dressing (9 × 15 cm)
- Surgical mask
- Clean sheet/Tray scissors
- Clean sheet/Tray
- Scissors
- Non-sterile gauze (4" × 4")
- Drugs/Sterile syringe with needles (if required)
- Unsterile receiver for soiled dressing
- Drip stand
- Weighing scale (hanging)
- Plastic apron
- Amuchina solution
- Three blue clamps
- Two small sterile containers.

Procedure

1. Wash and dry hands.
2. Bring the prepared trolley with all equipment to the patient's bedside.
3. Screen the bed to provide privacy. Encourage the patient to observe the procedure.
4. Wear surgical masks.

5. Wash and dry hands with HiBiSCRUB.
6. Wipe the top shelf of the trolley and the sides with non-sterile gauze soaks in spirit.
7. Arrange Freka-DERM, Freka-SEPT and Amuchina solution on top shelf at one corner.
8. Open a sterile gauze pack with aseptic technique and place the pack near the edge of the top shelf with the gauze exposed.
9. Check the new CAPD fluid bag for:
   - Leakage
   - Correct type
   - Amount
   - Expiry date
   - Clarity color
   - Place it at one corner of the trolley.
10. Place the drip stand near the patient.
11. Place the clean tray on the floor near the patient.
12. Place small disposal bin near the patient.
13. Place the patient in a comfortable position—sitting or recumbent and expose Tenckhoff catheter site.
14. Wash and dry hands.
15. Remove empty drainage bag from the patient and spray it around the connecting site with Freka-DERM and place the bag on the tray below the level of the patient.
16. Release both Tenckhoff catheter clamp and transfer set clamp and allow fluid to drain into the bag.

    Note: As the fluid flows out the tubing will be warm, if no flow, check the tubing to see whether it is linked or not. Check the position of the patient, encourage the patient to turn gently from side to side (if lying) or stand up (if sitting). Once the fluid has drained out, the tubing will be cool and drainage bag will be filled.
17. While the fluid is drained out, check the new CAPD fluid bag again for volumes type, clarity, expiry date and leakage.
18. Remove the outer pack using aseptic technique (do not touch the connecting tube site, place back on top shelf near the edge with the connecting site hanging freely).
19. Place the drainage bag beside the new bag in the same way.
20. Disinfect hands with Freka-SEPT (away from the trolley).
21. Place one piece of sterile dry gauze on the clean surface of the opened gauze pack and pour some Betadine antiseptic on it.
22. Disinfect hands again with Freka-SEPT.
23. Wrap the Betadine-soaked gauze around the connecting site of the drainage bag and leave it for at least 3 minutes.

24. Clean and dry fingers gauze and discard gauze into the dustbin.
25. After 3 minutes, discard Betadine-soaked gauze into the dustbin.
26. Disinfect hands again with Freka-SEPT.
27. Remove the cap of the connecting site of the new bag and spray all around the exposed site with Freka-DERM (avoid spraying the lumen) disinfect hands.
28. Wipe Betadine-soaked site of the old bag with sterile dry gauze.
29. Disconnect transfer set from the old bag holding the connecting site of the drainage bag with the thumb and forefingers (rest of the fingers facing the bag to prevent contamination) and quickly connect transfer set to the connecting site of the new CAPD bag using the same non-touch technique.

    Note: Do not hesitate to change the new bag, if the exposed connecting site of the new bag has been accidentally by the hands or any other objects.
30. Break the cone of the new CAPD bag and on the drip stand.
31. Release both clamps and allows fluid to flow in.
32. When the fluid completely drained in clamp or both clamps.
33. Fold the empty bag and coil the tubing around it and place with the patient.
34. Check the filled drainage by holding it up under direct light for:
    - Clarity
    - Fibrin
    - Blood.
35. Arrange all items back on the bottom shelf of the trolley. Clean top shelf with spirit and leave it in the one corner of the room.
36. Remove mask.
37. Make the patient as comfortable as possible.
38. Measure the drained out fluid in the dirty utility room using gloves.
39. Wash and dry hands.
40. Document the procedure in the CAPD chart and patient file.
41. Warm a new CAPD fluid bag under the tight of the patient for the next exchange.

    Note: If drained out fluid is cloudy, turbid or with blood or fibrin, informs the physician first and sends a specimen for culture and sensitivity and cell count, reserve the bag of fluid for the physician to see before measuring the amount.

Disconnecting a Patient from Peritoneal Dialysis Machine

Purposes

- To disconnect the patient from the machine on completion of dialysis
- To investigate malfunction in the system.

Policy

- All nursing staff working in the renal unit should be competent in disconnecting patients from PD
- Two nurse, of whom one should be on trained and experienced nurse, should carry out this procedure
- A strict aseptic technique should be maintained throughout the procedure in accordance with the policy and procedure of aseptic technique
- Handwashing should be performed according to policy and procedure on handwashing.

Equipment

- Trolley washed with soap, water and wiped with 70% spirit
- On and off pack
- Betadine solution with spirit
- Micropore tape
- Specimen containers
- Specimen bags
- Investigation forms
- Peritoneal catheter cap
- Syringe 10 mL: 1
- Syringe 5 mL: 1
- Injection heparin: 100 IU/mL
- Intravenous normal saline ampules
- Mask
- Sterile gloves
- Sterile gauzes.

Procedure

- Clean the trolley with 70% spirit
- Ensure that the prescribed number of liters is completed
- Ensure that all fluid has been drained from the patient's peritoneum
- Explain the procedure to the patient
- Place the patient in a comfortable position
- Both nurses wear masks and wash their hands
- The first nurse wears sterile gloves
- Place a sterile drape on the trolley
- Instruct the second nurse (assisting nurse) to:
  - Open the PD on and off pack, sterile 10 mL syringe, catheter cap and hand them over using aseptic technique
  - Pour Betadine solution into the gallipot.

- Clamp the peritoneal catheter with a sterile clamp
- Ask the second nurse (assisting nurse) to remove the bridging tape, while holding the tube to prevent it from being pulled out
- Clean the catheter with Betadine solution from exit site to wipe, scrub for 3 minutes
- Disconnect the catheter from PD line
- Aspirate a peritoneal fluid specimen from the line using 10 mL syringe, transfer the specimen aseptically into the specimen tube
- Flush the catheter with heparinized normal saline (2,000, i.e. 5 mL)
- Replace a new catheter cap, remove the clamps and apply required dressing
- Apply bridging tape
- Secure the catheter and dressing with adhesive tape
- Check vital signs
- Dispose the equipment appropriately
- Wash and dry hands
- Document the procedure in the nursing notes.

Maintenance and Cleaning of Peritoneal Dialysis Machine

Purpose

- To keep dialysis machine clean and trouble free, during the treatment.

Policy

- The procedure should be performed by qualified dialysis engineer
- Service the machine, should be serviced every 6 months including:
  - Complete electronic calibration
  - Changing the parts needing replacement with the test equipment
  - Checking the function of the machine with test equipment.
- The performance test should be performed every 2 months:
  - Checking the function of the machine with test equipment
  - Checking the overall performance of the machine.
- The service and performance record should be entered into the respective file of the machine.

Equipment

- Tools for maintenance
- Test equipment
- Cleaning solution.

Procedure

Cleaning the exterior parts of the machine is performed by a renal nurse:
- Prepare the solution (0.5% Milton)
- Soak the cloth in the solution
- Wipe the exterior parts of the machine.

PLASMAPHERESIS

Purpose

To remove any antibodies circulating in the plasma.

Requirements

- The procedure is performed on patients requiring renal transplant, but who have high levels of antibodies on the instructions of the attending physician
- Two nurses of whom one should be trained and experienced dialysis nurse should carry out this procedure
- A strict aseptic technique should be maintained throughout the procedure in accordance with the policy and procedure of aseptic technique
- Handwashing should be performed according to policy and procedure on handwashing.

Equipment

- Trolley washed with soap, water and wiped with 70% spirit
- Hemodialysis on and off pack
- Sterile drape: 2
- Fenestrated sterile drape: 1
- Forced vital capacity (FVC) pack, if no access
- Fistula needles: 2, if fistula is present
- Three-way tap
- Betadine 105 with 70% spirit
- Sterile spirit swabs/Mediswabs
- Sterile gloves
- Plaster/Micropore for dressing
- Local anesthesia injection
- Sterile syringes of various size
- Specimen bottles
- Plasma flux kidney (plasma separator)

- When the plasma is observed coming through the outlet line, then fix replacement plasma from the blood warmer on the replacement line. Open the clamp and slowly commence replacement
- As soon as the plasma starts coming through the outlet line, start the replacement of plasma. If heparin is contraindicated, so saline wash every 30 minutes
- Adjust the replacement according to the output
- Record vital signs
- Watch for any signs of anaphylaxis
- Continue the procedure
- Record the amount of plasma and exchanges
- When the amount of plasma prescribed by the physician has been removed and replaced, discontinue the procedure
- Switch off the pump, which has been used for replacement and clamp the line
- Do the normal wash back for regular hemodialysis with physiological saline
- When all the blood in the lines has been given to the patient, clamp all lines and disconnect from the fistula needles or catheter
- If any postplasmapheresis drugs are to be administered do so, before removing fistula needles or catheter
- If fistula needles are used, remove by applying pressure over the site until bleeding has stopped and then apply fresh dressing and firm plaster. If catheter is issued apply dressing and heparinized catheter
- Check the record of vital signs
- Make patient comfortable
- Remove all lines from the machine and discard into appropriate receptacle
- Dispose plasma into sink
- Allow the patient to relax after the procedure, check and record postplasmapheresis weight
- Send specimen to the laboratory
- Leave the room neat and tidy.

PREOPERATIVE PREPARATION OF PATIENT FOR INSERTION OF TENCKHOFF CATHETER

Purpose

To prevent postoperative infection at the incision sites.

Equipment

- Trolley washed with soap and water with 70% spirit
- Disinfectant
- Sterile sheet

- Razor/Clipper/Scissors
- Tenckhoff catheter
- Kidney basin
- Sharp box.

Requirements

1. Patient should be admitted at least 1 day prior to operation.
2. Written consent for the insertion of the Tenckhoff catheter should be obtained by the attending physician.
3. Phosphate enema should be given in the evening prior to surgery followed by two glycerin suppositories in the morning of the surgery.
4. The skin should be prepared from sternum (xiphoid) to mid-thigh. The evening prior to surgery in accordance with the policy and procedure on skin preparation.
5. Patient should be given a Betadine scrub bath and hair shampoo on the evening prior to surgery.
6. On the day of surgery, patient has to take a body bath. Then prepared area is painted with Betadine antiseptic and the area is draped with sterile sheet. Patient should wear operating theater gown.
7. A strict aseptic technique should be maintained throughout the procedure in accordance with the policy and procedure of aseptic technique.
8. Nasal swab is taken for *Staphylococcus aureus.*
9. Prophylactic antibiotic therapy is prescribed by the physician.
10. As surgery is usually done under local anesthesia.

POSTOPERATIVE CARE OF PATIENT WITH TENCKHOFF CATHETER

Purpose

To prevent postoperative infection at the incision and excision sites.

Equipment

- Trolley washed with soap, water and wiped with 70% spirit
- Betadine antiseptic
- Sterile gauze packs
- Sterile cotton swabs
- Dressing set
- Surgical mask
- Sterile gloves
- Micropore 1
- Non-sterile receiver.

Requirements

1. A strict aseptic technique should be maintained throughout the procedure in accordance with the policy and procedure of aseptic.
2. The dressing must be done by physician or a CAPD trained nurse
3. Culture and sensitivity swab should be taken, if there is any signs of infection, the physician should be informed.
4. If there is no bleeding from the wound site, dressing is left for 5 days.
5. Handwashing should be performed according to policy and procedure on handwashing.
6. The patient must rest in bed for 2 days, after insertion of the tube, as early mobility causes leakage.
7. The weight of the patient is to be checked daily to detect edema.
8. The bowel action of the patient is monitored daily as constipation causes pain and drainage problems.
9. The wound is inspected by the physician on the 5th postoperative day, unless there is bleeding or signs of infection.
10. Once Mepore is removed, it should be checked for any stains of discharge, note the color.
11. The catheter exit site is observed for discharge, bleeding or over granulation of tissue if present, culture swabs are taken for culture and sensitivity. The physician should be informed for further management.
12. Stitches at the incision site are removed on the 7th postoperative day.

Postoperative Care

Dressing of Incision Site

Refer to aseptic technique.

Dressing at Exit Site (Catheter Site)

1. Check the old dressing for any discharge, note the color.
2. Observe the exit site for discharge. Bleeding of over granulation of tissue, if present take swab for culture and sensitivity, inform the physician.
3. Clean the area around the catheter site in one direction with one swab and then discard swab into non-sterile receiver.
4. Wrap Betadine-soaked gauze around the tubing at the exit site and leave it for 3 minutes.
5. Clean the catheter from bottom to top with Betadine.
6. Discard the gauze around the tubing after 3 minutes.
7. Dry the catheter with sterile dry gauze and also exit site.
8. Clean abdominal area around exit site with Betadine antiseptic and dry the area with sterile gauze.

9. Place the catheter upward toward sternum and place sterile Mepore over the exit site.
10. Secure the catheter over the abdomen with Micropore.

Advice on Discharge

1. When the incision has healed and the exit site is clean and dry, the patient is advised to clean around the catheter with soap, while bathing.
2. Immediately after bath, the patient has to dry the area gently and clean with Betadine and apply the Mepore.
3. Check daily for discharge and tissue granulation.
4. The patient is advised to see the physician if, any symptoms of infection are noticed, e.g. redness, discharge and/or any leakage.

CONTINUOUS VENOUS HEMOFILTRATION WITH HEMODIALYSIS

Purposes

- To remove large molecular weight substances
- To facilitate intravenous feeding, total parenteral nutrition (TPN)
- To administer medication and fluid (intravenous).

Equipment

- Blood (artery venous)
- Hemofilter
- Drainage tube with graduated bag
- Sterile gloves
- Surgical spirit
- Betadine
- Heparinized saline (5,000 IU in 500 mL)
- Micropore tape
- Drip stand
- Normal saline: 5
- Sterile bottles
- Line clamps: 3
- Hemodialysis on and pack.

Requirements

1. The procedure is performed:
    - When hemodialysis is contraindicated

- For patient who are hypercatabolic
- For patient who need large amount of fluids to be removed.

2. The procedure should be performed by two nurses one of whom is an experienced senior nurse.
3. A strict aseptic technique should be maintained throughout the procedure on handwashing.
4. Handwashing should be performed according to policy and procedure on handwashing.
5. Written consent must be obtained prior to the procedure.
6. Clotting screen, if hemodialysis is available in the unit, clotting time is checked 2 hourly, otherwise it is checked 4–6 hourly by the laboratory.
7. Replacement fluid:
   - One hemofiltration (HF): 12
   - Two HF: 25
   - 31 intermittent peritoneal dialysis (IPD) solution (when HF is not available).
8. Syringe pump.
9. Imed volumetric pump (Gemini).
10. Sterile gauze.

Heparin Regime

1. If hyalinization is contraindicated, add injection heparin 500 IU in 500 mL normal saline and use it for priming the lines as well as the hemofilter.
2. Flush the extracorporeal circuit with a small amount of saline during the treatment however, this additional fluid has to be taken into consideration when totaling the balance at the end of 34 hours, e.g. if fluid is removed at the rate of 1,000 mL/h and infused at the rate of 900 mL/h, then the balance will be about 2,400 mL after 24 hours. If saline is given 2 hourly approximately 100 mL then replace only 800 mL. A target loss is achieved at the end of 24 hours.
3. If the patient is on heparin free during the procedure with a saline flushed of 100 mL hourly. Replacement should be 900 mL of HF 12 (hemofiltration solution) fluid at the end of 24 hours. The target loss of 2,400 mL is achieved.
4. If heparin is ordered, initially give four loading doses and follow with an hourly dose through the syringe pump. The physician prescribes the heparin dose.

Chapter 14 Stress and Adaptation

Stress is an universal phenomenon, all people experience it. Parents refer to the stress of missing children, working people talk of the stress of their jobs and at school level talk is about stress of students. The concept of stress is important because it provides a way of understanding the person as unified being, who responds in totality (mind, body and spirit) to a variety of changes that take place in daily life.

CONCEPT OF STRESS

Stress can have physical, emotional, intellectual, social and spiritual consequences. Usually, the effect are mixed because stress affects the whole person, physically stress can threaten a person's physiologic homeostasis. Emotionally, stress can produce negative or non-constructive feelings about self. Intellectually, stress can influence a person's perceptual and problem-solving abilities. Socially, stress can alter a person's relationship with others. Spiritually, stress can challenge one's beliefs and values. Many illnesses have been linked to stress.

DEFINITION

Stress is defined in a number of ways:

- Stress as a stimulus
- Stress as a response
- Stress as a transaction.

Stress as a Stimulus

Stress may be defined as a stimulus of life event (something called 'life change') or set of circumstances causing a disrupted response that increase the individual's vulnerability to illness. Both positive and negative events are considered stressful. Research has shown that people who have a high level of stress are often more prone to illness and have lowered ability to cope with illness and subsequent stress.

Stress as a Response

Hans Selye defined stress as "the specific response of the body to any kind of demand made upon it." To differentiate the cause of stress from the response of stress, the term stressor to denote any factor that produces stress and disturbs the body's equilibrium. Since stress is a state of the body, it can be observed only by the changes, which are produced in the body.

General Adaptation Syndrome

Stress syndrome or general adaptation syndrome (GAS) is the response of the body that occurs with the release of certain adaptive hormones and subsequent changes in the structure and chemical composition of the body.

Local Adaptation Syndrome

In addition to adapting globally, the body can also react locally that may be an organ or a part of the body reacts alone. This is referred to as the local adaptation syndrome (LAS), e.g. inflammation.

Stages of General and Local Adaptation Syndrome

General adaptation syndrome and LAS has three stages:

- Alarm reaction
- Resistance
- Exhaustion.

Alarm reaction: The initial reaction of the body is the alarm reaction (AR), which alerts the body's defenses against the stress; Selye divided this stage into two parts:

- Shock phase
- Counter shock phase.

During the shock phase, the autonomic nervous system (ANS) reacts. The person is then ready for 'fight or flight.' The second part of the alarm reaction is called counter shock phase. During this time, the changes produced in the body during the shock phase are reversed.

Stages of resistance: It is during the second stage in the GAS and LAS syndromes that the stage of resistance (SR), the body's adaptation takes place, in other words, the body attempts to cope with the stressor and to limit the stressor to the smallest area of the body that can deal with it.

Stages of exhaustion: During the third stage, the adaptation that is the body made during the second stage cannot be maintained. This means that the ways used to cope with the stressor have been exhausted.

MANIFESTATION OF STRESS

Manifestation of the stress experiences both physiological and psychological, may be considered as coping strategies or mechanisms. Coping is 'the cognitive and behavioral effort to manage specific external and/or internal demands that are appraised as taxing or exceeding the resources of the person.' Coping can be adaptive or maladaptive. Adaptive coping helps the person to deal effectively with stressful events and minimize stress. Ineffective coping results in maladaptation.

Physiological Manifestation

Physiological manifestations may or may not occur in clients experiencing stress, depending on the way the client perceives the stressful event and on the effectiveness of the client's coping strategies. Specific physiological manifestations are:

- Pupils dilate to increase visual perception
- Sweat production (diaphoresis)
- The heartbeat increases, which leads to an increased pulse rate to transport nutrients
- Skin is palled because of constriction of peripheral blood vessels, an effect of norepinephrine
- Blood pressure (BP) increases because of constriction of vessels in blood reservoirs
- The rate and depth of respirations increase because of dilation of the bronchioles, promoting hyperventilation
- Urinary output decreases
- Mouth may be dry
- Peristalsis of the intestine decreases, resulting in possible constipation and flatus
- Muscle tension increases to prepare for rapid motor activity or defense
- Blood sugar increases because of release of glucocorticoids and gluconeogenesis
- Lethargy, mental lassitude and inactivity
- There may be decreased physiologic functioning and loss of skeletal muscle tone (parasympathetic dominance).

Psychological Manifestation

Psychological manifestations of stress include anxiety, fear, anger, depression, cognitive behaviors, verbal and motor responses, and unconscious ego defense mechanisms.

Cognitive Manifestations

Cognitive manifestations of stress are thinking responses that include problem solving, structuring, self-control or self-discipline, suppression, fantasy and prayer. The person assesses the situation or problem, analyses or defines it, chooses alternatives, carries out the selected alternative and evaluates whether the solution was successful.

Verbal and Motor Manifestations

Verbal or motor manifestations of stress may be the first responses evident. These responses are crying, verbal abuse, laughing, screaming, hitting and kicking, and holding and touching.

NURSING MANAGEMENT OF STRESS

Assessment

Determine on a scale of 1–10, how would the client rate the stress? He/She is experiencing in the following areas:

- Home
- Work or school
- Finance
- Recent illness or loss of loved one
- Family responsibilities
- Ethnic or cultural group
- Religion
- Relationships with parents or children
- Relationship with partner
- Recent hospitalization
- How long has the client been dealing with the above stressor(s)?
- How does the client usually handle stressful situations?
  - Cry
  - Get angry
  - Become verbally abusive
  - Talk to someone (who)
  - Withdraw from the situation
  - Go for walk or physical exercise
  - Try to arrive at a solution
  - Pray for wisdom and courage
  - Laugh, joke or use some other relaxation techniques such as yoga guided imagery, etc.
- How does the client performs usual coping strategy work?

  Assess clinical manifestations indicating stress:
- Physiologic manifestations:
  - Restlessness
  - Pacing
  - Tremors
  - Muscle tension
  - Rigid posture
  - Purposeless activity
  - Rapid pulse
  - Increased respiratory rate
  - Hyperventilation

- Heart palpitations
- Diaphoresis
- Pallor
- Clammy hands
- Dry mouth.

- Perceptual change:
  - Increased awareness and attended or narrowed focus of attention
  - Inability to focus on, what is really happening?
- Verbalization changes:
  - Increased questioning or information seeking
  - Seeking help
  - Expressions of concern
  - Feeling of tension
  - Apprehension
  - Nervousness
  - Voice tremors and pitch changes
  - Anger.

Nursing Diagnosis

- Anxiety related to perceived threat to self-concept, health status and socioeconomic status
- Ineffective individual coping related to situational crises such as natural disasters or loss of loved ones through separation
- Fear related to anticipated treatment (e.g. surgery and chemotherapy) or language barrier
- Defensive coping
- Ineffective family coping disabling
- Decisional conflict related to conflict with personal values/beliefs or an ethical dilemma.

Planning

The nurse develops plans in collaboration with the client and significant support of persons, when possible. According to the client's state of health, the nurse and client set goals to change the existing client responses to the stressor(s). The overall client goals for persons experiencing stress related responses are:

- Decrease anxiety and fear
- Increase the ability to manage, cope with stressful events or circumstances.

Suggested Outcome Criteria

The client:

- Verbalize a reduced level of anxiety
- Develops realistic goals
- Expresses feelings in a positive way
- Verbalizes feelings to another
- Develops effective coping mechanisms in managing stress.

Implementation

Although stress accompanies every disease and illness, it is also highly individualized; a situation that to one person is a major stressor, may not affect another. Some methods help to reduce stress will be effective for one person, other methods will be appropriate for a different person. A nurse who is sensitive to client's needs and reactions can choose methods of intervention that will be most effective for each individual.

Minimizing Anxiety

Clients must first recognize that they are anxious. After clients realize that they are anxious, it is important to discuss all the possible reasons for their anxiety. When clients can identify the cause of their anxiety, they may find it helpful to explore the cause with the objective of learning better coping strategies. General guidelines to minimize the client's anxiety and stress are:

1. Support the client and family at the time of illness, by conveying caring and understanding, the nurse can help clients reduce their stress. Feeling that someone else cares is a source of support to stressed people.
2. Orient the client to the hospital or agency; the nurse helps the clients adjust to the role change from independent wage earner to relatively dependent client. The nurse can help family members by giving information for instance, about visiting hours and specific unit policies.
3. Maintain identity, nurses can identify clients by addressing them by the name as they prefer and by assisting them to wear their own clothes in hospital setting, when it is possible.
4. Provide information when the client has insufficient information. Fear of unknown and incorrect information can frequently cause stress. Additional information or clarification can ally stress.
5. Repeat information when the client has difficulty remembering. Nurses can assist client by repeating information, when it is requested/required.
6. Encourage the client to participate in the plan of care. Loss of right to determine their own destiny can be very stressful to some people.
7. Give the client time to express feelings and thoughts, allow time for clients to describe their feelings and worries, if they wish.

8. Ensure that expectations are within the clients capabilities; whatever the activity, whether an exercise or recreation, the nurse should make sure that it is possible for the client to accomplish it.
9. Be sensitive to specific situations and experiences that increase anxiety and stress for clients.
10. Assist a client to make a correct appraisal of a situation, sometimes through a lack of knowledge, people draw incorrect conclusions, having valid information nurse might relieve the client's stress.
11. Provide an environment in which a person can function independently to some degree without assistance.
12. Reinforce positive environmental factors and recognize negative ones to help reduce stress.
13. Arrange for other clients with similar experiences to visit the clients, e.g. colostomies or similar condition.
14. Bring clients and their support persons into contact with people in community with competence, understanding and empathy rather than stress and anxiety.
15. Communicate with competence, understanding and empathy rather than stress and anxiety.

Evaluation

To evaluate the achievement of client goals, the nurse collects data in accordance with the outcome criteria established earlier. Examples of evaluative statements indicating goal achievement are as follows:

- The client identified four personal strengths for coping with stressful events
- The client verbalized the ability to channel feelings of anger into assertive behaviors and exercise.

Chapter 15 Defense Against Injury

PHYSICAL BARRIERS AND THE IMMUNE SYSTEM

Physical barriers and the immune system defend the body against organisms that can cause infection. Physical barriers includes the skin, mucous membranes, tears, earwax, mucus and stomach acid. Also, the normal flow of urine washes out microorganisms that enter the urinary tract. The immune system uses white blood cells (WBCs), antibodies to identify and eliminate organisms that get through the body's physical barriers.

Physical Barriers

Usually, the skin prevents invasion by microorganisms unless it is damaged, e.g. by an injury, insect bite or burn. Other effective physical barriers are the mucous membranes such as the linings of the mouth, nose and eyelids. Typically, mucous membranes are coated with secretions that fight microorganisms. For example, the mucous membranes of the eyes are bathed in tears, which contain an enzyme called lysozyme that attacks bacteria and helps to protect the eyes from infection.

The airways filter out solid particles that are present in the air before breathed in. The walls of the passages in the nose and airways are coated with mucus. Microorganisms in the air become stuck to the mucus, which is coughed up or blown out of the nose. Mucus removal is aided by the coordinated beating of tiny hair-like projections (cilia) that line the airways. The cilia sweep the mucus up the airways, away from the lungs.

The digestive tract has a series of effective barriers including stomach acid, pancreatic enzymes, bile and intestinal secretions. The contractions of the intestine (peristalsis) and the normal shedding of cells lining the intestine help to remove harmful microorganisms.

The bladder is protected by the urethra, the tube that drains urine from the body. In males older than 6 months, the urethra is long enough that bacteria are seldom able to pass through it to reach the bladder, unless the bacteria are unintentionally placed there by catheters or surgical instruments. In females, the urethra is shorter, occasionally allowing external bacteria to pass into the bladder. The flushing effect as the bladder empties is another defense mechanism in both sexes. The vagina is protected by its normal acidic environment.

Blood

One way the body defends against infection is by increasing the number of certain types of WBCs (neutrophils and monocytes), which engulf and destroy invading microorganisms. The increase can occur within several hours, largely because WBCs are released from the bone marrow, where they are made. The number of neutrophils increases first. If an infection persists, the number of monocytes increases. The blood carries WBCs to sites of infection. The number of eosinophils, another type of WBC, increases in allergic reactions and many parasitic infections, but usually not in bacterial infections. Certain infections such as typhoid fever, actually lead to a decrease in the WBC count. How these infections cause the decrease of WBCs is not known.

Inflammation

Any injury including an invasion by microorganisms, causes inflammation in the affected area. Inflammation, a complex reaction, results from many different conditions. Through the release of different substances from the damaged tissue, inflammation directs the body's defenses to do the following:

- Wall off the area
- Attack and kill any invaders
- Dispose of dead and damaged tissue
- Begin the process of repair.

However, inflammation may not be able to overcome large numbers of microorganisms. During inflammation, the blood supply increases. An infected area near the surface of the body becomes red and warm. The walls of blood vessels become more porous, allowing fluid and WBCs to pass into the affected tissue. The increase in fluid causes the inflamed tissue to swell. The WBCs attack the invading microorganisms and release substances that continue the process of inflammation. Other substances trigger clotting in the tiny vessels (capillaries) in the inflamed area, which delays the spread of the infecting microorganisms and their toxins. Many of the substances produced during inflammation stimulate the nerves, causing pain. Reactions to the substances released during inflammation include the chills, fever and muscle aches that commonly accompany infection.

Immune Response

When an infection develops, the immune system responds by producing several substances and agents that are designed to attack the specific invading microorganisms. For example, the immune system may create killer T cells, a type of WBC, which can recognize and kill the invading microorganism. Also, the immune system produces antibodies that are specific to the invading microorganism. Antibodies attach to the immobilize microorganisms, killing them outright or helping the neutrophils target and kill them.

Fever

Body temperature increases as a protective response to infection and injury. The elevated body temperature (fever) enhances the body's defense mechanisms, although it can cause discomfort. However, certain people (such as alcoholics, the very old and the very young) may experience a drop in temperature in response to severe infection because fever helps the body defend against infection and fever itself is not dangerous [unless it is higher than about 106°F (41.1°C)], there is some debate as to whether fever should be routinely treated. However, people with a high fever generally feel much better when the fever is treated.

Microorganisms are tiny living creatures, such as bacteria and viruses. Microorganisms are present everywhere. Despite their overwhelming abundance, relatively few of the thousands of species of microorganisms invade, multiply and cause disease in people. Many microorganisms live on the skin and in the mouth, upper airways, intestine and genitals (particularly the vagina) without causing disease. Whether a microorganism lives as a harmless companion to a person or invades and causes disease depends on the nature of the microorganism and on the state of the person's natural defense.

Chapter 16

Fluid, Electrolyte and Acid-base Balance

Fluid and electrolytes are necessary to maintain good health and their relative amounts in the body must be maintained within a narrow range. The balance of fluid and electrolytes in the body is a part of physiologic homeostasis.

BODY FLUID DISTRIBUTION

The body's fluid is divided into two major reservoirs, intracellular and extracellular:

- The intracellular fluid (ICF) also referred to as the cellular fluid, is found within the cell of the body
- It constitutes two thirds to three quarters of total body fluid
- The extracellular fluid (ECF) is found outside the cells
- It is subdivided into two components:
  - Intravascular (plasma)
  - Interstitial.
- Plasma is a fluid, found within the vascular system
- Interstitial fluid is the fluid that surrounds the cells and it includes lymph, which the transparent slightly yellow fluid found within the lymphatic vessels
- Extracellular fluids constitute one third to one fourth of the total body fluids
- Normal body fluids functioning require that the volume of each fluid compartment remains relatively constant
- Total body fluid represents 40 L in an adult male weighing 70 kg.

Proportions

1. The proportion of fluid in the human body varies with age (Table 16.1), body fat and sex.

Table 16.1: Fluid percentage of body weight by age

Developmental stage	Percentage of water (approximate)
Newborn infant	75%
Adult male	57%
Adult female	55%
Elderly adult	55%

Note: As age increases, the proportion of body water decreases

2. As age increases, the proportion of body water decreases. For example, whereas 77% of a body weight is fluid, only 55% of an adult female's body weight is fluid.
3. Body fat is essentially free of fluid. The amount of fat substantially alters the total volume of fluid in proportion to a person's weight.

Composition

All body fluids contain important substances such as:

- Salts
- Oxygen from the lungs
- Dissolved nutrients (glucose, fatty acids and amino acids) from the digestive tract
- Waste products of metabolism (e.g. carbon dioxide).

The salts in solution break into one or more electrically charged particles called ions or electrolytes. For example, sodium chloride (NaCl) breaks into one ion of sodium (Na^+) and one ion of chloride (Cl^-). Ions that carry a positive charge are called cation and those carrying negative charge are called anion. Examples are given in Table 16.2.

In a solution, positive and negative ions are attracted to one another until a balance is attained. For example, the electrolyte composition of the fluid compartments varies from one to another (the principal ions of the extracellular compartment are Na^+ and Cl^-, while the principal ions of the intracellular compartment are potassium and phosphate).

Just as the fluid volumes within the compartments, electrolyte composition of the various compartments must be maintained. Although, the specific numbers of cations and anions may differ in the fluid compartments. In a state of homeostasis, the total number of cations equals to the total number of anions within each compartment.

Sources of Fluid and Electrolyte

The healthy person obtains fluid and electrolytes from these major sources (Tables 16.3 and 16.4):

- Solid foods account for about half of the fluid requirement of the average adult (750 mL)
- The water content of fresh vegetables is approximately 90% and of fresh fruits about 85%
- Electrolytes are also found in foods
- Ingested fluids such as water and juices, account for most of the other half of the fluid

Table 16.2: Cations and anions

Cation	Anion
Sodium (Na^+)	Chloride (Cl^-)
Potassium (K^+)	Bicarbonate (HCO_3)
Calcium (Ca^{2+})	Phosphate (PO^{3-}_4)
Magnesium (Mg^{2+})	Sulfate (SO^{2-}_4)

Table 16.3: Major sources of selected electrolytes

Electrolytes	Sources
Sodium (Na)	Table salt, cheese, ham, processed meats, canned foods and fish
Potassium (K)	Dark leaf greens, bananas, oranges, nuts, meat, fish and liver
Calcium (Ca)	Milk, cheese and yoghurt
Magnesium (Mg)	Nuts, peanut, butter and whole grains
Phosphorus (P)	Milk, poultry, fish and cereals

Table 16.4: Sources of adult average daily fluid intake

Sources	Amount	Ratio
Water consumed as a fluids	1,500 mL	4
Water present in food	750 mL	2
Water produced by oxidation	350 mL	1
Total	2,600 mL	7

- Oxidation of food within the body also produces water; oxidation is a chemical process by which a substance combines with oxygen, energy is released and other substances.
- The ill person who cannot ingest food, may receive fluids through unusual routes that are:
  - Intravenous fluids
  - Nasogastric tube feeding
  - Gastrostomy/Jejunostomy feeding.
- Age-specific fluid-intake requirements include:
  - Newborn: 80–100 mL/kg/24 h
  - Infant: 120–130 mL/kg/24 h
  - Age 2 years: 115–125 mL/kg/24 h
  - Age 6 years: 90–100 mL/kg/24 h
  - Age 15 years: 70–85 mL/kg/24 h
  - Age 18 years: 40–50 mL/kg/24 h.

Fluid and electrolyte disturbances (e.g. diarrhea, vomiting and fever) occur more frequently and develop more rapidly in infants and young children than in older children and adults.

Infants and young children are more vulnerable to alterations in fluid and electrolyte balance due to:

- A relatively larger percentage of fluid volume as a percentage of body weight
- A greater body surface area in proportion to body mass
- Higher metabolic rates, which increase the body's fluid demands
- Immature kidney function.

Disturbances in Fluid and Electrolytes Balances

Fluid Imbalances

1. Fluid imbalance occurs, when the body's compensatory mechanisms are unable to maintain homeostatic state.
2. Fluid imbalance may relate to either volume or distribution of water or electrolytes.
3. Fluid volume deficit (FVD) is a deficiency in the amount of both water and electrolytes in ECF, but the water and electrolytes proportions remain near normal. The state is commonly known as hypovolemia (Box 16.1).
4. The FVDs result from the loss of body fluids, especially if fluid intake is simultaneously decreased.
5. Fluid volume excess (FVE) is excessive retention of water and sodium in ECF in near normal proportions. It is also called overhydration, refers only to above normal amounts of water in extracellular spaces (Box 16.2).
6. Malfunction of kidneys causing an inability to excrete the excess amount of urine, is the most common cause.
7. The excessive ECF may accumulate in tissue spaces is known as edema.
8. Edema is most frequently seen around the eyes, finger, ankles and sacral space.
9. It may result in a weight gain in excess of 5%.

Box 16.1: Clinical signs of fluid volume deficit

Observation
• Postural hypotension • Weight loss • Dryness of mucous membranes • Decreased tissue turgor • Weak, thready, rapid pulse • Sunken eye balls • Oliguria, i.e. urine output < 30 mL/h • Pale skin
Laboratory findings
• Increased specific gravity of urine • Elevated hematocrit • Decreased central venous pressure

Box 16.2: Clinical signs of fluid volume excess

Observation
• Peripheral edema (face, hands, feet or dependent areas) • Weight gain: – Mild: 2% in an adult – Moderate: 5% in an adult – Severe: 8% in an adult • Distended neck veins when sitting at 45° • Moist crackles in lungs • Distended peripheral veins • Ascites • Bounding full pulse
Laboratory findings
• Decreased hematocrit due to plasma dilution • Decreased blood urea nitrogen (BUN) due to plasma dilution

Acid-base Disturbances

Acid-base imbalances are common complications of diarrhea, vomiting and febrile conditions in infants and young children, as well as possible complications of respiratory, endocrine, renal and metabolic disorders.

Acid-base disturbances (Table 16.5) include acidosis, resulting from either accumulation of acid or loss of base and alkalosis; resulting from either accumulation of base or loss of acid.

Respiratory acidosis: Results from diminished or inadequate pulmonary ventilation, leading to an elevated practical pressure of carbon dioxide (pCO_2) level and a decreased plasma pH.

Metabolic acidosis: Results from a gain of non-volatile acids or the loss of base and leads to decreased plasma pH and decreased plasma bicarbonate (HCO_3) concentration.

Respiratory alkalosis: It results from an increase in the rate and depth of pulmonary ventilation leading to a decreased pCO_2 level and an elevated plasma pH.

Metabolic alkalosis: It is produced by a gain in base or loss of acid, results in elevated urine pH, elevated plasma pH and elevated plasma HCO_3 concentration.

Compensatory mechanisms refer to the body to attempt the correct acid-base imbalance through compensatory changes in the component of the acid-base equilibrium, which is not primarily affected.

Interventions that can sustain a child with an acid-base imbalance until the primary disorder has resolved includes:

- Providing adequate hydration
- Replacing electrolytes
- Correcting the acid-base imbalance.

FLUID IMBALANCE: DEHYDRATION

Description

Excessive loss of fluid from body tissues that exceeds the total intake.

Table 16.5: Acid-base disturbances

Disturbance	Initial metabolic change	Effect on blood pH	Compensatory reaction
Metabolic alkalosis	Decreased HCO_3* Increased HCO_3	Increased	Increased pCO_2†
Metabolic acidosis	Decreased HCO_3	Decreased	Decreased pCO_2
Respiratory alkalosis	Decreased pCO_2	Increase	Decreased HCO_3
Respiratory acidosis	Increased pCO_2	Decreased	Increased HCO_3

*HCO_3, bicarbonate; †pCO_2, pressure of carbon dioxide.

Etiology

1. Dehydration most commonly results from abnormal fluid losses such as excessive vomiting or diarrhea.

2. Other possible causes include insufficient fluid intake, diabetic ketoacidosis, severe burns, prolonged high fever and hyperventilation.

Pathophysiology

Depending on the cause and nature of fluid loss, a client will lose water and various electrolytes. Dehydration is classified as isotonic, hypertonic or hypotonic.

Isotonic Dehydration

- In isotonic dehydration, electrolyte and water deficits occur in approximately balanced proportions
- This is the most common type, accounting for about 70% of dehydration cases linked to diarrhea in infants
- The major loss involves extracellular components and circulating blood volume, making the child susceptible to hypovolemic shock
- Serum Na^+ is decreased or within the normal range; Cl^- is decreased; and potassium (K^+) is normal to increased
- Deficits should be corrected over a 24-hour period.

Hypertonic Dehydration

- In hypertonic dehydration, water loss exceeds electrolyte loss
- This type accounts for about 20% of cases, resulting from severe diarrhea in infants
- It results in fluid shifts from the intracellular compartment to the extracellular compartment, which can lead to neurological disturbances such as seizures
- The Na^+ is increased, K^+ varied and Cl^- increased.

Hypotonic Dehydration

- In hypotonic dehydration, electrolyte deficit exceeds water deficit
- It may be caused by excessive perspiration, severe diarrhea or administration of oral/intravenous (IV) fluids without electrolytes added; it accounts for 10% of cases in infants resulting from severe diarrhea
- In response to hypotonic dehydration, water shifts from osmotic equilibrium, which further increases ECF loss and commonly results in hypovolemic shock
- Here Na^+ is decreased, Cl^- is decreased and K^+ variable
- Volume and Na^+ should be replaced within 24–36 hours
- The degree of dehydration can be estimated by comparing the child's current weight with his/her preillness body weight
- Dehydration can be classified by severity:

- Mild: Loss of up to 5% of preillness body weight
- Moderate: Loss of up to 10% of preillness body weight
- Severe: Loss of up to 15% of preillness body weight.

Assessment Findings

Common clinical manifestations include:

- Weight loss
- Dry mucous membranes
- Decreased tear production
- Poor skin turgor
- Sunken eyeballs
- Depressed fontanels (in infants)
- Decreased urine output
- Tachycardia
- Tachypnea
- Decreased blood pressure
- Excessive thirst.

Laboratory study results may reveal:

- Concentrated urine with high specific gravity (> 1.03) and high osmolarity
- Elevated hematocrit
- Elevated blood urea nitrogen (BUN)
- Decreased urine sodium concentration
- Altered serum electrolyte values (Na^+, K^+ and Cl^-)
- Low serum pH, if the child is acidotic.

Nursing Diagnosis

- Altered family processes
- Fluid volume deficit
- Hyperthermia
- High risk for infection
- Knowledge deficit
- Altered nutrition: Less than body requirements
- Impaired tissue integrity.

Planning and Implementation

1. Obtain an accurate initial weight and monitor for changes indicating fluid gains and losses. Evaluate the client health history, physical assessment findings and laboratory study results to help identify the underlying cause of dehydration.
2. Administer clear liquids orally, as ordered to correct fluid deficiency.

3. Offer oral fluids in small quantities (e.g. 1–2 oz every hour); withhold a full diet until the child is well-hydrated and the underlying problem is under control.
4. If the client is unable to ingest sufficient fluid orally, start an IV line and administer appropriate replacement solution, as ordered.
5. Monitor IV replacement therapy, checking the IV site frequently.
6. Instruct client an IV on positioning, moving and care.
7. Evaluate the hydration status by assessing for signs and symptoms of dehydration.
8. Monitor, record intake and output, and note urine specific gravity.
9. Help to maintain skin integrity by providing good hygiene and skin care turning frequently, changing damp or soiled linen as indicated, carefully washing and drying the diaper area with every change, using aseptic technique when inserting IV catheters, and monitoring the IV infusion site for signs of infiltration.
10. Prevent infection by maintaining good hygiene and handwashing, and instituting necessary isolation techniques appropriate to the cause of dehydration.
11. Reintroduce the client to a regular diet gradually, as ordered; monitor the child's response to diet changes by noting his/her ability to retain orally ingested food and fluids.
12. Provide support to the family and explain all tests and therapeutic measures.
13. Encourage family members to participate in the child's care as appropriate.
14. Provide patient and family teaching, covering diet and oral fluid instructions.
15. Causes of dehydration signs and symptoms of dehydration to watch for an report.
16. Handwashing and hygiene instructions as indicated.
17. Follow-up appointments.

Evaluation

1. The client displays no signs of dehydration and tolerates a regular diet.
2. The family verbalizes knowledge of home diet and fluid intake instructions, causes of dehydration, signs, and symptoms of dehydration, the importance of handwashing and good hygiene and scheduled follow-up appointments.

ELECTROLYTE IMBALANCE

1. **Sodium (Na):** Hyponatremia and hypernatremia (Table 16.6).
2. **Potassium (K):** Hypokalemia and hyperkalemia (Box 16.3).
3. **Calcium (Ca):** Hypocalcemia and hypercalcemia (Tables 16.7 and 16.8).

Table 16.6: Disturbances in sodium balance

Risk factors	Clinical signs	Nursing intervention
Hyponatremia		
• Excessive loss of sodium through gastrointestinal fluids (e.g. diarrhea, sweating, use of diuretics) • Excessive gain of water through hypotonic tube feeding and drinking water • Conditions such as head injury and stroke	• Feeling of apprehension and lethargy • Muscle cramps • Anorexia, nausea and vomiting • Postural hypotension • Seizures, coma *Laboratory findings* • Serum sodium below 135 mEq/L	• Monitor fluid intake and output • Assess clinical signs • Monitor laboratory data (e.g. serum sodium) • Encourage food and fluid high in sodium, if permitted (e.g. table salt, bacon, ham, processed cheese) • Assess client closely, if administering hypertonic saline solution
Hypernatremia		
• Excessive losses of fluid through insensible water loss through hyperventilation diarrhea • Deprivation of water • Excessive salt intake through parental administration of sodium, hypertonic tube feeding without adequate water • Condition such as diabetes insipidus, heat stroke, excessive use of table salt (1 table spoon contains 2,300 mg of sodium)	• Extreme thirst • Dry, sticky mucous membranes, tongue red, dry, swollen • Severe hypernatremia • Agitated behavior, fatigue, • Restlessness • Disorientation • Hallucinations *Laboratory findings* • Serum sodium above 145 mE/L	• Monitor fluid intake • Monitor behavior changes (e.g. restlessness, disorientation) • Monitor laboratory findings (e.g. serum sodium) • Encourage fluids as ordered • Monitor diet as ordered (e.g. restrict intake of salt and foods high in sodium)

Box 16.3: Potassium rich foods

- Vegetables: Baked potato, raw carrot and tomato
- Fruits: Dried fruits, raisins, dates, bananas, apricots, cantaloupe, orange and apple
- Beverages: Milk, orange juice, apricot nectar and tender coconut
- Others: Chocolate, poultry and honey

Sodium

- Normal serum sodium ranges from 135 mEq/L and is the most abundant cation (positively charged) electrolytes in the ECF
- Normal sodium concentrations in the ECF are regulated by antidiuretic hormone (ADH) and aldosterone.

Table 16.7: Disturbances in potassium balance

Risk factors	Clinical signs	Nursing intervention
Hypokalemia		
Excessive loss of potassium through: • Vomiting and gastric suction, urine diarrhea, heavy perspiration • Poor intake of potassium (as with debilitated clients, alcoholics, anorexia nervosa)	• Muscle weakness, leg cramps, fatigue, anorexia, nausea, vomiting • Decreased bowel sounds and motility • Cardiac arrhythmias • Depressed deep tendon reflexes *Laboratory findings* Serum potassium below 3.5 mEq/L	• Monitor clients receiving digitalis closely, because hypokalemia enhances digitalis toxicity • Administer oral potassium as ordered with food or fluid to prevent gastric irritation • Monitor heart rate and rhythm • Teach client about potassium rich foods • Closely monitor clients receiving intravenous potassium • Teach client how to prevent excessive loss of potassium (e.g. rough abuse of diuretics and laxatives)
Hyperkalemia		
• Decreased loss of potassium through the kidneys due to renal failure, hypoaldosteronism; intake of potassium conserving diuretics • High potassium intake through excessive use of potassium containing salt substitute • Excessive or rapid IV potassium • Conditions in which potassium moves out of the tissue cells into the plasma (e.g. infections and burns)	• Gastrointestinal hyperactivity, diarrhea, irritability, apathy, confusion, cardiac arrhythmia, bradycardia, cardiac arrest, muscle weakness, areflexia (absence of reflexes) • Parethesia and numbness in extremities *Laboratory findings* Serum potassium above 5.0 mE/L electrocardiogram (ECG) abnormalities	• Closely monitor clients receiving diuretics; before administering intravenous potassium, determine serum potassium levels and follow protocol for administration carefully • Teach clients to avoid foods high in potassium • Draw blood specimens carefully to avoid false hyperkalemia • Do not take the specimen from a site near an intravenous (IV) insertion

- Aldosterone, a hormone produced by the adrenal cortex, acts to maintain sodium concentrations
- Sodium not only moves into and out of the body but also moves in careful balance among the three fluid compartments
- Sodium is found in most body secretions, e.g. saliva, gastric and intestinal secretion, bile and pancreatic fluids

Table 16.8: Disturbance in calcium balance

Risk factors	Clinical signs	Nursing intervention
Hypocalcemia		
• Condition such as hypoparathyroidism, acute pancreatitis, hyperphosphatemia, thyroid carcinoma • Inadequate intake of vitamin D • Excessive loss of intestinal secretions • Alcohol abuse	• Numbness, tingling of extremities and around the mouth • Muscle tremors, cramps, if severe can progress to tetany and convulsions • Cardiac arrhythmias, decreased stroke volume and ventricular contractions *Laboratory findings* Serum calcium < 4.0 mEq/L (total)	• Monitor the client's breathing closely, because of possible laryngeal stridor; take precautions to protect a confused client • Teach postmenopausal women about food sources • Calcium supplements as ordered • Value of regular exercise
Hypercalcemia		
• Prolonged immobilization • Condition such as hyperparathyroidism • Malignancy of the bone • Paget's disease	Flank pain secondary to urinary calculi lethargy, weakness, reduced muscle tone, anorexia, nausea, vomiting, depressed deep tendon reflexes, constipation polyuria, cardiac arrest may occur in hypercalcemia crisis *Laboratory findings* Serum calcium above 5.5 mEq/L (total)	• Increased client movement and exercise • Encourage oral fluids as permitted to maintain dilute urine • Teach clients to limit intake of food and fluid high in calcium • Encourage ingestion of fiber to prevent constipation • Protect a confused client • Encourage intake of acid ash fluids, e.g. prune or cranberry juice • To counter act deposited calcium salts in the urine • A urinary pH of > 6.5 predisposes to calcium deposits

- Continuous excretion of any of these fluids via intestinal suction can result in a sodium deficit
- Sodium ions function largely in the control and regulation of the body fluid (i.e. water balance)
- With potassium, sodium helps to maintain the electrolyte balance of ICF and ECF
- Sodium is also involved in transmitting nerve impulses and contracting muscles.

Hyponatremia

- Hyponatremia is a sodium deficit in the blood plasma
- It causes water to move out of the vascular space into the interstitial space and then into the intracellular space
- Water retention in the brain cell accounts for many of the clinical signs of hyponatremia (e.g. confusion)
- A sign of hyponatremia is pitting edema over the bony prominence such as the ankles
- Cells swell as water is pulled from ECF, whereas cells shrink when water is pulled out into ECF.

Hypernatremia

- Hypernatremia is excess sodium in the blood plasma
- Because of the increased extracellular osmotic pressure, fluid moves out of the cells into the ECF
- As a result, the cells have insufficient fluid and become dehydrated.

Potassium

- Potassium is the major cation in ICF
- The normal adult serum potassium range 3.5–5.0 mEq/L
- Potassium balance is regulated by the kidneys
- Potassium affects the function of most body systems, including:
  - Cardiovascular system
  - Gastrointestinal system
  - Neuromuscular system
  - Respiratory system.
- Potassium plays a role in the acid balance of the body
- It transmits electrical impulses to the heart and other muscles, to lung tissues and to intestinal tissues
- Most of the body's potassium found inside the cells, a small amount is found in the plasma and interstitial fluids
- Potassium is usually excreted by the kidneys
- It is found in many fruits and vegetables regularly.

Hypokalemia

- Hypokalemia is the condition potassium deficit in the blood plasma
- It can develop quickly in people who are starving
- The combined effects of inadequate potassium intake and excessive potassium loss due to prolonged diarrhea can deplete potassium stores acutely

- A common cause of hypokalemia is the use of potassium wasting diuretics such as thiazide diuretics.

Calcium

- The normal total serum calcium in an adult is 4.5–5.5 mEq/L
- Calcium functions in:
  - Bone formation
  - Transmission of nerve impulses
  - Muscle contraction
  - Blood coagulation
  - Activation of certain enzymes such as pancreatic lipase and phospholipase.
- It is equivalent for vitamin absorption
- Only 1% of the body's calcium is found in ECF
- The richest sources of calcium are milk and milk products
- Calcium is excreted in urine, feces, bile, digestive secretions and sweat
- The concentration of the body calcium is controlled indirectly by the effect of the parathyroid hormone on bone reabsorption
- Calcitonin, another hormone, has an effect nearly opposite to that of the parathyroid hormone and it reduces the concentration of calcium ions in the blood.

Hypocalcemia

- Hypocalcemia is a calcium deficit in the blood plasma
- Severe depletion of calcium can cause tetany (muscle spasm and sharp flexion)
- The clients at risk for hypocalcemia include those who have hypomagnesemia (low-serum magnesium levels)
- Chronic alcohol abuse can cause hypocalcemia as a result of intestinal malabsorption of calcium and hypomagnesemia
- Many drugs also predispose to hypocalcemia, loop diuretics (furosemide) and anticonvulsants (phenytoin).

Hypercalcemia

Hypercalcemia is an excess of calcium in the blood plasma.

NURSING PROCESS: FLUID AND ELECTROLYTE IMBALANCE

Assessment

Assessment of clients with or at risk for developing fluid and electrolyte disturbance includes (Box 16.4):

Box 16.4: Assessment interview of fluid and electrolyte balance

Fluid and food intake
• What amount and type of fluids do you drink each day? • What type of food do you eat each day? *Note:* The nurse may focus on protein, sodium and potassium rich foods • Has there been any recent changes in food or fluid intake, e.g. as a result of taking part in a weight loss program? • Have you experienced any nausea, pain or loss of appetite that has altered your intake?
Fluid output
• Have you noticed any recent changes in the frequency or amount of urine output?
Fluid imbalance
• Are you losing body fluids in any major way, e.g. vomiting, diarrhea, excessive perspiration, other route? • Have you noticed any signs that indicate the body is experiencing too little hydration, e.g. excessive thirst, dry skin, dry mucous membranes, concentrated urine, reduced urine output? • Have you had any signs indicating that the body is experiencing too much hydration swollen ankles, difficulty in breathing and weight gain?
Electrolyte balance
• Have you noticed any of the following: Signs that indicate an electrolyte imbalance, loss of mental alertness, disorientation? • Faintness, muscle weakness, twitching, cramps, fatigue pain or spasm abnormal sensations such as burning, prickling, tingling, abdominal cramps or distention heart palpitations
Disease process
• Have you experienced any long term or recent disease processes that might disrupt fluid or electrolyte balance, such as kidney disease, heart disease, high blood pressure, diabetes insipidus, thyroid or parathyroid disorders, severe trauma or other chronic disease states (e.g. cancer colitis and ileitis)?
Medications
• Are you taking any of the following: Medications that could affect the fluid and electrolyte balance, diuretics, steroids, potassium supplements, salt substitute, antacids and aldosterone inhibitor agents
Treatments
• Have you recently had any treatments such as dialysis, total parenteral nutrition (TPN), tube drainages' (e.g. nasogastric or intestinal suction) or tube feeding

- Taking a nursing history
- Obtaining clinical measurements
- Assessing skin turgor and neuromuscular irritability
- Performing a physical examination

- Reviewing results of laboratory tests performed to evaluate fluid and electrolyte balance
- The nurse needs to elicit specific data about many aspects of the client's needs and functional health patterns
- Data must be obtained about the clients are following:
  - Fluid and food intake
  - Fluid output
  - Recent fluid loss
  - Signs of fluid deficit or excess
  - Common signs of electrolyte problems
  - Long term and recent disease processes
  - Medications and treatments that alter fluid and electrolyte balance.

Nursing Diagnosis

- High risk for fluid volume deficit, related to increased urinary, output frequency, thirst and altered intake
- Fluid volume deficit related to increased urine output greater than intake of fluid volume, excess related to compromised regulatory mechanisms, excess fluid and intake sodium
- Alteration in sodium balance (hyponatremia) related to excessive sodium loss and water gain
- Alteration in sodium balance (hypernatremia) related to inadequate water intake
- Alteration in potassium balance (hypokalemia) related to excessive potassium loss in diarrhea
- Alteration in potassium balance (hyperkalemia) related to decreased potassium excretion
- Alteration in calcium balance (hypocalcemia) related to inadequate vitamin D consumption and magnesium deficiency
- Alteration in calcium balance (hypercalcemia) related to immobilization.

Planning

Client Goals

Nursing care for any client supports the following client goals, the healthy adult client will:

- Maintain an approximate balance between fluid intake and fluid output
- Maintain a urine specific gravity within normal range (1.010–1.025)
- Practice self-care behavior to promote fluid, electrolyte and acid-base balance
- When an imbalance exists, the client will relate relief of symptoms (specify) after implementation of treatment regimen.

Implementation

Nursing interventions to prevent or correct fluid electrolyte and acid-base imbalances includes:

- Preventing fluid imbalance
- Modifying fluid intake
- Developing a dietary plan
- Administering medications
- Preparing electrolyte and mineral food
- Administering IV fluids as prescribed.

Preventing Fluid Imbalance

An adequate fluid intake and well-balanced nutritious diet with appropriate adjustments throughout the life cycle are basic essentials to promote fluid balance, the following are some of the basic items that the nurse needs to be consider for help and prevent the fluid imbalances:

1. Be familiar with common events in life that lead to fluid imbalances and observe the client carefully.
2. Note the client's present fluid and food intake, and learn what his/her previous eating and drinking patterns have been. Learn whether the client has used fad diets, which may lead to imbalances.

Modifying Fluid Intake

Simple dietary changes may help to resolve fluid and electrolyte disturbances. After doing a nutritional assessment to identify actual potential imbalances and food preferences, the nurse can initiate teaching.

Increasing fluids: The care plan should specify the amount of fluid to be ingested in 24 hours for hospitalized clients, shift totals are helpful (e.g. 7–3 for 1,200 mL, 3–11 for 900 mL, 11–7 for 300 mL) and the client's food preference. Fluids should be chosen that best provide the calories and electrolytes needed by the client.

Restricting fluids: A variety of technique is recommended to help the client who has a restricted fluid intake:

- Serve ice tube instead of water from time to time
- Use of small glasses or cups, so that the container appear to contain more fluid than it actually does
- Avoid offering the client salty or sweet foods and fluids, because they tend to increase thirst.

Developing a Dietary Plan

Simple dietary changes may help to resolve fluid and electrolyte disturbances. After doing a nutritional assessment to identify actual or potential imbalances and food preferences, the nurse can initiate teaching.

Food: Specific fluid and electrolyte imbalance may require simple dietary changes. For example, clients receiving potassium depleting diuretics are commonly given potassium supplements. Nurses can often help clients by giving them a list of foods and fluid high in the electrolytes, which they require or need to avoid.

Administering Medications

Clients with fluid, electrolyte and acid-base imbalance are often prescribed medications as part of the therapeutic regimen. Nurses need to be, knowledgeable about the therapeutic effects of mineral electrolyte preparations and diuretics.

Nurse's responsibilities include accurate administration consistent with manufactures guidelines (e.g. dilute oral potassium supplements to disguise the unpleasant taste and decrease gastric irritation).

Diuretics: These are drugs that increase renal excretion of water, sodium and other electrolytes. Although, helpful in treating client's fluid volume excess (FVE) they have the potential to cause dehydration and serious electrolyte deficiencies. Client needs careful monitoring and education, while on diuretic therapy.

Administering Intravenous Therapy

A relatively common form of therapy for handling disturbances is the use of various solutions infused IV. The physician is responsible for prescribing the kind and amount of solution to be used. The nurse is responsible for:

- Initiating, monitoring and discontinuing the therapy
- Understanding the client's need for IV therapy, the type of solution being used, its desired effect and untoward reactions that may occur.

Evaluation

Expected Outcomes

The client will be:

- Oriented to time, place and person
- Excrete normal urine volume with normal concentration and specific gravity
- Consume food and fluids as prescribed
- Exhibit moist skin and mucous membranes
- Adhere to diet therapy
- Exhibit normal cardiac function with regular pulse rate, normal electrocardiogram.

Chapter 17 Management of Patients in Pain

Pain disables and distressed more people than any single disease entity. It is probably the most common reason for a person to seek health care. More medical surgical problems are associated with pain resulting from:

- Disease process
- Diagnostic test
- Treatment modalities.

COMPONENTS OF PAIN

Three components of pain appear as:

- A stimulus, physical or mental
- A bodily sensation of hurting
- The reaction of a person experiencing it.

The nurse spends more time with the patient with pain than any other members of the healthcare team and therefore has the opportunity to make a significant contribution towards increasing the patient's comfort and relieving pain.

DEFINITION

Pain is a subjective, unpleasant sensory and emotional experience associated with actual or potential tissue damage. It is whatever the experiencing person says it is, existing whenever he/she says it does.

TYPES OF PAIN

Acute Pain

Acute pain is a very common occurrence. It indicates that some degree of damage has occurred within the body that requires some form of treatment or intervention. Healing may also be accompanied by acute pain. As healing progresses, the pain subsides and gradually disappears. Acute pain is accompanied by muscle tension and anxiety.

Chronic Pain

Chronic pain is sometimes defined as pain that lasts for 6 months or longer. An episode of pain may assume the characteristics of chronic pain before 6 months have elapsed or some types of pain may remain primarily acute in nature for longer than 6 months. Nevertheless after 6 months, the majority of pain experiences are accompanied by problems associated with chronic pain (Table 17.1).

Referred Pain

Referred pain is felt in areas other than those stimulated. It may occur when stimulation is not perceived in the primary areas. For example, the person having a heart attack may complain only of pain radiating down the left arm, when in fact the tissue damage is occurring in the myocardium. Referred pain occurs most often with damage or injury to visceral organs and the pain is referred to cutaneous surfaces.

Psychogenic Pain

The term 'psychogenic pain' has been used to describe pain where no physical pathology has been found or where the pain appears to have a greater psychological basis than a physical one. A caution here is that diagnostic tests are not definitive measures and may not be sophisticated enough to detect pathophysiological changes. Distinguishing between physical and emotional components of pain is difficult and it is important to remember that all pain is real.

Table 17.1: Comparison of acute pain and chronic pain

Acute pain	Chronic pain
Mild to severe	
Sympathetic nervous system responses: • Increased pulse rate • Increased respiration rate • Elevated blood pressure • Diaphoresis • Dilated pupils	Parasympathetic nervous system responses: • Vital signs normal • Dry, warm skin • Pupils normal or dilated Depressed and withdrawn
Related to tissue injury	
Resolves with healing	Continues beyond healing
Client appears restless and anxious	Client appears depressed and withdrawn
Client report pain	Client often does not mention pain unless asked
Client exhibits behavior indicative of pain: • Crying • Rubbing area • Holding area	Pain behavior often absent

CLINICAL MANIFESTATION OF PAIN

The patient's response to the pain may be any one or a combination of possible reactions. These may include:

- Physiologic manifestation (Table 17.2)
- Verbal statements
- Vocal behavior
- Facial expression
- Body movements
- Physical contact with others
- These behaviors vary greatly from one person to another and may differ within the same person from one time to the next.

FACTORS THAT INFLUENCE RESPONSES TO PAIN

- Meaning of pain to individual person
- Degree of pain perception
- Past experience
- Cultural values
- Social expectations
- Physical and mental health
- Parental attitudes toward pain
- Setting in which pain occurs
- Fear, anxiety
- Usual way of responding to stressors
- Age
- Preparation for pain context
- Health professionals response.

Table 17.2: Objective signs of acute pain

Physiological signs	Behavioral signs
Pulse: Increased rate	Rigid body position
Respiration: Increased depth and frequency	Restlessness
Blood pressure: Increased systolic and diastolic pressure	Frowning
Diaphoresis: Pallor	Clenched teeth
Dilated pupils	Clenched fists
Muscle tension, face and body	Crying
Nausea and vomiting, if pain is severe	Moaning

GUIDELINES FOR ASSESSMENT OF THE PATIENT IN PAIN

1. **Assess the characteristics of the patient's pain:**
   a. Severity of pain (intensity scale: 0 means no pain and 10 is most intense pain).
   b. Type, location, duration and rhythmicity of pain.

c. Tolerance of pain.
d. Harmful effects of pain on patient's recovery.
e. Strategies that patient believes will help to relieve pain.
f. Concern the patient has about the pain.
g. Precipitating factors.
h. Alleviating factors.

2. **Assess the patient's behavioral response to the pain experience:**
   a. Determine if the pain is acute or chronic.
   b. Observe for the following behavioral responses:
      - Physiological manifestations (changes in pulse, blood pressure, respiratory rate, etc.)
      - Verbal statements
      - Vocal responses
      - Facial expressions
      - Body movements
      - Alteration in response to the environment
      - Physical contact with others
      - Adaptation of physiological and behavioral responses
      - Effect of pain on ability to communicate and carry out usual activities of daily living.
3. **Assess factors that influence responses to pain:**
   a. Ethic and cultural factors.
   b. Previous pain experiences.
   c. Meaning of the pain experiences.
   d. Patient's responses to pain relief strategies.

NURSING DIAGNOSIS

The nursing diagnosis given to clients experiencing pain are acute pain and chronic pain. When writing the diagnostic statement, the nurse may further specify the type or location of the pain (e.g. postoperative, chest, abdominal, back), etiologic factors and precipitating factors. When known, must be part of the diagnostic statement. Because the pain experience affects so many facets of human functioning, pain itself maybe the etiology of other nursing diagnoses. Examples of such nursing diagnoses are:

- Ineffective airway clearance related to postoperative incisional chest pain
- Anxiety related to past experiences of poor control of pain and to anticipation of pain
- Ineffective breathing pattern related to postoperative abdominal pain
- Ineffective individual coping related to prolonged continuous back pain, ineffective pain management and inadequate support systems
- Fear related to anticipated pain after surgery
- Altered health maintenance related to chronic pain and fatigue

- Hopelessness related to ineffective pain management strategies
- Knowledge deficit (pain control measures) related to lack of exposure to information resources
- Impaired physical mobility related to arthritis pain in knee and ankle joints
- Self-care deficit: Bathing/Hygiene, dressing/grooming, toileting related to pain in the joints
- Sleep pattern disturbance related to increased pain perception at night.

Planning

The nurse identifies nursing interventions that will assist the client in achieving the overall client goals of preventing, modifying or eliminating pain, so that the client is able partially or completely to resume usual daily activity and be able to cope more effectively with the pain experience. When planning, nurses need to choose pain relief measures appropriate for the client. Nursing interventions may include a variety of pharmacological and non-pharmacological intervention.

Implementation

Pain management is the alleviation of pain or a reduction in pain to a level of comfort that is acceptable to the client. It includes two basic types of nursing interventions:

- Pharmacological
- Non-pharmacological interventions.

Generally speaking, combinations of strategies are available for the client in the pain. Sometimes, strategies need to be tried and changed, until the client obtains effective pain relief.

General Strategies for Pain Management

- Assess patient's pain status based on patients past experience
- Incorporate the following factors in the assessment of patient's pain status:
  - Location/Characteristics
  - Onset
  - Frequency
  - Intensity
  - Quality
  - Precipitation factors
  - Effective pain control measures
  - Pain expression style (verbal, crying and moaning)
  - Impact of quality of life
  - Effect of pain on daily activities
  - Effect on sleep/wake pattern
  - Effect on energy level.

- Apply previous strategies that have controlled pain
- Explore strategies that have been successful in the past
- Assess patient's willingness to incorporate non-pharmacological pain control measures
- Administer medication as per physician's orders
- Immobilize or rest the affected area
- Relieve pressure areas with turning or pressure reduction devices such as air fluidized support systems
- Suggest and instruct patient in relaxation techniques; short simple technique with nurse directing for acute pain and more complex techniques for chronic pain
- Encourage patient's attention to proper posture and alignment
- Provide therapeutic positioning
- Provide distraction
- Use hypnotic strategies as prescribed
- Provide music therapy
- Use counter stimulation, pressure, massage, vibration, heat/cold external analgesics and transcutaneous nerve stimulation
- Provide a supportive environment
- Help patient to identify activities that may enhance pain
- Discuss strategies to reduce enhancement of pain
- Discuss strategies to avoid these activities within patient's lifestyle
- Provide touch, especially for infants or for disoriented or unresponsive patients.

Evaluation

Example of evaluative statement, indicating goal achievements are:

- Reports lower intensity of pain
- Accepts pain medications as prescribed
- Exhibits decreased physical and behavioral signs of pain and discomfort
- Identifies effective pain relief strategies.

Section 3

Critical Care for Neonates and Children

Chapter 18 Neonatal Critical Care

TERMINOLOGIES

Born before arrival: Delivery of any part of the baby or the placenta that takes place before the women arrives in the labor room.

Indirect obstetric death: Those resulting from the previous existing disease or disease that developed during pregnancy, which are due to direct obstetric causes.

Large for gestational age: Birth weight, above the 90th percentile for gestation.

Live birth: Any baby, which at birth shows any evidence of life such as breathing, beating of the heart, pulsation of cord or definite movement of voluntary muscle, irrespective of the duration of gestation.

Low birth weight: A baby-born with a birth weight of less than 2.5 kg (up to and including 2.499 kg) irrespective of the gestation.

Maternal death: It is defined as the death of women, while pregnant or within 42 days of termination of pregnancy.

Post-term: From 37 to 42 completed weeks of gestation or more (294 day or more).

Preterm: Less than 37 completed week's gestation (< 259 day).

Small for gestational age: Birth weight, which is below the 10th percentile for gestation.

Stillbirth: A child, which is born after the 28th week of pregnancy, at the time of birth and after being completely expelled from the mother, shows no signs of life.

Term: From 37 to 42 completed week's gestation (259–293 day).

ORGANIZATION OF NEONATAL UNIT

All staff involved in the care of newborn, i.e. staff in labor room, postnatal wards, nurseries and special care baby unit (SCBU) should undergo regular training. Training should be organized under the following main heading:

- Resuscitation of the newborn
- Basic care of the newborn and low-birth weight babies
- Management of the sick neonate
- Transport of the sick newborn
- Breastfeeding
- Immunization.

Staffing

The staff working in the nursery or SCBU must have been trained to care for the newborn. The nurse in charge of the nursery on each shift must have been trained to know how to care for the newborn baby. Neonatal nurses should not be posted anywhere else except with neonates. Close liaison between the nursing officers and the pediatrician is required to ensure that there are always trained staffs in charge of the nursery or SCBU and postnatal ward.

Equipment and Drugs

All delivery institutions should have basic equipment and drugs for use in the care of the newborn. The equipment should be checked regularly and any repairs done immediately. The following is a guideline list of minimal equipment (resuscitation equipment) required in each delivery hospital:

- Radiant warmer
- Mucus extractor
- Suction machine
- Oxygen cylinder
- Oxygen analyzer
- Weighing scales
- Incubator
- Phototherapy unit
- Transport cot
- Emergency box
- Emergency drugs
- Breast pump
- Blood pressure apparatus
- Infusion pump
- Exchange transfusion set
- Respiratory and apnea monitor, transport incubator/ventilator.

HEALTH EDUCATION

Health education will be given to mothers daily by nurses and doctors.

BREASTFEEDING

A breastfeeding, nurse/midwives responsible to ensure the following that:

- Baby stay with mothers, day and night, unless they require special care
- No unauthorized bottle or pacifiers (dummies) are used in the wards
- All mothers should know why breast milk is the best
- Encourage all mothers to breastfeed their babies
- Encourage all other staff, to promote breastfeeding.

PROVISION OF INFECTION CONTROL

Hand washing must be done before and after handling every baby. Avoiding using outside equipment, ideally each baby should have its own cot, bowl for washing and set of equipment to ensure that cross-infection does not take place.

AIM AND OBJECTIVES

Aim

- To ensure the health and well-being of mothers and their babies
- To reduce the mortality and morbidity in the perinatal period
- To promote optimal growth and development of the infant and his/her family
- To strengthen mother-infant bonding
- To subject the neonate to minimal stress
- To minimize or prevent complications.

Objectives

1. During the neonatal period the baby is adjusting to new life outside the womb and mother is recovering from delivery, and learning about the needs of her new baby. The majority of babies are normal and well, and is cared for in the postnatal wards. Some are unwell and have to be cared for in the nursery or in SCBU, but in all places the tasks of caring for the newborn baby are the same.
2. To ensure the baby is born in the best condition and that he/she remains well and healthy.
3. To avoid any adverse conditions that may harm the baby and mother.

ADMISSION TO NEONATAL CARE UNIT

Babies with the following problems should be admitted to the neonatal unit.

From Labor Room

- Preterm baby < 35 weeks
- Weight < 2.0 kg
- Meconium aspiration syndromes
- Birth asphyxia
- Respiratory distress syndrome
- Central cyanosis
- Shock, hypotension and pallor
- Convulsions

- Congenital heart disease
- Major congenital heart disease and malformation.

From Postnatal Ward

- Hypothermia (temperature < 35°C)
- Hypoglycemia not corrected by feeding
- Apnea
- Tachypnea (respiratory rate > 60 beats per minute)
- Central cyanosis rapid rising bilirubin
- Persistent vomiting
- Suspected infection
- Severe jaundice
- Bleeding disorder.

Perinatal asphyxia is still a very important cause of neonatal morbidity and mortality. Good planning and management in the first few minutes of life of a newborn is of long-term benefit and will prevent long-term handicap. Quick and effective resuscitation is the single most important aspect of neonatal care and more cost and time effective contribution to child health.

CHILD MORBIDITY AND MORTALITY

UN informed India over its high infant mortality rate information comes from UN weeks after UNICEF revealed that one in every 21 children being born in India is dying before reaching their fifth birth day.

Mexico, UNICEF has projected that if current trends of fewer than five mortality rate continue, by 2030 just five countries will account for more than half of all under five deaths—India (17%), Nigeria (15%), Pakistan (8%), Democratic Republic of the Congo (7%) and Angola (5%).

According to UNICEF, if mortality rates stay at the present day levels, 69 million children will die before the age of 5 during the next 15 years, about half of those children will die within their first month of life. According to their latest estimates, released on the sidelines of the global maternal health conference in Mexico, 5.9 million children will die before the age of 5 (Globally in 2015). Based on current population projections, 6.6 million will die worldwide in 2030, if rates remain at 2015 levels of these under five deaths, nearly a third will die in South Asia.

The warning comes weeks after UNICEF revealed that one in every 21 children being born in India is dying before reaching their fifth birth day as the country recorded the highest number of fewer than five deaths in 2015 globally. The less than five mortality rate (U5MR) in India is about seven times higher than in high income countries where 1 in 147 is dying. A study published in the lancet showed that 1 in 5 under 5 deaths took place in India in 2015 (20%) of the global deaths numbering to 1.2 million children.

There was also a silver lining to it, U5MR in India dropped from 126 deaths 1,000 live birth in 1990 to 48 in 2015—a 62% reduction. This is higher than the average global reduction of 53%.

Infectious diseases such as pneumonia and diarrhea are still main killers of children under age five in India. In 2015, pneumonia is estimated to account for about 15% of the 1.2 million under five deaths in India. Diarrhea accounts for about 9%. UNICEF says that 70% of the global decline in under-five deaths since 2000 and 2015. The annual number of under-five deaths fell from almost 10 million to 5.9 million.

Child Mortality—Common and Largely Preventable

According to United Nations International Children's Emergency Fund (UNICEF), 9.2 million children under age of five died worldwide in 2007. Tragically, an estimated two third of childhood deaths are preventable with existing tools and interventions. Existing vaccines alone can prevent an estimated 25% of death under age of five. In fact, researchers predict that the utilization of existing tools and interventions around the world could save > 6 million young lives every year. The main causes of child death are as neonatal, pneumonia, diarrhea, malaria, measles, human immunodeficiency virus (HIV)/acquired immunodeficiency syndrome (AIDS) and injuries.

World's Goal to Reduce Child Deaths

In 2000, leaders from 189 countries signed the United Nation Millennium Declaration, signaling a worldwide commitment to eradicating extreme poverty by the year 2015, aim to decrease child mortality by two third, from an incidence of 93 deaths per 1,000 children under age of five in 1990 to 31 per 1,000 in 2015, while some countries are on mortality rates.

The good news is that solutions exist to improve child health and survival. However, a greater worldwide effort, commitment and investment will be needed to bring life-saving track to meet Millennium Development Goal (MDG) by 2015, many lag behind and some have even shown increasing child interventions to the most vulnerable children, prevent more child deaths.

Pneumonia: A Major Cause of Child Morbidity and Mortality

Pneumonia is the number one killer of children under age of 5. One child dies from pneumonia every 15 seconds, i.e. 5,500 children every day and 2 million children every year. Most of these children are dying in poor countries, many of the same countries that are in danger of failing to meet the MDG child survival goal. Pneumonia prevention and treatment is therefore essential to increase child survival.

CHANGING TRENDS IN HOSPITAL CARE: PREVENTIVE, PROMOTIVE AND CURATIVE ASPECTS OF CHILD HEALTH

Disease Prevention and Health Promotion

Nurses must remember that 'prevention is better than cure'. The pediatric nurse practitioner (PNP) role was evolved as a result of this trend. The PNP program led to the development of several specialized ambulatory or primary care roles for nurses. The practitioner programs have expanded to prepare school nurse practitioners and hospital nurse practitioner. The clinical nurse specialist's (CNS) role has been developed for providing expert nursing care.

Health Teaching

Health teaching is inseparable from advocacy and prevention. Informing parents and children for a diagnosis or medical treatment, encouraging children to ask questions about their bodies, referring families to health-related professional groups or lay groups and supply appropriate literature are all considered as health education. Anticipatory guidance is one of the most important types of health teaching.

Support Counseling

Attention to emotional needs requires support and sometimes, counseling. The role of child advocate or health teacher is often supportive by the very nature of the individualized approach. Support can be offered in many ways, the most common of which include listening, touching and physical presence. Touching and physical presence are most helpful with children, because they facilitate non-verbal communication.

Counseling involves a mutual exchange of ideas and opinions that provides the basis for mutual problem solving. It involves support, teaching and techniques to foster the expression of feelings or thoughts and approaches to help family to cope with stress. Optimally, counseling not only helps to resolve a crisis or problems, but also enables the family to attain a higher level of functioning, greater self-esteem and closer relationships.

Restorative Role

The most basic of all nursing roles is the restoration of health through care giving activities. Nurses are involved with meeting the physical and emotional needs of children including feeding, bathing, toileting, dressing, security and socialization. Although they are responsible for instituting physician's orders, they are also held singularly accountable for their own actions and judgments regardless of written orders.

A significant aspect of restoration of health is continual assessment and evaluation of physical status. The nurse must be aware of normal findings in order to intelligently identify and document deviations; in addition, the pediatric nurse never loses sight of the emotional and developmental needs of the individual child, which can significantly influence the course of the disease process.

Coordination/Collaboration

The nurse as a member of the health team collaborates and coordinates nursing services with the activities of other professionals. Working in isolation does not service the child's best interest to achieve holistic care. An interdisciplinary approach is necessary.

Ethical Decision-making

The nurse is forced to determine the most beneficial or least harmful action within the framework of social morales. Professional practice standards, the law institutional rules, religious traditions, family's value system and the nurse's personal values, while giving care to children.

Research

Practicing nurses are in key position to contribute to research, because they are the ones observing human responses to health and illness. Nurses can systematically record or analyze such observations. If these interventions are clinically evaluated and shared with other nurses, then body of knowledge on nursing practice develop. Research also implies questioning why something is effective or if there is a better approach. Evaluation is essential to the nursing process and research is one of the best ways to accomplish this. Therefore nurses need to be more involved in research and in applying research findings to their practice.

Healthcare Planning

The nursing role has expanded and includes the community-based health driven system of the future, traditionally, nurses have been in public healthcare on either a continuous or an episodic basis. Nurses have been involved in healthcare planning occasionally the nursing role has expanded to include community-based involvement. Healthcare planning involves not only providing new services, but also promoting the highest quality of existing ones.

Future Trends

The present shift in healthcare settings, the focus has turned from treatment of disease to promotion of health through health teaching. As more support is provided outside the hospital, the need for home care and community health services will necessitates that nursing is the traditional care setting with increased emphasis on prevention through anticipatory guidance. Child health and family assessment, discharge planning, care in the home and community.

Technological advances also influence pediatric nurse's roles. Increasing technical skills related to patient care, as well as the demand for computer knowledge in the work setting are inevitable future trends. As more positions not requiring a nursing background, such as patient care educator, are created in the healthcare system, nurses will required to continually update their knowledge and prove their unique contribution.

CHILD HEALTH ASSESSMENT

History Taking and General Physical Examination

History taking and examination in child health assessment is detailed in Box 18.1.

Box 18.1: Child health assessment

Child Health History

Informant's relationship to child: .... Date of admission: ....

Name of the child............ Inpatient number: ....

Age in months, if under 3 years: .... Gender: ....

.... Ordinal position of the child: ....

Language spoken: .... Nationality: ....

Income of the parent: .... Religion: ....

Education status (if school-age child): .... Home town/City address: ....

Provisional diagnosis: .... Reason for admission: ....

Treatment received on arrival to hospital: ....

Nursing History

Family: .... Home environment: ....

Name of family members in home (e.g. parents, siblings, grandparents and others)	Inpatient number	Health status	Education	Occupation

Hereditary illness: ....

Child

If both parents are working, who take the care of the child: ....

Any significant vital statistics in the family: ....

Bottle feed: ....

Breastfeed: ....

Cup or spoon, if cup or spoon is being used how is this being done? ....

Contd...

Contd...

Age of weaning, type of formula: ....

Amount of milk per day: ....

Amount of water per day: ....

Feeding or eating problems: ....

Elimination: ....

Number of bowel movements daily: ....

Use training chair: ....

Time taken in bath room: ....

Method used, if toilet training is being done: ....

Problem regarding elimination: Diarrhea/Constipation/Incontinent urine/feces

Urinary stream/frequency of voiding: ....

Sleeping

Sleep in crib/bed/alone Special bedtime rituals: ....

Usual bedtime: ....

Fears for dark: ....

Problem related to sleep: ....

Nightmares: ....

Sleep walking: ....

Bedwetting: .... If yes, how handled? ....

Personal hygiene

Care by another: ....

Need assistance for personal hygiene: Dressing/Brushing teeth

Problem related to personal hygiene: ....

Dental hygiene and problem: ....

Behavior

How does child react to distress, crying/temper tantrum/withdraw/run away?

Disciplinary measure: ....

Behavior problems: ....

Plays: Usually alone/parallel play/play activity and toys enjoyed: ....

Handicaps

Vision: ....

Hearing: ....

Speech: ....

Dental: ....

Gait: ....

Contd...

Contd...

Other handicaps: ....
Supportive devices: ....
Communication and socialization/problem with communication, explain: ....

Health History

Ask any or all of the following as appropriate and write summary below: ....
What problem made to bring to hospital?...
When this symptoms started? ....
Any precipitating factors/aggravating (what were you doing at that time?): ....
Was the onset of sudden or gradual? ....
How often does the problem occur? ....
Where is the exact location of the problem? ....
Has the problem occurred before? ....
Significant area affected: ....
Direct admission: ....
Referred by others: ....
Any relevant information: ....
Neonatal history: Gestation normal/Deviation from normal
Birth: Normal/Deviation normal
How soon bonding taken place? ....

Newborn Examination

Alive/Stillbirth: ....
Sex of the baby: ....
Weight of the baby: ....
Activity: Active/Dull

Head-to-toe examination
Head: Distribution of hair ....
Condition of the hair ....
Condition of the scalp ....
Face or essence of edema ....
Neck rigidity ....

Ears
Hearing capacity: ....
Eyes
Any discharge/Swelling/Redness: ....
Color of the conjunctiva/Pink/Pale: ....
Nose: Any discharge, polyp: ....
Lips: Moist or any cracks: ....
Neck: ....
Tongue: ....

Chest and thorax
Symmetry of movement: ....
Auscultation of breath: ....
Sounds: ....
Extremities
Full range of movement: ....

Contd...

Contd...

Maternal History

Last menstrual period: .... Expected date of delivery (EDD): ....
Gestation: .... Weeks: ....
Tetanus toxoid: ....

Pregnancy complications
Pregnancy induced hypertension (PIH): ....
Diabetes mellitus (DM): ....
Preterm/Post-term: ....
Antepartum hemorrhage: ....

Investigation
Blood group and Rh ....
Hemoglobin (Hb) ....
Venereal disease research laboratory (VDRL) ....

Labor
Admitted in labor room: ....
Date: .... Time: ....
Presentation: ....

Delivery
Normal/Instrumental: ....
Membrane: Ruptured spontaneously/ Artificially: ....

Amniotic fluid:
Normal/Excessive/Decreased/Absent/ Clear/Yellow/Meconium-stained/Foul-smelling

Placenta: Healthy/Unhealthy

Duration of labor
1st stage: ....
2nd stage: ....
3rd stage: ....

Maternal complication
....
....
....

Neonatal Examination History

Condition at birth: .... Resuscitation: ....

Throat suction: .... Oxygen: ....

Bag and mask ventilation: .... Endotracheal intubation: ....

Apgar: 1 minute/5 minute Drug used: ....

Gestational age: .... Birth weight (kg): ....
Week: .... Length (cm): ....
Term/Preterm/Post-term: ....

Abdominal girth: .... Chest circumference: ....

Physical assessment

Temperature: .... Heart rate: ....

Respiration: ....

Muscle tone/Activity

- Activity: Quite/Lethargic/Flaccid/Paralysis/Tremors/Seizure activity
- Cry: Vigorous/Week/High pitched/Difficulty to elicit
- Skin color: Pink/Jaundice/Pallor/Cyanosis; Central and peripheral rashes/Birthmark
- Skin turgor: Lost/Good

Contd...

Contd...

Reflexes
Moro: ....
Rooting: ....
Sucking: ....
Grasp: ....
Babinski: ....
Tonic neck: ....

Facial feature
- Asymmetrical
- Symmetrical
- Injuries

Eyes
- Position
- Size and shape
- Subconjunctival hemorrhage
- Clear
- If discharge, specify: ....
- Heart
- Normal/Ectopic/Murmur

Abdomen
- Soft /Firm/Flat/Distended

Abdominal girth (cm)
- Liver
- Palpable/Not palpable
- Umbilicus
- Normal/Inflamed

Spine

Normal/Abnormal, specify: ....

Extremities

Movement: Limited range of motion/ Unable to assess
- Length of upper limbs/Lower limbs/Equal/Unequal/Extra digit (specify)
- Talipes
- Hips: Normal/Abnormal/Unable to assess

Genitals
- Normal/Male/Female/ Ambiguous/Term/Preterm

Anus
- Patent/Imperforate

Head neck
Anterior fontanel: Soft/Bulging/Firm/Flat/ Depressed

Sagittal suture:
Approximation/Separated/Overriding

Ears
- Size
- Position
- Shape
- Development of cartilage

Nose
- Patent
- Obstructed
- Flaring

Mouth
- Lips
- Color
- Cleft
- Palate

Thorax
- Asymmetrical/Symmetrical

Clavicle
- Normal/Abnormal

Lungs
- Breath Sounds: Equal/Unequal/ Bilateral
- Rhonchi/Rales/Wheeze/Grunting/ Secretion/Spontaneous/Rate

REFLEXES IN THE NEONATE

Sucking reflex: Sucking motion begins when a nipple is placed in the neonate's mouth.

Moro reflex: When the neonate is lifted above the crib and then suddenly lowered, then arms and legs symmetrically extend, then abduct the fingers spread, forming 'C.'

Rooting reflex: Stroking the cheek makes the neonates turn the head in the direction of the stroke.

Tonic neck (fencing position): When the neonate is supine and the head is turned to one side, extremities on the same side straighten, while those on the opposite side flex.

Babinski: Stroking the sole on the side of the small toe makes the toes fan upward.

Grasping: Placing a finger in each hand makes the neonate grasps the fingers tightly enough to be pulled to a sitting position.

Stepping: Holding the neonate upright with the feet touching a flat surface elicit dancing or stepping movements.

Startle: A loud noise such as hand clap, elicit arm abduction and elbow flexion, the hands stay clenched.

Trunk incurvature: When a finger is run down the neonate's back laterally to the spine, the trunk flexes and pelvis swings toward the stimulated side.

Chapter 19 High-risk Neonate

HYALINE MEMBRANE DISEASE

Hyaline membrane disease also called respiratory distress syndrome. It is a complex disorder manifested by signs of respiratory distress.

Clinical Manifestations

- Tachypnea
- Nasal flaring, grunting, retraction.

Assessment

Use Silverman-Anderson index to evaluate the neonates' respiratory status. Five areas such as upper chest, lower chest, xiphoid retractions, nares dilation and expiratory grunt; each graded from 0 to 10.

Medical and Nursing Management

- Ventilatory therapy
- Maintenance of acid-base balance
- Temperature regulation
- Adequate nutrition
- Oxygen monitoring and protection from infection.

TRANSIENT TACHYPNEA OF THE NEWBORN

Transient tachypnea of the newborn is also known as type II respiratory distress syndrome.

Etiology

Aspiration of amniotic or tracheal fluid compounded either by delayed clearing of the airway or by excess fluid entering the lungs.

Clinical Manifestations

- Expiratory grunting
- Nasal flaring
- Slight cyanosis
- Tachypnea.

Medical and Nursing Management

- Oxygen administration
- Ventilatory assistance (rarely needed)
- Maintenance of acid-base balance
- Thermoregulation
- Adequate nutrition
- Oxygen monitoring
- Protection from infection.

MECONIUM ASPIRATION SYNDROME

Etiology

Asphyxia in utero leads to increased fetal peristalsis, relaxation of the anal sphincter passage of meconium into the amniotic fluid and reflex gasping of amniotic fluid into the lungs.

Clinical Manifestations

- Fetal hypoxia as indicated by altered fetal activity and heart rate
- Meconium staining of amniotic fluid noted on rupture of membranes
- Signs of distress at delivery such as Apgar score below six, pallor cyanosis and respiratory distress.

Medical and Nursing Management

- Immediate endotracheal suctioning of the neonate at delivery
- Respiratory assistance via mechanical ventilation
- Maintenance of a neutral thermal environment
- Postural drainage
- Chest physiotherapy
- Administration of antibiotics.

SEPSIS

Etiology

Sepsis can occur before, during, or after delivery, most common causative agents are the gram-negative *Escherichia coli* and *Aerobacter proteus, Klebsiella* and gram-positive-β-hemolytic streptococci.

Clinical Manifestations

- Lethargy, hypotonia
- Temperature instability

- Feeding pattern changes such as poor sucking or decreased intake
- Apnea
- Hyperbilirubinemia
- Abdominal distention.

Medical Management

- Collection of specimen to identify causative organisms
- Lumbar puncture
- Urine, skin blood and nasopharyngeal culture
- Gastric aspiration.

Nursing Management

- Administration of broad-spectrum antibiotics before culture report is received
- Maintenance of neutral thermal environment
- Respiratory support
- Evaluation of signs and symptoms of sepsis
- Monitoring of fluid and electrolyte balance
- Evaluation of metabolic disturbances
- Provision for cardiovascular support.

HYPERBILIRUBINEMIA

Condition characterized by:

- A bilirubin level that exceeds 6 mg/dL within the first 24 hours after delivery and remains elevated beyond 7 days in a full term neonate and 10 days in a premature neonate
- A bilirubin level that rises by > 5 mg/dL/day
- A level that is > 12 mg/dL in premature or term neonates
- Conjugated (direct) bilirubin level that exceeds 1.5–2.0 mg/dL.

Clinical Manifestation

- Kernicterus may occur with serum bilirubin level at or above 20 mg/dL (full term) at lower levels (approximately 14 mg/dL) in premature neonates
- Jaundice, elevated bilirubin levels and hepatosplenomegaly.

Medical and Nursing Management

- Treatment for hemolytic anemia
- Increased serum albumin levels
- Removal of maternal antibodies and sensitized red blood cells (RBCs) via exchange transfusion and phototherapy.

Signs of Kernicterus

Lethargy, decreased reflexes, seizures opisthotonos and high-pitched cry:

- Causes
- Hemolytic disease of the neonates
- Sepsis
- Impaired hepatic functioning
- Polycythemia
- Enclosed hemorrhage
- Hypothermia
- Hypoglycemia and asphyxia neonatorum.

ISOIMMUNE HEMOLYTIC DISEASE OF THE NEONATE

Hemolytic disease of the newborn is also called erythroblastosis fetalis (breakdown of RBCs).

Causes

Transplacental passage of maternal antibodies that cause RBC breakdown.

Clinical Manifestations

- Hemolytic anemia
- Hyperbilirubinemia and jaundice.

Medical and Nursing Management

- Drug therapy, family support
- Phototherapy
- Exchange transfusion
- Monitoring of bilirubin levels.

ABO Incompatibility

1. Incompatibility of ABO blood type can occur when fetal blood type differs from maternal blood type.
2. The most common incompatibility occurs when a type O mother carries a type A or type B fetus. Type O blood contains anti-A and anti-B antibodies that travel transplacental to the fetus, causing jaundice and hepatosplenomegaly.
3. The ABO incompatibility can occur with the first pregnancy and is usually milder and of shorter duration than Rh-positive incompatibility (Rh is rhesus).

Rhesus Incompatibility

- It occurs when an Rh-negative mother carries an Rh-positive fetus
- Leakage of fetal Rh-antigen commonly occurs during delivery at the time of placental separation
- Maternal antibodies are produced in response to a subsequent pregnancy with an Rh-positive fetus, maternal antibodies enter the fetal circulation transplacental causing erythroblastosis
- Signs and symptoms include hemolytic anemia, hyperbilirubinemia, jaundice, direct Coombs' test and hepatosplenomegaly.

Prevention

Prevention involves administration of Rh immune globulin (RhoGAM) within 72 hours of delivery:

- RhoGAM prevents antibody formation
- It is ineffective, when the woman is already sensitized
- RhoGAM should be administered to Rh-negative D-negative women, who has had an abortion or whose newborn is Rh-D-positive
- During pregnancy Rh-sensitization can occur if the cellular layer separating maternal and fetal circulation is disrupted
- RhoGAM can be administered at 28 weeks of gestation to decrease the incidence of maternal isoimmunizations.

SEXUALLY TRANSMITTED DISEASE

Syphilis

Congenital syphilis is diagnosed with serologic tests at 3–6 months, the development of antibodies is necessary to make a diagnosis.

Clinical Manifestations

- Vesicular lesions on the soles and palms irritability, small for gestational age, failure to thrive rhinitis and red rash around mouth, and anus
- Copper rash on face, soles and palms.

Management

- Penicillin therapy
- Isolation technique initially followed by general care
- Covering of hands to minimize trauma from scratching.

Gonorrhea

Etiology

Exposure to lesions during vaginal delivery.

Clinical Manifestation

Ophthalmia neonatorum.

Management

- Penicillin therapy
- Prophylactic medication administration such as erythromycin to the eyes after delivery
- Isolation measures
- Culture specimen of eye discharge, if present.

HYDROCEPHALY

Abnormal increase in the amount of cerebrospinal fluid (CSF) in the ventricles of the brain, leading to cerebral ventricle enlargement.

Cause

Alteration in production (increased) flow, obstructed or reabsorption of CSF.

Clinical Manifestations

- Head enlargement
- Forehead prominence, sunset eyes
- Irritability, weakness and seizures.

Medical and Nursing Management

- Skin care to prevent breakdown and infection
- Careful head support during handling
- Emotional support and education for the parents
- Assessment of neurologic status and progression of symptoms
- Shunt insertion to eliminate excess CSF
- Management of shunt and prevention of infection at the surgical site.

PHENYLKETONURIA

Causes

Inborn metabolic error resulting in a deficiency of phenylalanine hydroxylase, a liver enzymes essential for the conversion of phenylalanine to tyrosine.

Clinical Manifestations

- Accumulation of phenylalanine and its abnormal metabolites in the brain, possibly leading to mental retardation

- Failure to thrive
- Vomiting and rashes
- Decreased pigmentation.

Medical and Nursing Management

- Infants are placed on low phenylalanine formula (Lofenalac) and on a continued special diet that limit phenylalanine intake
- Central nervous system damage can be minimized if treatment is initiated before the age of 3 months.

TORCH SYNDROME

Group of maternal infectious disease [toxoplasmosis, rubella, cytomegalovirus (CMV) and herpesvirus type 11] that can lead to serious complications in the embryo, fetus and neonate.

Toxoplasmosis

- The disease is transmitted to the fetus primarily via the mother's contact with contaminated cat box filler
- A therapeutic abortion is recommended if the diagnosis is made before the 20th week of gestation
- Effects include increased frequency of stillbirth, neonatal deaths, severe congenital anomalies, seizures and coma.

Rubella

- Rubella is a chronic viral infection lasts from the first trimester to months after delivery
- The greatest risk occurs within the first trimester
- Effects include congenital heart disease, intrauterine growth retardation, cataracts, mental retardation and hearing impairments.

Management

- Therapeutic abortion, if the disease occurs during the first trimester and emotional support for parents
- Women of childbearing age should be tested for immunity and vaccinated, if necessary.

Cytomegalovirus

Cytomegalovirus is a member of the herpesvirus group that can be transmitted from an asymptomatic mother transplacentally to the fetus or via the cervix to the neonate at delivery:

- It is the most frequent cause of viral infections in the fetus
- The CMV may be the most common cause of mental retardation
- Principal sites of damage are the brain, liver and blood
- Other effect includes auditory difficulties and a birth weight that is small for gestational age
- Antiviral drugs cannot prevent CMV or treat the neonate.

Herpesvirus Type 11

- The fetus can be exposed to the herpesvirus through indirect contact with infected genitals or via direct contact with those tissues during delivery
- Affected neonates may be asymptomatic for 2–12 days, but then may develop jaundice, seizures increased temperature and characteristics vesicular lesions
- A cesarean delivery can protect the fetus from infection.

PREMATURITY

Delivery before the end of the 37th week of gestation.

Problems

- Immaturity of all systems extent depends on gestational age and level of development at delivery
- Premature neonates between 28 and 37 weeks have the best chance of survival.

Medical and Nursing Management

- Respiratory assessment
- Maintenance of fluid and electrolyte balance
- Prevention of infection
- Assessment of neurologic status
- Maintenance of body temperature
- Renal function monitoring
- Emotional support to parents
- Assessment of glucose and bilirubin level.

Small for Gestational Age

Birth weight at or below the 10th percentile on Denver growth chart, also referred to as small for dates and intrauterine growth retardation.

Causes

Maternal causes: Poor nutrition, advanced diabetes, pregnancy-induced hypertension, smoking age over 35 and drug use.

Placental causes: Partial placental separation and malfunction.

Fetal causes: Intrauterine infection, chromosomal abnormalities and malformations.

Problems Related to Small for Gestational Age

- Perinatal asphyxia
- Hypoglycemia
- Hypocalcemia
- Aspiration syndromes
- Increased heat loss
- Feeding difficulties
- Polycythemia.

Large for Gestational Age

Birth weight at or above the 90th percentile on the intrauterine growth chart.

Etiology

- Mother with poorly controlled diabetes
- Multiparty
- Infant with transposition of the great vessels (unknown cause)
- Genetic predisposition
- Problems associated with large for gestational age
- Increased incidence of cesarean deliveries, birth trauma and injury
- Hypoglycemia
- Polycythemia.

POSTMATURITY

Delivery after 42 weeks of gestation.

Etiology

Etiology not well-understood, but associated with primigravida anencephalic fetus, history of postmaturity and delayed ovulation, and fertilization.

Problems Associated with Postmaturity

- Meconium aspiration placental insufficiency
- Hypoxia
- Hypoglycemia
- Polycythemia
- Seizures and cold stress.

Chapter 20

Nursing Care of Newborn

Care of the newborn at birth is primarily aimed at helping the newborn to adapt to the extrauterine environment and physiological adaptation, it includes:

- Initiating respiration and oxygenation of the arterial blood
- Temperature adaptation
- Initiation of feeding.

PREPARING FOR BIRTH

Make sure that the following things are available for the newborn:

1. Two clean and warm towels/cloths for keeping the baby warm; one for drying and wrapping the baby initially, the other one for covering the newborn to prevent heat loss.
2. The room, where the delivery takes place should be clean, warm, well-lighted and ventilated, but draught-free.
3. Ensure the 'five clean's during' delivery such as soap, water, new razor blade, a clean plastic sheet and a clean piece of thread:
   - A clean delivery kit for cord care
   - An oral mucus extractor
   - A blanket
   - A watch to note the time of delivery.

ADMISSION ROUTINE

1. On arrival in the postnatal ward, the baby should have his/her birth weight, length and head circumference taken.
2. The temperature, pulse, respiration, blood glucose, color and activity should be recorded.
3. Note should be made if baby has passed urine or meconium.
4. Identity band and sex of the baby should be checked against admission notes and with staff from labor ward.
5. Keep the baby with the mother, in this ways she can learn to respond and manage the demands and needs of the baby.
6. Establish breastfeed early.

OBSERVATIONS

All babies in the postnatal ward should have their observations charted on the maternal health card at least once daily. Any abnormalities detected must be reported to the doctor for further evaluation.

General Condition of the Baby

Assess Baby's Color

The baby should be pink; note presence of cyanosis, jaundice, pallor or plethora.

Activity

Note activity movements and response to handling.

Cardiorespiratory Pattern

The normal baby has a pulse rate of 120–160/min and a respiratory rate 35–45/min.

Skin

Note the skin for rashes, lumps, swelling, bruised or inflamed area.

Passage of Urine and Meconium

1. The majority of infants pass urine and meconium in the first 48 hours. If the baby has not passed meconium or urine in the first 48 hours, contact the referral unit for advise on management.
2. Do not perform a rectal examination or pass thermometer rectally.
3. Do not discharge a baby until meconium and urine have been passed. However, if she has to leave, ask her to bring the baby back if the body has not passed urine or meconium after 48 hours.

CARE

Clamping of the Cord

The umbilical cord should be clamped 2–3 minutes after the neonate is delivered completely. Wait till the cord has stopped pulsating before clamping and cutting it. This will result in an extra amount of blood being transfused in the neonate and prevent neonatal anemia. However, early and immediate clamping of the cord is recommended in newborn with severe birth asphyxia.

Care of the Cord in Hospital

The umbilical cord must be cut with a pair of sterile scissors/blade 3.5 cm from the abdominal skin surface. Note the following:

1. Nothing needs to be applied to the cord. The cord is frequently infected because many mothers apply substances, which may not be clean. The cord will dry and fall off on its own.
2. Tell the mother to prevent the cord from getting soiled with newborn urine or stool.

3. The mother should wash her hands with soap and water after cleaning the baby every time, when it passes stool.
4. Inspect the cord for bleeding 2 hours after tying.
5. Do not apply anything on the stump. Keep the cord clean and dry.
6. Inspect for discharge or infection till the healing occur.

After Discharge from the Hospital

1. If the parents complains about the cord, the area around and base of the cord should be cleaned with spirit. Nothing else should be used.
2. Refer to the pediatrician, if there are signs of infection such as:
   - Area of redness or tenderness around the cord
   - Cord is smelly or there is discharge
   - If the baby is ill or has a temperature above or below normal.

Temperature

Take the temperature of the baby in the axilla.

How to Measure Body Temperature in the Newborn?

The simplest way to measure body temperature in a newborn is by placing a thermometer in the axilla of the child. The thermometer should be kept for at least 5 minutes before taking the reading of the thermometer. The normal temperature of the baby is between 36.5 and 37°C. Axilla temperature is comparable to rectal temperature and is safer (less chances of injury and/or infection).

Hypothermia results in increased oxygen consumption and hypoxemia, increased glucose consumption, hypoglycemia and metabolic acidosis. Hypoxemia and hypoglycemia can result in death of the newborn. Among survivors, it can lead to permanent impairment of the brain resulting in developmental handicap.

Preventing Heat Loss

Heat loss at birth can be prevented by the following simple intervention:

1. Receive the baby in a dry, warm and clean towel, dry the baby well. While drying, make sure that the head is in a neutral position. Neither too flexed nor too extended. Discard the wet towel immediately and wrap/cover the baby (except for the face and upper chest) in a fresh, clean and dry towel. The baby should be kept wrapped during the assessment and suction ventilation applied (if required) to prevent heat loss.
2. Wrap the baby in loose multiple layer of light, but warm cloth. Blood meconium and some of the vernix will have been wiped off during drying at birth. The remaining vernix does not need to be removed as it is harmless, may reduce heat loss and is reabsorbed through the skin during the first few days of life.

3. Place the baby near a source of warmth. A normal baby, who is crying well after birth, can be placed in skin-to-skin contact with the mother's abdomen and covered with a dry cloth. The maternal body heat will provide the extra warmth required. It is also an additional assurance to the mother of the baby's well-being.
4. Ensure that during and after the delivery, no fans are running in the delivery room, and no windows are open through which air currents blow into the room.
5. While the baby needs to be kept clean, discourage the mother from giving a bath to the baby on the first day after birth. The mother or the birth attendant can clean the baby by wiping with a soft moist cloth. When the baby is given a bath, it should be done quickly in a warm room, using warm water in summer, depending upon the environmental temperature, the baby should be dressed in loose cotton cloths and kept indoors as far as possible. Low-birth-weight infants should not be given a bath. Instead, clean the baby with a soft clean cloth soaked in lukewarm water.

Airway and Breathing

If the baby is crying and the breathing is normal, then there is no need for resuscitation, provide normal care, and clear the upper airway by wiping the nose and mouth of the baby, and removing the secretions present there in. If the baby is not crying, assess the breathing, if the chest is rising symmetrically and the respiratory rate is > 30/min, no immediate action is needed. Remember, occasional gaps are not considered breathing.

Care of the Skin

Clean the blood, mucus and meconium on the baby before presenting to the mother. Bathing the babies soon after birth is not recommended. Postpone the first bath for the next day. Ensure that the baby's temperature is normal before giving a bath to the baby.

Care of the Eyes

- Do not clean eyes routinely
- It is common for a newborn baby to have some crusting or a little discharge
- The eyes should be bathed with clean water and cotton wool after handwashing
- Antibiotic eyedrops should not be used routinely
- Show the mother, how to bathe the eyes with clean water, if there is a discharge
- Ask the mother to the healthcare provide, if the eyes have not improved after 24 hours

- If the eyes are red or there is purulent discharge, a swab should be taken for culture and sensitivity from each eye and sent to the nearest laboratory, refer the baby to the doctor.

Feeding

Initiate breastfeeding within half-an-hour of a normal delivery. Ensure that the baby is sucking well. If suckling is poor, ensure correct positioning and attachment of the baby to the breast. Pregnancy is the ideal time to council the mother regarding the benefits of breastfeeding her baby, though breastfeeding is almost universal in India, a few points would need to be emphasized to mother.

Initiation of Breastfeeding

Counsel the mother that breastfeeding should ideally be initiated within half-an-hour of a normal delivery (or within 2 hour of a cesarean section or as the mother regains consciousness, in case she undergoes a cesarean section).

It is common practice in India to delay initiation. Colostrum (the first milk) is thrown away and prelacteal feeds are given instead. This has obvious disadvantages. First, the prelacteal feed may not be hygienic and can cause an intestinal infection in the baby. Second, the baby is deprived of colostrum, which is very rich in protective antibodies. Most importantly, the sucking and rooting reflex in the child, which are essential for the baby to successfully start breastfeeding, are the strongest, immediately after delivery making the process of initiation much easier for the mother and the baby. These reflexes gradually become weaker over the span of few hours, thus making breastfeeding difficult later on.

Exclusive Breastfeeding for 6 Months

It should be emphasized to the mother that only breast milk and nothing, but breast milk should be given to the baby for the first 6 months; not even water. The mother should be assured that breast milk has enough water to quench the baby's thirst (even in the peak of summer) and satisfy its hunger for the first 6 months. Take special care in the case of a female child to ensure that she is adequately breast fed and not discriminated against because of her sex.

Demand Feeding

Demand feeding refers to the practice of breastfeeding the child, whenever he/she demand it, as can be made out by the child crying. The practice of feeding the child by the clock should be actively discouraged. After few days of birth, most children will develop their own hunger cycle and will feed every 2–4 hours. Remember that each child is different as far as the feeding requirements and timing are concerned.

The practice of giving night feeds should be actively encouraged. Often there is a misconception that breastfeeding the baby at night disturbs the mother's sleep, thus depriving her of adequate rest inform the women and her husband that this is not so. Night feeds help the baby to sleep more soundly.

Rooming In

Rooming in refers to the practice of keeping the mother and baby in the same room and preferably on the same bed. This is usually practiced in the Indian setting. The practice should be encouraged, as it has certain advantages:

- Makes demand feeding easier to practice, as the mother can here the child cry
- Keep the baby warm, thus preventing hypothermia in the newborn
- Helps build a bond between the mother and baby.

Weight Changes

The baby should be weighed at birth. It is normal for the baby to loose weight in the first 3–4 days of life, primarily due to water loss from extracellular fluid. However, the weight loss in the first few days should not exceed 10% of the birth weight.

Immunization

1. All babies should be given bacille Calmette-Guérin (BCG), polio and hepatitis B vaccination immunization before discharge, if mother is found hepatitis B antigen positive or is infectious, the baby should be given hepatitis B immunoglobulin within the first 24–48 hours.
2. Babies who are admitted for long period in the nursery or special care baby unit (SCBU) should be immunized as soon as they are well-enough.
3. According to the expanded program on immunization (EPI) schedule, the dates should be filled in on the pink card and the due date for the next dose must be interred in the card and pointed out to the mother.

Chapter 21 Examination of the Newborn by the Pediatrician

All newborn babies should be examined by the pediatrician within the first 24 hours of birth, preferably in front of the mother, so that her questions can be answered.

HISTORY

The following should be checked before the examination:

- Mother medical obstetric and social history
- Outcome of previous pregnancies
- Information on labor, delivery and resuscitation
- Apgar score.

  Inquiry about the following:
- Feeding pattern, vomiting, frothing or choking
- Breathing difficulties
- Onset of jaundice
- Meconium and urine passage time.

FORMAL EXAMINATION

General Condition

Observe the baby's spontaneous behavior.

Skin

- Pallor
- Jaundice
- Cyanosis
- Good perfusion and abnormal skin lesions.

Head and Face

- Facial feature are normal
- Measure and record occipitofrontal circumference of the head
- Check fontanel's including size and tension of anterior fontanel
- Examine the eyes for cataracts, corneal opacity purulent discharge
- Check the red reflex
- Look at the ear for accessory skin tag, malformation or low set ears

- Check the mouth for presence of cleft palate, cleft lip and tongue tie
- Check the neck for swelling, cysts or tumor.

Heart and Lungs

- Record heart rate, normal heart rate should be between 120 and 160 beats per minute
- Listen for murmurs, accentuated second heart sound or crepitations
- Check for presence of femoral pulses and note the presence of hepatomegaly
- Check shape and symmetry of the chest
- Respiration rate should be between 35 and 45/min
- Check breathing pattern—tachypnea, apnea, stridor and recession
- Auscultate for air entry.

Abdomen

- Observe for any distension or visible vein inflammation, swelling and genitalia
- Palpate gently for any masses and/or presence of big liver, spleen or kidneys
- Check the genitalia and exclude undescended testes, hydrocele hypospadias or epispadias ambiguous genitalia, imperforated anus, enlargement of the clitoris or increased pigmentation.

Hips

Examine the hip for evidence of congenital dislocation in all babies especially girl baby born by breech delivery, post-term or large babies, this examination should be done at the end, since it may upset the baby and mother.

Skeletal System

- Full range of motion in all joints
- Note any deformities.

Hands and Feet

- Examine the arms, hands and legs
- Note any asymmetry or abnormalities, i.e. talipes, equinovarus, extra digits abnormalities of limb movement suggest neurological lesions, fracture, etc.

Back and Spine

- Turn the baby over and examine the back and spine
- Check the spina bifida occulta, hairy patches and for dermal sinus.

OBSERVATION

- Try to observe in quite awake state
- Check for abnormal posture including neck retraction frog-like posture and asymmetry
- Check tendon reflexes look for clonus, note any exaggeration or asymmetry
- Look for abnormal involuntary movements, i.e. jitteriness and seizures
- Check reflexes (moro, rooting, sucking and grasps)
- Assess visual fixation and reaction to sound
- When the examination is over, the mother should either be reassured that her baby is normal or if any abnormalities have been detected these should be explained to the mother
- All the findings (normal and abnormal) should be recorded
- If baby has any abnormalities that require admission to the nursery, full details of the condition should be kept in the neonatal record
- Explain to the parents, the reasons for admission into the nursery.

Chapter 22 Common Parental Questions/ Concerns and its Answers

Parents often worry about the appearance of their babies; following are the parents concern and need an explanation.

FONTANEL

The fontanel is the soft patch on top of the baby's head. This is where the skull bones have not yet fused together; the bones take more than a year to close over. The fontanel moves as the baby breathes. Under the skin is a tough layer of membrane.

BREASTS

A newborn baby's breast is often a little swollen and oozes some milk irrespective of whether the baby is a boy or a girl. Girls also sometimes bleed a little or have a white cloudy discharge from the vagina. All of this are the result of hormones passing from the mother to baby before birth. There is nothing to worry about this and it will stop after a few days, if left alone, the nipples should not be squeezed as it certainly does not help and may harm the baby by causing an infection.

BUMPS AND BRUISES

It is quite common for a newborn baby to have some swelling and bruises on the head and even to have bloodshot eyes. This is just the result of being born the marks fade very soon.

BIRTHMARKS AND SPOTS

Once the parents begin to look closely at their baby, they may find different marks and little spots, mainly on the head and face. This spots and rashes are very common in newborn babies and may appear and go. They should be left as such alone. Sometimes the marks are larger and may make worry the parents. Many of them fade gradually, but the parents should ask the doctor advice.

JAUNDICE

Some babies develop a yellow color to their skin after birth. This is normal and usually fades within 10 days or so, if it increases they need to bring the baby back to a doctor, a baby that is severely jaundiced will need treatment.

CRADLE CAP

It is quite common for babies to have scaling on their heads, this does not require any treatment and will gradually disappear, if the parents are worried they should be reassured and then advised to soften the scalp with oil before bath.

ECZEMA

Some babies have a more sensitive skin than others. Breastfed babies have fewer problems with eczema; the mother should be advised to add a little oil to the water in which she bathes the child and to avoid using too much soap. Moisturizing cream can be massaged into the skin. Steroid creams should not be used.

BONDING AND BREASTFEEDING

1. The most important function of the postnatal ward, nursery and special care baby unit (SCBU) is to assist the bonding between the mother and baby, to teach the mother, how to care for her baby both by giving breastfeeds and by keeping the baby clean and warm.
2. Bonding is important as all the other routine things done on these wards. The baby should be with mother all the time—day and night, unless the baby needs to be in the special care unit.

Recent research has revealed and still is revealing the many advantages to the mother who suckles and the infant who is suckled.

Breastfeeding

Advantages

1. Many pediatrician/senior nurses/elderly women recommends breastfeeding for 2 years, breastfeeding is the best and most natural way of feeding the newborn baby.
2. It is very satisfying and rewarding for a mother to feed her own baby. Breast milk and breastfeeding have many unique advantages for the mother and baby; new advantages are being discovered all the time.
3. Breastfeeding develops a loving relationship between the mother and baby.
4. Breast milk:
   - It has easily digested proteins, lactose or milk sugar and fat
   - It gives the baby all the nourishment required
   - Also contains antibodies to protect the babies against infections
   - It has a reduced risk of contamination
   - It is readily available.
5. Breastfeeding is advantages to the mother in the following ways:
   - It causes the uterus contract, which prevents prolonged blood loss

- The pelvic muscle regains their tone quicker
- The extra weight put on during pregnancy is used up in breastfeeding
- Birth spacing.

Establishing Breastfeeding

1. All normal full-term babies should be breastfed exclusively for the first 4 months.
2. Preterm and low-birth weight babies should be breastfed if the sucking reflex is developed, if they are unable to suck, a nasogastric tube should be passed and expressed breast milk is given.
3. It is very important to establish breastfeeding early and to emphasize to the mother, the importance of giving breast milk to her baby, so that the baby will have the best advantage of growing strong and healthy.
4. Explain to the mother, the importance of giving the colostrum to the baby.
5. Explain that no other feeds should be given and that is natural for there to be little milk in the breasts for the first few days after delivery. However, this colostrum is all the baby requires, so it is very important to breastfeed the baby on demand.
6. Babies should only be given expressed breast milk from his/her own mother in correct position; if the correct position for breastfeeding is used the women should have no serious problems.

Frequency of Feeds

The baby should be fed on demand. It is important to remember that every mother and baby are different, and some will feed faster and some slower. Encourage the mother that she will know best, what to do for her baby.

Ensuring Good Supply of Milk

1. Encourage the mother to breastfeed on demand, the more frequently the baby sucks, the more milk is produced.
2. Tell the mother that night feeding helps to develop a good milk supply and stimulates hormones that inhibit ovulation. The mother should be encouraged to keep her baby close to her at night and always breastfeed during the night.
3. Reassure the mother that, all breast, even they are small or soft, produce plenty of milk when the baby sucks.
4. Never give glucose water, other milk, other fluids or foods between, breastfeeds to normal baby until the baby has completed the 4th month of life.
5. If the mother feel there is insufficient milk, reassure her and encourage her to breastfeed frequently to increase the milk production.
6. Encourage the mother to drink plenty of liquids every day and eat extra food to make more milk.

7. Explain to her the importance of taking regular iron and folic acid tablets for 3 months following the delivery.
8. Advise her to rest whenever possible. This is often very difficult for the busy mother, but suggests that she lies down to breastfeed sometimes.

Bonding

The most important function of the postnatal ward is to assist the bonding between the mother and baby. The mother must be encouraged to care for the baby at all times.

Cleanliness

Before express milk, mothers must wash their hands thoroughly with water. If they are using a breast pump, make sure it is clean before begin. Follow directions supplied with the pump for advice on proper cleaning. Make sure that the collection containers are sterile.

Refrigerating Breast Milk

- Always express milk into a sterile bottle
- Cover mark and date the bottle
- Breast milk can be kept in a refrigerator on the top shelf for up to 24 hours
- Discard if not used in that time.

Breast Care

Washing

Advise the mother that her breasts only require washing once a day with clean water and advise her not to use soap too often because soap dries out the skin, which can cause painful nipples, advise her to wash her hands thoroughly with soap and water before feeding.

Hardness of Breast

Explain the mother that breasts often become enlarged and hard when the milk comes in around the 3rd day:

1. This is quite normal and is due to venous congestion following the increased blood flow to the breasts.
2. The mother should be advised and encouraged to give frequent breastfeeds in early days, which will help to reduce the hardness.
3. Some women find warm or cold cloths applied to the breasts will be helpful, others find gentle massage with olive oil helpful.
4. Sometimes it is necessary to hand express some milk before a feed. This softens the breast, so that the baby can take the areola into his/her mouth.

Sore Nipples

The nipples should not become sore, if the mother is shown how to breastfeed correctly. However, if they do become sore, the following may be helpful:

- Check that the baby has the nipple and areola well into baby mouth, failure to ensure this is the most common cause of cracked nipples
- Advise the mother to breastfeed more often and to limit sucking to about 10 minutes on each side
- Encourage her to relax and get into a comfortable position before starting to feed, so that the milk flows more easily
- Suggest that she starts the flow by hand expressing some milk before the feed
- Advise the mother to start breastfeeding on the side, which is less sore as sucking is strongest at the beginning of a feed
- Teach the mother how to take the baby off the breast, by either putting a finger in the baby's mouth or by pressing down on baby's chin
- Never pull the baby off the breast
- Advise the mother to breastfeed in different positions to see, which is the most comfortable.

Blocked Milk Duct

Blocked milk duct is diagnosed when there is localized hardness of breast without reddening, it is not normal, if it is detected then the following steps have to be followed:

- Advise the mother to breastfeed more often, so that the breast is as empty as possible
- Hand express the milk between feeds, if the baby is full
- Before feeds, put a warm, wet cloth on the tender area or soak the breast in a bowl of warm water and gently stroke the lump toward the nipple whilst the baby is feeding
- If a fever develops or if the pain persists, the mother should see a doctor
- Frequent breastfeeding, rest and application of warm cloths should continue during any treatment with antibiotics.

BATHING A BABY

1. The vernix protects the baby, so the baby should not be bathed for the first 24 hours. However, the baby should be cleaned off blood and meconium with clean cotton wool or towel.
2. The mother should be shown, how to bath a baby before she goes home, this can be done in groups by a trained nurse.
3. The baby must be well enough and warm enough to have a bath.
4. The room should be warm and free of draughts and doors should be closed.

5. All the preparations should be made before the baby is undressed. The water should be in the right temperature. Soap washed clothes and clean warm towels should be within easy reach. Ensure that the nappy area is clean before the baby is put in the bath.
6. The infant should be bathed before a feed and after checking that the temperature is normal.

Equipment

- Mediswabs
- Nappy
- Clean cloths
- Sterile cotton balls/face towel
- Soap
- Disposal bag.

Directions

1. Wash hands thoroughly with Hibiscrub.
2. Undress the baby except for the nappy and wrap in a clean towel.
3. Prepare the bath water and test the temperature with fingers, if it feels pleasantly warm to you then it will be safe for the baby.
4. Using the sterile cotton wool, clean the face and ears avoiding the eyes completely.
5. Dry the face with sterile cotton wool.
6. Wash the head with baby soap and rinse well, dry thoroughly.
7. Unwrap the baby in the cot and remove the nappy and clean only perineum, if baby has passed meconium.
8. Soap your hands and wash the arms, trunk and legs ensuring that all the skin folds, and between the fingers and toes are included.
9. Role the baby toward you and apply soap to back and buttocks.
10. Grasp the baby firmly, but gently using left arm to support baby's shoulders and the left hand to hold baby's upper arm.
11. The right hand should support the baby's buttock, while having a firm grip on the left thigh.
12. Immerse the baby in the bathtub and rinse off with the right hand, while still supporting the baby with the left arm, then remove the baby from the bathtub and dry with a towel in the cot ensuring that all the skin folds and creases are thoroughly dried.
13. Dress the baby and wrap up warmly.
14. As far as possible the mother should give bathing and caring for their own baby. The role of the nurse is to first demonstrate the procedure and supervise the mother until she is confident and relaxed when handling her baby.

Chapter 23 Neonatal Resuscitation

IMMEDIATE NEWBORN CONDITIONS OR PROBLEMS

1. The newborn has serious conditions or problems:
   - Gasping or not breathing
   - Breathing with difficulty (< 30 or > 60 breaths per minute, indrawing of the chest or grunting)
   - Central cyanosis (blueness)
   - Preterm or very low birth weight (< 32 week gestation or < 1,500 g)
   - Lethargy
   - Hypothermia [axillary temperature < 35°C (95°F)]
   - Convulsions.
2. The newborn has other conditions or problems that require attention in the delivery room:
   - Low birth weight (1,500–2,500 g)
   - Possible bacterial infection in an apparently normal newborn, whose mother had prelabor or prolonged rupture of membranes or amnonitis
   - Possible congenital syphilis in newborn whose mother has a positive serologic test for syphilis or is symptomatic.

MANAGEMENT

Two situations require immediate management:

1. Gasping or not breathing.
2. Cyanosis (blueness) or breathing with difficulty.

Cyanosis or Breathing with Difficulty

1. If the baby is cyanotic (bluish) or having difficulty in breathing (< 30 or > 60 breaths per minute, indrawing of the chest or grunting), give oxygen by nasal catheter or prongs:
   - Suction the mouth and nose to ensure airways are clear
   - Give oxygen at 0.5 L/min by nasal catheter or nasal prongs.
2. When using oxygen, remember:
   - Supplemental oxygen for difficulty in breathing or cyanosis
   - If the baby is having severe indrawing of the chest, is gasping for breath or is persistently cyanotic, increase the concentration of oxygen by nasal catheter, nasal prongs or oxygen hood.

Note: Indiscriminate the use of supplemental oxygen for premature infants has been associated with risk of blindness.

Gasping or Not Breathing

General Management

- Dry the baby, remove the wet cloth and wrap the baby in a dry warm cloth
- Clamp and cut the cord immediately, if not already done
- Move the baby to a firm, warm surface under a radiant heater for resuscitation
- Observe standard infection prevention practices when caring for and resuscitating newborn.

RESUSCITATION

Objectives

1. The primary objectives of resuscitation are prevention and correction of:
   - Hypoxia
   - Hypercapnia
   - Acidosis.

   This is achieved by restoring and maintaining respiration and circulation.
2. Secondary objectives are to prevent:
   - Hypothermia
   - Hypoglycemia and hypovolemia
   - Hypovolemia and shock.

Equipment and Drugs

1. All delivery and neonatal care units must have a full set of resuscitation equipment.
2. If there are any deficiencies, the pediatrician should identify and noticed concerned person.
3. The equipment must be checked daily and in each shift.
4. A notebook or register must be kept on the trolley to keep a record of the equipment and the drugs, and should be counter signed daily after checking all the items:
   - Equipment is functioning
   - Missing items are replaced
   - Outdated supplies are replaced.

Equipment

- Resuscitaire with overhead heating and lighting
- Oxygen source with a flowmeter

- An extra oxygen cylinder should be available, check that the cylinder is always full
- Ambu or Laerdal bag with a functioning pop-off valve
- Facemask
- Mucus extractor
- Suction catheters size (68 and 10 Fr)
- Oropharyngeal airway
- Endotracheal tube (ETT) of internal diameter
- Pediatric laryngoscope with straight neonatal blades
- Malleable wire stylet with blunt tip stabilizes ETT during insertion
- Nasogastric tubes, size 6 FG and 8 FG for gastric decompression
- Pediatric stethoscope
- Sterile syringes of size 1 mL, 2 mL, 5 mL,10 mL, 20 mL and 50 mL with needles
- Umbilical vein catheter sizes
- Intravenous cannula
- Scissors, cord clamp and adhesives
- Containers of blood sample
- Dextrostix
- Transport incubator gloves to be used in suspected hepatitis B or human immunodeficiency virus (HIV) cases.

Drugs

- Adrenaline 1:10,000 solution (3–10 mL ampules)
- Sodium bicarbonate 8.4% solution
- Volume expanders (50 mL)
- Plasma protein fraction
- Albumin (5%)
- Normal saline 0.9% or Ringer's lactate
- Dextrose 10% solution
- Naloxone hydrochloride (infant 0. 2 mg/mL)
- Vitamin K injection.

Resuscitation Procedure at Birth

Evaluation

Evaluation is primarily based upon:

- Heart rate (if single most important sign)
- Respiration
- Color.

Apgar score: It is an objective assessment of the degree of asphyxia or lack of it. It is not used to determine when to initiate resuscitation or to make decision regarding the course of resuscitation. It may be helpful in assessing the infant's condition and the effectiveness of resuscitative effort. The decision on intervention needed depends upon the condition of the infant.

The Apgar score of the baby indicates baby's well-being. It should be calculated at 1 minute and at 5 minutes after birth. The criteria for judging the Apgar score is given in Table 23.1. An Apgar score greater than 7 is considered satisfactory.

Table 23.1: Apgar score

Parameter	0	1	2
Respiratory effort	Absent	Gasping	Good cry
Heart rate	Zero	< 100/min	> 100/min
Color (cyanosis)	Central cyanosis	Peripheral cyanosis	Pink
Muscle tone	Flaccid	Partial flexion of the extremities	Complete flexion
Reflex (response to nasal catheter)	None	Grimace	Cry, cough, sneeze
Color	Pale blue	Body; pink, extremities; blue	Completely pink

Prevention of Hypothermia

No matter, how flat the baby is invest a few seconds, before commencing resuscitation to dry the baby and prevent hypothermia:

1. Turn on the clock at the birth.
2. Transfer the baby to the Resuscitaire, place baby under the warmer.
3. Wipe off all the excess liquor with a dry, warm towel to avoid heat loss. Special attention to the head and face.
4. Remove the wet sheets and cover the baby with dry warm sheets.
5. Clear the airway with gentle suction, ensuring that only mouth and upper airway are cleared. Mouth is suctioned first before the nose, in order to ensure that nothing is aspirated from the mouth. Be careful that suction near the vocal cords tends to cause spasm and reflex bradycardia.
6. Assess the condition of the baby very quickly.
7. If the baby is severely asphyxiated, immediate resuscitation is needed.

Score: Each baby should have a score for each of the signs. These are added together to give the Apgar score. This is done at 1 minute, 5 minutes and at 10 minutes:

- Severe birth asphyxia: 0–3
- Mild to moderate asphyxia: 4–6
- Normal: 7 and more.

Intervention

1. Normal baby (Apgar score > 7).
2. If the heart rate is above 100 beats per minute (bpm) and the baby is pink, active and with a good cry, and breathing spontaneously within second then:
   - Dry the baby, wrap in prewarmed sheets
   - Handover to the mother to cuddle
   - Advise the mother to immediately start breastfeeding
   - Observe and begin routine care.
3. Mild to moderate asphyxia (Apgar score 4–6):
   - If the heart rate is above 100 bpm and the baby is blue, but breathing then clear the airway and give facial oxygen
   - If the heart rate above 100 bpm, the baby is blue and is not breathing spontaneously or respiratory effort is poor or not well-established then:
     - Clear the airway
     - Stimulate gently by rubbing on the back
     - Give oxygen by facial mask or with artificial ventilation using resuscitation bag and mask
     - Do not pinch.
4. Severe birth asphyxia (Apgar score 0–3):
   - If the heart rate is below 100 bpm, the baby is blue, apneic or gasping then:
     - Begin artificial ventilation (bag and mask)
     - Reassess baby after 2 minutes.
   - If preterm baby, consider in intubation
   - If the heart rate is below 60 bpm, the baby is blue/white, apneic and limp, then:
     - Begin cardiac massage
     - Call for help.
   - If there is thick particulate meconium present in the upper airway, then:
     - Suck the upper airway, intubate and suck below the cords
     - Give oxygen and artificial ventilation as needed.
   - If maternal pethidine/morphine or omnopon is given, then use neonatal naloxone intravenously (naloxone 0.02 mg/kg early)
   - Consider giving an additional dose intramuscularly, as the half-life is longer in the baby and respiratory depression can occur in the postnatal ward.

TECHNIQUE OF ARTIFICIAL VENTILATION

Tactile Stimulation

1. **Foot slap or flick:** Stimulating the soles of the feet either by slapping or flicking the feet, often initiates respiration in the mildly depressed infant.
2. **Back rub:** Quickly and firmly rubbing the infants back is another safe method of attempting to initiate respiration.

Bag and Mask

1. Select appropriate size of infant mask and connect it to the Ambu resuscitation bag, connect this bag to oxygen. Set the flow of oxygen at 4-6 L/min.
2. Position infant with the head slightly downward and neck extended slightly.
3. Place a folded towel under the shoulders for support and to maintain position.
4. Suck the upper airway.
5. Apply mask to face covering the nose and mouth.
6. Ensure adequate pressure seal.
7. Hold the lateral edges of the mask with thumb and index finger.
8. Give positive pressure ventilation by compressing the bag with the other hand at a rate of 40–60/min. Set the flow of oxygen at 4–6 L/min.
9. Decompress the stomach by inserting a nasogastric tube, if bagging is required for > 2 minutes or if there is abdominal distension.
10. Use a correct technique of bag and mask, ensuring good seal around the face and checking for:
    - Symmetrical chest expansion.
    - Increase in heart rate.
    - Improvement in color.

Major Steps on Orogastric Catheter Procedure

1. Always measure the length of the catheter, which is going to insert. It must be long enough to reach the stomach, but not so long as to perforate it. The length of the inserted catheter should be equal to the distance from the bridge of nose to the earlobe and from the earlobe to the xiphoid process (the lower tip of the sternum). To minimize interruption of ventilation, measurement of the orogastric tube can be approximated with the mask in place.
2. Insert the catheter through the mouth rather than the nose. The nose should be left open for ventilation (ventilation can be resumed as soon as the catheter has been placed).

3. Once the catheter is inserted to the desired distance, attach a 20 mL syringe and quickly, but gently remove the gastric contents.

Endotracheal Intubation

1. Prepare the correct size of ETT (with or without a stylet, stylet must not be beyond tip of tube).
2. Position the infant with the head downward and chin extended slightly.
3. Introduce the laryngoscope blade into the right corner of the mouth and push the tongue slightly to the left.
4. Visualize the mouth structures and the vocal cord.
5. Suck out any secretions.
6. Identify the epiglottis, place the tip of the blade between the base of the tongue and the epiglottis (vallecular space). Lift blade and visualize the epiglottis opening.
7. A slight pressure downward on the anterior neck may be required.
8. Pass the ETT into the glottis avoiding trauma.
9. Connect the Ambu resuscitation bag to the ETT.
10. Begin intermittent positive pressure ventilation (IPPV).
11. Ventilate the baby at a rate of about 40–60 minutes using 5 L oxygen flow in a minute. Use sufficient pressure to produce adequate chest expansion.
12. Check that tube has not entered the right main bronchus by listening, with a stethoscope for equal air entry.
13. Check for effectiveness of bagging, it includes:
    - The heart rate rapidly increases
    - The color of the skin returns to normal
    - The breath sounds are heard all over the lungs fields
    - Spontaneous movement returns
    - The baby begins to breath spontaneously and the chest movements are equal.

Failure to Improve In Spite of Adequate Ventilation

If the baby is not improving, in spite of adequate artificial ventilation consider the following:

1. Recheck the equipment being used (oxygen flow is on, oxygen cylinder not empty, Ambu/Laerdal bag not leaking).
2. Endotracheal tube wrongly placed. The tube may be in the main bronchus or in the esophagus. Confirmation of correct tube position can obtained by chest X-ray.
3. The tube is blocked by secretions.
4. Severe blood loss.

5. Pneumothorax.
6. Circulatory collapse: Call for help, transfer to special care baby unit (SCBU), if available.

Correction of circulatory collapse: After 30 seconds of adequate ventilation with 100% oxygen, if the heart rate remains < 60 bpm, additional measures must be initiated and it includes:

- Ensure adequate ventilation has been established
- External cardiac massage
- Emergency drugs.

External Cardiac Massage

- Place the infant on a firm surface in a level position
- Place the tips of first and second fingers perpendicularly on the lower one third of the baby's sternum
- Compress the baby's chest wall by 1.27–1.90 cm at a rate of approximately 100 per minute with steady rate and depth
- Do not use excessive force and do not lift off fingers from chest
- Continue with artificial ventilation simultaneously, discontinue when heart rate > 80 bpm
- Excessive and misplaced force can cause liver laceration, fractures of ribs and pneumothorax.

EMERGENCY DRUGS

1. Might be required, if heart rate is < 80 bpm after 30 seconds with 100% oxygen and external cardiac massage.
2. In majority of resuscitation situations, drugs are not required. The most important is oxygen.
3. The easiest way to give drugs is through an umbilical venous catheter.
4. A drug dose chart should be stuck on every Resuscitaire for quick reference.

When to Stop

1. Irreversible brain damage will occur, if the infant remains profoundly asphyxiated and unresponsive.
2. Repeat the cycle of evaluation, ventilation, chest compressions and drugs three times.
3. If the infant remains unresponsive after full resuscitative measures, do not continue resuscitation.
4. Do not continue resuscitation after 10 minutes if:

- There is no heartbeat
- There is no spontaneous response
- The pupils are fixed and dilated.

5. It is important to tell the mother that what is happening to her baby:
   - Whether or not resuscitation is successful, the baby should be wrapped in a towel and given to the mother, so that she can see and hold her baby
   - She may want to see the whole body and her wishes must be respected.

Chapter 24

Nursing Care in Different Conditions

CARE OF THE NEWBORN INFANT FROM HIV- OR HBSAg-POSITIVE MOTHER

Adequate facilities must be available for the resuscitation of all infants in this group; however certain procedures must be modified:

1. The use of unprotected mouth suction using mucus extraction, should be abandoned for these deliveries. A portable suction or bulb suction should be used.
2. The receiving nurse should wear gloves, an apron and a gown. Face protection should not be necessary if proper suction equipment is available, but facial splashing should be avoided. After the resuscitation, the non-disposable equipment including mattresses must be cleaned with sodium hypochlorite solution, then washed with detergent and hot water.
3. After the baby is born, he/she should be bathed in the labor room and hair washed. Great care must be taken to avoid hypothermia. The baby should then be cared for with and mainly by the mother at all times. Gloves should be worn whilst handling the infant.
4. The infant should be breast fed normal way.
5. Blood should be sent from the infant to check for the infant's human immunodeficiency virus (HIV) or hepatitis B (HB) status as necessary. The presence of a positive enzyme-linked immunosorbent assay (ELISA) test for HIV.

Acquired Immunodeficiency Syndrome

Description

Acquired immunodeficiency syndrome (AIDS) is an immune disorder spread by the HIV through contact with blood and body secretions.

Etiology/Incidence

- Exposure through infected mother
- Exposure to contaminated blood (transfusion).

Pathophysiology

- Generalized dysfunction of the immune system
- Deficiencies in both cell mediated (screening and removal of infectious organisms) and humoral (development of antibodies) immunities.

Assessment Findings

1. Symptoms develop within the first 24 months of life.
2. General symptoms include:
   - Failure to thrive
   - Fever
   - Chronic lymphadenopathy
   - Profuse diarrhea
   - Anemia
   - Enlargement of lymph nodes, spleen and liver.
3. Opportunistic infections develop (recurrent upper respiratory tract infections, oral candidiasis and chronic diarrhea).
4. Neurologic symptoms include the progressive encephalopathy, developmental delay and loss of developmental milestones.

Diagnostic Evaluation

1. Children aged 13 months to 13 years, should meet one or more of the following criteria:
   - Confirmed HIV in blood or tissue (ELISA or Western blot tests)
   - Symptoms meeting centers for disease control (CDC) case definition
   - Evidence of HIV antibody.
2. Children younger than 13 months should meet one or more of the following criteria:
   - Confirmed HIV in blood or tissue
   - Symptoms meeting CDC case definition
   - Evidence of cellular, humoral deficiency and HIV antibodies.

Nursing Diagnoses

- High risk for infection
- Altered nutrition
- Altered growth and development
- Ineffective family coping
- Pain
- Fear.

Planning and Implementation

1. Promote good health practices in the areas of nutrition and hygiene.
2. Protect child from contact with infection:
   - Isolate child from children, who have had poliomyelitis
   - Prepare foods safely.
3. Teach infection prevention measures to family members (hand washing and proper disposal of infected items).

4. Provide diet that is high in protein, calories and vitamins; provide supplements.
5. Provide stimulation to infant and occupational or physical therapy to older child.
6. Provide emotional support to family members.
7. Enhance parenting skills by encouraging parents to hold and cuddle the child.
8. Provide referrals to appropriate community services.
9. Administer medications as ordered, which may include zidovudine (Retrovir) that appears to slow disease progression.

Evaluation

- Child and family follow good health practices
- Child shows no sign of infection
- Child maintains adequate nutritional intake or diet as necessary
- Family feels supported and uses community services
- Child shows steady development progress
- Parental self-esteem increases.

HYPOGLYCEMIA IN NEWBORN

Rate of glucose utilization in preterm babies is 6–8 mg/kg/min, as compared to adult values of 2–4 mg/kg/min. This is the reason why neonatal brain is more prone to damage with low blood sugar level. Hypoglycemia is therefore a preventable cause of mental retardation and cerebral palsy. Recurrent and persistent hypoglycemia is usually due to serious metabolic or endocrine disorders. There is no consensus on what is low blood sugar in a newborn. Because of the potentially serious consequences, most people feel that any infant with blood glucose level less than 2.2 mmol (40 mg%) should be investigated and treated.

Etiology

- Limited glycogen supply
- Prematurity
- Perinatal stress
- Starvation
- Glycogen storage disease
- Hyperinsulinism:
  - Infant of diabetic mother (IDM)
  - Erythroblastosis fetalis
  - Maternal drug therapy.

- Diminished glucose production:
  - Small for date babies
  - Genetic metabolic disorders.

Symptoms

- Poor feeding
- Lethargy
- Cyanosis
- Tremors or jittery movements
- Seizures
- Recurrent apnea
- Hypothermia
- Weak- or high-pitched cry
- Asymptomatic.

Investigations

- Dextrostix
- Blood sugar
- Complete blood count (CBC) differential and hematocrit
- Serum electrolytes
- Investigate for sepsis.

Treatment

At risk well infant: Monitor dextrostix on arrival at 3, 6, 12, 24 hourly intervals, frequency would depend upon individual situation. Early feeding with 30–50% more than standard requirements via nasogastric (NG) feeds at 1–2 hourly intervals. Start breastfeeding and wean gradually, increasing feed intervals, while monitoring with dextrostix.

Symptomatic infants: About 2 mL/kg bolus of 10% dextrose followed by an infusion of 8 mg/kg/min until the blood sugar is normal. Do not give concentrated solutions of glucose. Reduce the amount of intravenous (IV) dextrose slowly whilst increasing oral feeds, to avoid rebound hypoglycemia.

CONVULSION IN THE NEWBORN

Only a small percentage of newborns experience classic adult type generalized tonic-clonic seizures, because of immaturity of the brain. Presentation in the newborn often takes a subtle form:

- Rhythmic eye movements (jerking or blinking)
- Gaze abnormalities
- Chewing or lip smacking

- Abnormal postures
- Apnea/Bradycardias
- Pedaling/Cycling movement.

Etiology

- Birth asphyxia
- Severe birth trauma
- Metabolic problems, e.g. hypoglycemia or hypocalcemia
- Hyponatremia
- Infections, e.g. meningitis
- Intracranial bleeding
- Cerebral malformation
- Genetic metabolic disorders.

History

- Unexplained neonatal deaths (genetic metabolic disorders)
- Diabetes in mother
- Fetal distress (meconium-stained liquor/type II dips)
- Traumatic (instrumental) delivery, shoulder dystocia less than 2.5 kg or greater than 4 kg
- Age at first convulsion
- Feeding prior to convulsion.

Investigations

Final choice will be guided by availability and clinical setting. The following should be considered:

- Estimation of blood glucose
- Hemoglobin (Hb), CBC—total, differential and platelets
- Lumbar puncture
- Culture [blood, cerebrospinal fluid (CSF) and urine]
- Cranial ultrasound.

Treatment

Supportive Treatment

- Clear the airway
- Ensure oxygenation
- Nutrition: Breast or NG feeding
- Restrict fluids to 40 mL/kg/day on 1st day of life following birth asphyxia.

Specific Treatment

Specific treatments include anticonvulsants:

1. **Phenobarbitone:** 20 mg/kg slowly IV over 15 minutes. Maintenance dose 3 mg/kg/day IV or oral as single dose, starting 24 hours after loading dose.
2. **Phenytoin:** 10 mg/kg slow IV injection and maintenance dose of 3 mg/kg/day oral or IV.
3. **Diazepam:** Not good for maintenance, effective for rapid control of seizures; risk of apnea.

Top priority in a seizing baby is to exclude hypoglycemia by a bedside dextrostix if low, draw blood sugar sample and immediately administer IV glucose. Second priority is to look for and to treat other treatable disorders, i.e. sepsis, hypocalcemia, hyponatremia and hypomagnesemia. Recognition of seizure is the most difficult aspect of treating seizures in newborn.

JAUNDICE IN THE NEWBORN

Types

1. **Pathological jaundice:**
   - Clinically visible in first 24 hours
   - Total bilirubin greater than 250 μmol/L at any time
   - Direct (conjugated) bilirubin greater than 30 μmol/L
   - Clinical jaundice persisting for more than 2 weeks.
2. **Early jaundice:** It is usually unconjugated hemolytic jaundice may appear in the first 24 hours. The common causes are:
   - ABO incompatibility
   - Glucose-6-phosphate dehydrogenase (G6PD) deficiency
   - Sepsis
   - Rhesus isoimmunization (less common)
   - Cephalohematoma
   - Polycythemia.
3. **Prolonged jaundice:** Often conjugated jaundice persisting more than 2 weeks. The common causes are:
   - Infection
   - Congenital hypothyroidism
   - Neonatal hepatitis.

History

- Jaundice in a sibling
- Unexplained illness during pregnancy
- Family history of anemia

- Traumatic delivery
- Delayed passage of meconium
- History suggestive of sepsis.

Examination

- Prematurity
- G6PD deficiency
- Sepsis
- Rhesus isoimmunization (less common)
- Cephalohematoma
- Polycythemia
- Petechiae
- Hepatosplenomegaly.

Basic Laboratory Data

- Mother blood group, antibody screen and indirect Coombs' test
- Hemoglobin, hematocrit and reticulocyte count
- Red cell morphology
- Serum bilirubin: Total and direct
- Treatment.

General Support

- Explain the mother about physiological jaundice
- Keep the baby warm
- Feeding: Give adequate fluid and nutrition via breast/gastrostomy tube or IV, depending upon severity and condition of infant.

Specific Treatment

- Plot the bilirubin on the graph and follow recommendation
- Phototherapy should be started according to the level of bilirubin
- Exchange transfusion may be required, if the jaundice is severe.

Phototherapy

1. Position the phototherapy unit 25–30 cm from baby in a cot or 5 cm above the top of the incubator.
2. Baby is nursed naked.
3. If the infant is in an incubator, light rays should be perpendicular to the surface of the incubator in order to minimize loss of efficacy due to reflectance.

4. Use appropriate eye shades (size and type) to protect the eyes:
   - Baby shades (small)
   - Baby shades (large) hydrogel adhesive is used to position on baby
   - Eye max (term infants).
5. Eye pads should be removed 4 hourly and eye cares attended with normal saline.
6. Use the phototherapy light meter to check the unit's light output each duty output should be over 10 mcW/nm/cm^2 on all body surfaces.
7. To avoid the possibility of burns, do not use baby lotions or creams on baby's skin.
8. Phototherapy lamps act as a source of radiant heat. Monitor the baby's temperature closely when commencing phototherapy and adjust incubator temperature as required to avoid overheating.
9. Decrease incubator temperature when phototherapy is commenced.
10. Recheck axilla temperature within half-an-hour of making adjustment.

Nursing Management

1. Do not expose babies to direct sunlight. The possible benefit is far outweighed by the risk of hypothermia or hyperthermia and dehydration.
2. Encourage the mother to feed frequently. This promotes peristalsis and therefore diminishes enterohepatic circulation of bilirubin. Keep the baby with the mother and encourage breastfeeding on demand and more frequently.
3. Do not give extra feeds of glucose water and breastfeeding, very rarely need to be stopped. This might be necessary when an exchange transfusion is about to be carried out.

NURSING MANAGEMENT OF A LOW-BIRTH-WEIGHT BABY

Low-birth-weight Babies

Definition

1. Low birth weight (LBW): A baby who weighs less than 2.5 kg at birth.
2. Babies may be born small because they are preterm (born early) or because they have not grown adequately in utero, small for gestational age (SGA), small for dates and dysmature.
3. About two third of the LBW are SGA and one third are preterm, infants who are LBW, are more prone to metabolic problems, require higher calorie intake and have more mature lungs. Preterm babies problems are more related to immaturity of organ system, i.e. lungs.

Problems of Preterm and Low-birth-weight Babies

- Respiratory distress
- Asphyxia
- Infections
- Apnea
- Hypoglycemia
- Hypocalcemia
- Hypothermia.

Management

Management of the premature or LBW baby can be divided into the following headings:

- General basic principles
- Warmth/Prevention of hypothermia
- Oxygen requirements
- Feeding and nutrition
- Treatment of specific problems
- Phototherapy (discussed earlier).

General basic principles

- Effective resuscitation at birth
- Minimal handling
- Nurse the baby prone or on the side
- Monitor the vital signs.

Warmth/Prevention of hypothermia

Newborn babies lose heat rapidly at birth due to a large surface area as the baby is wet and the delivery rooms are usually cold. Hypothermia increases the metabolic activity and therefore oxygen consumption, and can cause hypoglycemia. There is a direct relation between hypothermia and neonatal, mortality and morbidity. Prevention of hypothermia is therefore essential in the management of the sick and LBW and preterm babies:

- Keep labor, postnatal and nursery room warm (26–28°C)
- Exclude draught (close doors and windows)
- Dry the baby thoroughly at birth before commencing resuscitation and remove wet towels
- Cover the baby with prewarmed blankets
- Cover the head, 40% of the heat loss in the newborn is from the head
- Place infant under radiant warmer, if necessary (Fig. 24.1)
- Monitor the temperature regularly (axilla not rectal temperature)
- Nurse the baby in an incubator if the temperature is unstable, the birth weight is 1.5 kg or less
- Avoid making the baby hypoxic or hypothermic during procedures such as insertion of an IV line, suction, lumbar puncture, etc.

- The LBW baby can be dressed fully and nursed in an incubator or a cot, if the axilla temperature is within a normal range.

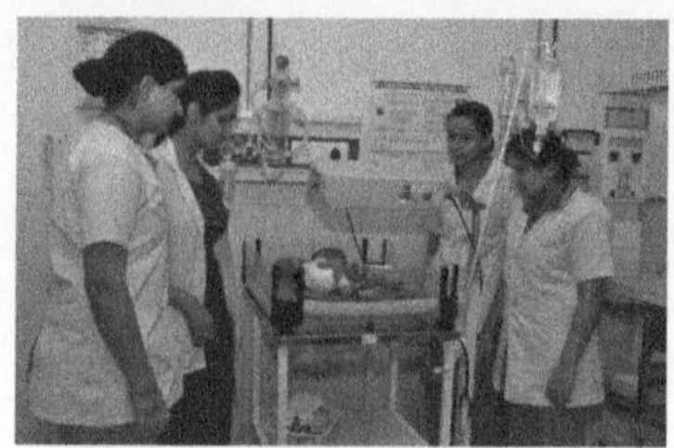

Fig. 24.1: Neonate in warmer (*Courtesy:* Anil Baghi, Multispecialty Hospital, Ferozepur, Punjab)

Oxygen requirements

- Be ready to resuscitate a LBW baby in the labor room
- Give adequate resuscitation at birth
- Give oxygen if required (cyanosis and/or hypoxemia)
- Do not routinely put babies in oxygen
- Remember the dangers of oxygen toxicity especially in the preterm baby.

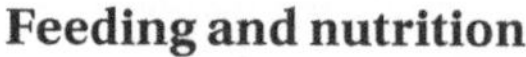

Feeding and nutrition

1. Babies who are able to suck and swallow should be breast fed on demand, if the suckling reflex has not yet developed, the baby should be fed with expressed breast milk (EBM) through a NG tube, breast suckling should still be attempted for 'let down reflex' and psychological advantages for short periods.
2. Nasogastric feeds should be introduced slowly then gradually increased according to the baby's tolerance.
3. If babies cannot tolerate oral feeds, an IV line should be inserted and IV fluids given.

CARE OF BABY IN INCUBATOR

Infants should be nursed in the neutral thermal environment and have a core body temperature between 36.5 and 37.2°C. The neutral thermal environment is the temperature range where heat production is at the minimum needed to maintain normal body temperature. It depends on birth weight, postnatal age and whether the infant is clothed or naked. Because heat production requires oxygen consumption and glucose use, persistent hypothermia may deplete these stores, leading to metabolic acidosis, hypoglycemia, decreased surfactant production, increased caloric requirements and if chronic, impaired weight gain. Infants lose heat through conduction, convection, radiation and evaporation. Nursing care is critical in supporting thermoregulation through ongoing assessments and environmental interventions to decrease heat loss for the infant being cared for in an incubator.

Indications

An infant may require an incubator for the following reasons:

- When they are not maintaining their own temperature with clothing and wrapping

- When they are acutely unwell and close observation is required
- When they are at risk of abnormal heat loss
- They have a known infection/or the potential to develop sepsis
- There are nutritional concerns (given that infants use a large proportion of their calorific intake for maintaining their temperature)
- They are SGA, they have a large wound site
- New stoma (not always indicated) or exposed bowel.

RESPIRATORY SYSTEM

Essential Concepts

Development

1. Appearance of the laryngotracheal groove around the 4th week of gestation is closely followed by development of the larynx and trachea.
2. Development of the bronchial tree occurs predominantly between 5 and 16 weeks of gestation.
3. In gestation period of 16–24 weeks, luminal and blood vessel growth occurs in bronchi and bronchioles.
4. Production of surfactant (a phospholipids protein complex that reduces surface tension of the alveoli, thereby decreasing tendency of alveoli to collapse during expiration) begins at about 24 weeks of gestation.
5. Two surface—tension reducing substances such as lecithin and sphingomyelin, can be detected in amniotic fluid and are useful predictors of lung maturity; a lecithin-sphingomyelin ratio of 2:1 or greater indicates fetal lung maturity.
6. The presence of phosphatidylglycerol in amniotic fluid also indicates fetal lung maturity.
7. At birth, the lungs contain fluid; this is replaced by air as the infant begins respiration.
8. Lungs continue to develop after birth and new alveoli are formed until about age of 8 years. Thus, a child with pulmonary damage or disease at birth may regenerate new pulmonary tissue and eventually attain normal respiratory function.

Function

1. The major respiratory system function is to oxygenate arterial blood and remove carbon dioxide (CO_2) from venous blood, a process known as gas exchange.
2. Normal gas exchange depends on three process:
   - Ventilation—movement of gases from the atmosphere to the alveoli
   - Diffusion—transfer of inhaled gases across the alveolar membrane to the lung

- Perfusion—movement of oxygenated blood from the lungs to body tissues.

3. Control respiration involves neural and chemical processes:
   - The neural system, comprising four parts located in the pons, medulla and spinal cord, coordinates respiratory rhythm and regulates depth of respirations
   - Chemical processes perform several vital functions including:
     - Regulate alveolar ventilation and maintain normal blood gas tension
     - Guard against hypercapnia (excessive CO_2 in the blood) as well as hypoxia [reduced tissue oxygenation caused by decreased arterial (oxygen PaO_2)]. An increase in arterial CO_2 inhibits ventilation
     - Help to the maintain respiration (through peripheral chemoreceptors) when hypoxia occurs.

The normal functions of gas exchange, O_2 and CO_2 tension, chemoreceptors are similar in children and adults. However, children respond differently from adults to respiratory disturbances; major areas of difference include:

1. Poor tolerance of nasal congestion, especially in infants, who are obligatory nose breathers until age of 2–4 months.
2. Increased susceptibility to ear infection due to shorter, broader and more horizontally positioned Eustachian tubes.
3. Increased severity of respiratory symptoms due to smaller airway diameters.
4. A total body response to respiratory infection, with symptoms such as fever, vomiting and diarrhea.

Assessment

1. Health history should determine whether the problem is acute or chronic, self-limiting recurrent or life-threatening. Other important points include alleviating or exacerbating factors, effects of prior treatments and family history of respiratory problems.
2. Physical assessment should focus on the following:
   - Alertness, changes in mental status
   - Activity level and complaints of fatigue
   - Skin color changes, particularly cyanosis
   - Respiratory rate and pattern, presence of apnea (Table 24.1)
   - Intercostal retractions: Presence, severity and location
   - Adventitious lung sounds (wheezes, crackles and rhonchi)
   - Cough (productive or nonproductive).

Laboratory Studies and Diagnostic Tests

1. Radiological evaluation may include:
   - Chest radiograph to visualize internal structures
   - Lung scan to visualize pulmonary blood flow.

2. Thoracentesis involves puncturing the chest wall with a needle to obtain a pleural fluid specimen for analysis.
3. Pulmonary function tests include a series of measurements to evaluate ventilatory function.
4. Blood gas analysis involves measuring PaO_2, $PaCO_2$ and blood pH.

Table 24.1: Respiratory assessment

Age	Breaths per minute
Birth to 6 month	30–50
6 month to 2 year	20–30
3–10 year	20–28
10–18 year	12–20

Psychosocial Implications

1. Acute respiratory illness is frightening to both the child and parents, calling for effective crisis intervention by the nurse.
2. Chronic respiratory illness in children often is accompanied by a history of acute crisis episodes and chronic stress.
3. The respiratory-impaired child's developmental needs can be met best by maintaining optimal exercise and activity levels.

Acute Laryngotracheobronchitis

Description

Acute laryngotracheobronchitis (ALTB) refers to severe inflammation and obstruction of the upper airway, the most common form of croup.

Etiology and Incidence

1. Laryngotracheobronchitis usually results from viral infection. Common causative organisms include parainfluenza viruses, adenoviruses, respiratory syncytial virus (RSV), influenza and measles viruses.
2. It also may be of bacterial origin (diphtheria or pertussis).
3. Laryngotracheobronchitis affects boys more than girls, typically between age 6 months and 3 years.
4. Incidence peaks in the winter months.

Pathophysiology

1. Laryngotracheobronchitis usually is preceded by an upper respiratory infection, which proceeds to laryngitis and then descends into the trachea, and sometimes the bronchi.
2. The flexible larynx of a young child is particularly susceptible to spasm, which may cause complete airway obstruction.

3. Profound airway edema may lead to obstruction and seriously compromised ventilation.

Assessment Findings

Health history and physical examination typically reveal one or more of the following:

- Upper respiratory infection
- Inspiratory stridor
- Substantial and suprasternal retractions
- Barking cough and hoarseness
- Pallor or cyanosis
- Restlessness and irritability
- Low-grade fever
- Crackles, rhonchi, expiratory wheezing and localized areas of diminished or absent breath sounds.

Diagnosis is based on symptoms. Laryngotracheobronchitis is differentiated from epiglottis by a lateral neck radiograph showing a normal epiglottis.

Nursing Diagnoses

- Ineffective airway clearance
- Anxiety
- Ineffective breathing pattern
- Family coping: Potential for growth
- Altered family processes
- High risk for fluid volume deficit
- High risk for injury
- Knowledge deficit.

Planning and Implementation

1. Assess for airway obstruction by evaluating respiratory status, color, respiratory effort, evidence of fatigue and vital signs. Keep emergency equipment at the bedside.
2. Administer oxygen therapy, as ordered to alleviate hypoxia.
3. Administer IV fluids, as ordered to ensure adequate hydration.
4. Administer prescribed medications as ordered, which may include:
   - Racemic epinephrine via nebulizer
   - Antibiotics, if LTB is bacterial in origin
   - Corticosteroids to reduce inflammation (this therapy is controversial).
5. Help to reduce the child's anxiety by maintaining a quiet environment, promoting rest and relaxation, and minimizing intrusive procedures. Encourage parents to bring a favorite toy for the child.

6. Support parents by answering questions and explaining all treatments, and procedures. Encourage them to be present and participate in their child's care, as appropriate.
7. Provide patient and family teaching by covering:
   - Medication dosages, administration techniques and possible side effects
   - Symptoms of croup to watch for and report
   - How to manage home vaporizer or mist treatments (e.g. when child awakens with barking cough and other symptoms of croup, put him/her in the bathroom, and run hot water to produce steam, which may help reduce symptoms).

Evaluation

1. The child exhibits no signs of respiratory distress and is afebrile, and well-hydrated.
2. Parents verbalize understanding of diagnosis, treatment, home care and follow-up.

Bronchiolitis

Description

Bronchiolitis is an inflammatory process affecting the bronchioles and alveoli.

Etiology and Incidence

1. Respiratory syncytial virus is the most common underlying cause of bronchiolitis.
2. Bronchiolitis affects boys more than girls, common in children under 2 years.
3. Incidence peaks in the winter months.

Pathophysiology

1. The inflamed bronchioles become edematous and respiratory secretions accumulate, thereby occluding the bronchial lumen.
2. The narrowing of the small airways compromises expiration and causes air to be trapped in the alveoli.
3. The trapped air, in turn induces lung hyperinflation and may lead to atelectasis.
4. Inadequate ventilation results in hypoxemia and hypercapnia.

Assessment Findings

Initially, the child may have clinical manifestations of an upper infection:

1. Nasal drainage, sneezing, coughing, poor appetite and a low-grade fever.
2. As these mild symptoms worsen, expect signs of respiratory distress such as tachypnea, shallow respiration, inspiratory crackles, expiratory wheezing, tachycardia, chest retractions, dyspnea and a productive or congested cough.
3. In infants, who are breast fed, an inability to suck may cause feeding difficulties from increased respiratory effort.
4. Diagnosis commonly depends on clinical findings and such defining characteristics as the child's age.

Nursing Diagnoses

- Activity intolerance
- Ineffective airway clearance
- Ineffective breathing pattern
- High risk for fluid volume deficit.

Planning and Implementation

1. Assess for respiratory distress by monitoring vital signs and respiratory status.
2. Ease respiratory effort by:
   - Administering oxygen therapy as ordered
   - Suctioning as needed
   - Changing position frequently and elevating the head of the bed.
3. Promote rest by maintaining bedrest and organizing nursing care to minimize disturbances.
4. Ensure adequate nutrition by providing small amount of feed at time.
5. Support the child's family by answering questions and explaining all treatments, and procedures; encourage parents to participate in their child's care, as appropriate.
6. Administer prescribed medications as ordered, which may include:
   - Antibiotic to secondary complications
   - Ventolin via nebulizer
   - Antipyretics to reduce fever.
7. Provide family teaching, covering home care and follow-up measures.

Evaluation

1. The child exhibits no signs of respiratory distress.
2. Parents verbalize understanding of diagnosis, treatment, home care and follow-up measures.

Pneumonia

Description

1. Pneumonia refers to acute inflammation of the lung parenchyma (the respiratory bronchioles, alveolar ducts and sacs, and alveoli) that impairs gas exchange.
2. Pneumonia is classified according to etiological agents.
3. According to location and extent of involvement pneumonia also may be classified:
   - Lobar pneumonia, involving a large segment of one or more lung lobes
   - Bronchopneumonia, begins in the terminal bronchioles and involves nearby lobules
   - Interstitial pneumonia is confined to the alveolar walls and peribronchial and interlobular tissues.

Etiology and Incidence

1. Pneumonia most commonly results from infection with viruses, bacteria, mycoplasma or from aspiration of foreign substances (this entry deals primarily with viral and bacterial pneumonia).
2. Viral pneumonia is the most common type with RSV, the most common causative organism. Others include influenza and parainfluenza viruses, psittacosis rhinovirus and adenovirus.
3. Major causative organisms in bacterial pneumonia include:
   a. Pneumococci: The most common usually results in lobular pneumonia. Most often affects children of age 1–4, with highest incidence in late winter or early spring.
   b. Streptococci: Infection usually results in lobar pneumonia; commonly occurs as complication of influenza and measles.
   c. Staphylococci: The most common cause of bronchopneumonia; most often affects children under age 2 years, with highest incidence in winter.
4. Pneumonia occurs in about 4% children under age 4; incidence decreases with advancing age.

Pathophysiology

1. Pneumonia typically begins as mild upper respiratory tract infection.
2. As the disorder progresses, parenchyma inflammation occurs.
3. Bacterial pneumonia most often causes lobular involvement and sometimes consolidation; viral pneumonia, inflammation of interstitial tissue.

Assessment Findings

1. Common clinical manifestations of viral pneumonia include:
   a. Signs and symptoms varying from mild fever, slight cough and malaise to high fever, severe cough, and prostration.
   b. Cough, nonproductive or productive with whitish sputum.
   c. Rhonchi or fine crackles.
2. In pneumococcal pneumonia, clinical manifestations vary with age and commonly include:
   a. Infants: Vomiting, seizures, poor feeding, fretfulness, fever, stiff neck, bulging anterior fontanel, circumoral cyanosis, respiratory distress, diminished breath sounds and rales, pleural friction rub.
   b. Older children: Headache, abdominal or chest pain. High fever with chills, intermittent drowsiness and restlessness, tachycardia, tachypnea, hacking non-productive cough, expiratory grunting, circumoral cyanosis, diminished breath sounds, tactile and vocal fremitus, tubular breath sounds and disappearance of crackles (indicating consolidation), moist crackles and cough productive of copious blood-tinged mucus (as the disease resolves).
3. Clinical findings in streptococcal pneumonia are similar to those of pneumococcal pneumonia, with sudden onset of:
   a. Fever and chills.
   b. Signs of respiratory distress.
   c. Listlessness or extreme prostration.
   d. Rales.
4. Clinical findings in staphylococcal pneumonia may include:
   a. High fever.
   b. Cough.
   c. Tachypnea.
   d. Cyanosis.
   e. Anorexia.
   f. Dyspnea.
   g. Subcostal and sternal retractions.
   h. Grunting respirations.
   i. Nasal discharge.
   j. Lethargy.
   k. Abdominal distention.
   l. Diminished breath sounds, crackles and rhonchi.
   m. As the child's condition deteriorates, signs of empyema (purulent fluid in the pleural cavity) or pneumothorax.

Radiological Findings

1. **Viral pneumonia:** Diffuse or patchy infiltration with peribronchial distribution.
2. **Pneumococcal pneumonia:** Areas of consolidation (usually patchy) in one or more lobes.
3. **Streptococcal pneumonia:** Disseminated infiltration.
4. **Staphylococcal pneumonia:** Patchy clouding in one or more lobes.

Laboratory Study Results

- Elevated white blood cell count
- Identification of the causative organism through blood cultures
- In streptococcal pneumonia, positive antistreptolysin-O titer is the diagnostical
- Diagnostic thoracentesis may be performed, if fluid in the pleural cavity is suspected.

Nursing Diagnoses

- Activity intolerance
- Ineffective airway clearance
- High risk for altered body temperature
- Ineffective breathing pattern
- Altered family processes
- Potential fluid volume deficit
- Knowledge deficit
- Altered nutrition; less than body requirements
- Pain.

Planning and Implementation

1. Assess for respiratory distress by monitoring vital signs and respiratory status.
2. Ease respiratory effort by:
   - Administering oxygen therapy as ordered (e.g. head box)
   - Performing chest physiotherapy and postural drainage
   - Suctioning as needed
   - Changing position frequently and elevating head of the bed.
3. Help to prevent dehydration by ensuring adequate oral or IV fluid intake; evaluate fluid status by monitoring intake and output, and weighing the child daily.
4. Promote rest by maintaining bedrest and organizing nursing care to minimize disturbances.

5. Ensure adequate nutrition by providing desirable high-calorie foods served in a pleasant and relaxed atmosphere.
6. Support the child's family by answering questions and explaining all treatments, and procedures. Encourage parents to participate in their child's care, as appropriate.
7. Administer prescribed medications as ordered, which may include:
   - Penicillin G to treat pneumococcal and streptococcal pneumonia
   - Synthetic penicillin to treat staphylococcal pneumonia
   - Antipyretics to reduce fever.
8. Provide patient and family teaching by covering:
   - Recommendations for the pneumococcal polysaccharide vaccine for children of age 2 years, who are at risk
   - Home care and follow-up measures.

Evaluation

1. The child exhibits no signs of respiratory distress and is a febrile, and well hydrated.
2. Parents verbalize understanding of diagnosis, treatments, home care and follow-up measures.

Bronchial Asthma

Description

Bronchial asthma is a chronic, episodic, reversible obstructive disorder characterized by airway narrowing due to bronchospasm, increased mucus and mucosal edema.

Etiology and Incidence

1. Asthma most commonly results from allergic hyperresponsiveness of the trachea and bronchi to irritants.
2. Common precipitants include respiratory viral infection, air pollution, animal dander, dust, molds, pollens, certain foods, exercise, rapid changes in environmental temperature and physical or psychological stress.
3. A familial tendency has been observed.
4. The most common chronic lung disease in children is asthma, which affects 2.5% children.
5. Before puberty, twice as many boys as girls are affected; at puberty, the incidence in girls increases.
6. Asthma tends to be more severe in younger children; improvement often occurs in adolescence.
7. Incidence is greater in urban dwellers.

Pathophysiology

1. Obstruction due to edema of the respiratory mucosa causes bronchiolar narrowing, secretion accumulation and bronchial, and bronchiolar smooth muscle spasm. This leads to air trapping, characteristic wheezing and respiratory distress.
2. If not treated promptly, status asthmaticus (an acute, severe, prolonged asthma attack that does not respond to usual treatment) may result, requiring hospitalization.

Assessment Findings

1. Health history and physical examination will reveal one or more of the following:
   - Dyspnea, air hunger
   - Anxiety
   - Coughing
   - Wheezing, particularly expiratory
   - Fatigue
   - Tachypnea
   - Complaints of chest tightness
   - Costal retractions
   - Cyanosis
   - Diaphoresis.
2. Improvement in respiratory function following use of a bronchodilator is a diagnosis of asthma.
3. Skin sensitivity tests may identify the causative allergen.

Nursing Diagnoses

- Activity intolerance
- Ineffective airway clearance
- Anxiety
- Body image disturbance
- Ineffective breathing pattern
- Altered family processes
- High risk for fluid volume deficit
- Altered health maintenance
- Health-seeking behaviors
- High risk for infection
- High risk for injury
- Knowledge deficit
- Noncompliance.

Planning and Implementation

1. Increase respiratory effectiveness by:
   - Administering medications as ordered
   - Elevating head of the patient's bed
   - Administering oxygen therapy as needed
   - Performing chest physiotherapy and suctioning as needed.
2. Assess respiratory status by closely evaluating breathing patterns and monitoring signs.
3. In an acute attack:
   - Administer prescribed medication as ordered, which may include inhaled bronchodilators, epinephrine or terbutaline subcutaneous (SC) or aminophylline IV
   - Assess respiratory and cardiovascular status closely
   - Monitor arterial blood gas results for pO_2, pCO_2 and pH (Table 24.2)
   - Administer oxygen or in severe cases, provide ventilatory assistance, as needed (Fig. 24.2)
   - Administer IV fluid therapy as ordered, to prevent dehydration.

Table 24.2: Normal arterial blood gas values by age

Parameters	Normal
pO_2	• At birth: 8–24 mm Hg • Age 1 day: 45–95 mm Hg • Thereafter: 83–108 mm Hg (decreases with age)
pCO_2	• Neonate: 27–40 mm Hg • Infant: 27–41 mm Hg • Thereafter: – Male: 35–48 mm Hg – Female: 32–45 mm Hg
pH	• Premature neonate (48 hour after birth): 7.5 • Term neonate (at birth): 7.11–7.36 • Age 1 day: 7.29–7.45 • Thereafter: 7.35–7.45

4. Promote rest by scheduling nursing activities to allow for periods of rest and encouraging activities appropriate to the child's tolerance level.
5. Prevent dehydration by encouraging oral fluid intake or monitoring IV fluid therapy, carefully monitoring intake and output, recording daily weights and assessing for signs of dehydration.

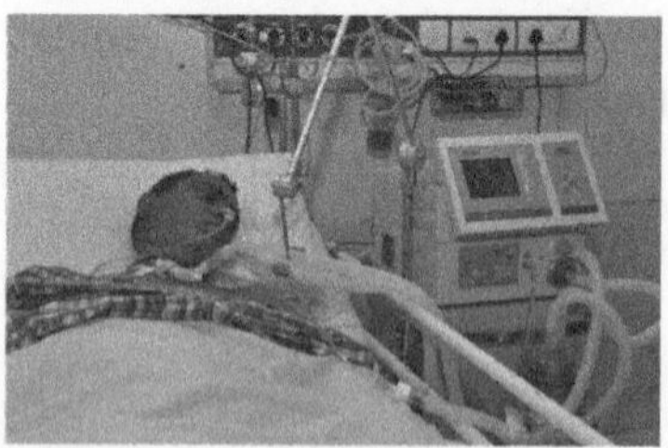

Fig. 24.2: Patient with ventilator (*Courtesy:* Anil Baghi, Multispecialty Hospital, Ferozepur, Punjab)

6. Administer prescribed medications as ordered, which may include:
   - Methylxanthines, especially theophylline and aminophylline, to provide bronchodilator for both daily maintenance and acute attacks
   - Sympathomimetics (β-adrenergics) to promote bronchodilator in acute attacks: Epinephrine, isoetharine, isoproterenol, metaproterenol, albuterol and terbutaline.
   - Cromolyn sodium can be administered via inhaler four times per day, as a prophylactic agent
   - Corticosteroids to reduce airway inflammation during acute attacks or as prophylactic therapy
   - Antihistamines to decrease postnasal drip-induced cough that may lead to bronchospasms
   - Antibiotics, if respiratory tract infection is present.
7. Monitor for effectiveness and side effects of medication therapy.
8. Help the child and family identify possible ways to limit exposure to these factors.
9. Teach the child and family to prevent respiratory infection by avoiding exposure to infection and maintaining good hygiene and sound health practices.
10. Encourage physical activity based on the child's tolerance level. Explain that the child may require pretreatment wit bronchodilator inhalation before exercising.
11. Encourage chest physiotherapy, breathing exercises and inhalation therapy to help strengthen the respiratory musculature, and develop more efficient breathing patterns.
12. Help the child cope with poor self-esteem by encouraging him/her to ventilate feelings and concerns; listening actively as the child does so; focusing on his/her personal strengths and helping him/her assume an active role in identifying both the positive and negative aspects of his/her situation.
13. Help alleviate the child's anxiety by remaining calm and staying with him/her in emergency and anxiety-producing situations. Provide explanations and preparation for all treatments and procedures.
14. Support the family by answering questions, providing reassurance, explaining treatments and procedures, and apprising them of their child's condition.
15. Encourage family members to participate in the child's care when hospitalized, if appropriate.
16. Encourage family members to express their feelings and concerns in acute situations related to asthma's chronic nature, and its effects on family functioning; assess the family to identify maladaptive behaviors undue stress; refer for counseling, if needed.
17. Discuss the need for periodic pulmonary function tests to evaluate and guide therapy, and monitor the course of the disease.

18. Provide patient and family teaching by covering:
    - Ways to identify and prevent contact with known precipitants of asthma attacks
    - The importance of promoting overall physical and psychological well-being in the child
    - The need for adequate hydration to keep secretions from thickening
    - Physical activities commensurate with the child's capabilities
    - Breathing exercise, inhalation therapy and chest physiotherapy
    - Dosage administration and side effects of all prescribed medications
    - Signs and symptoms of acute asthma attack and appropriate treatments.

Evaluation

- The child exhibits a normal breathing pattern with lungs clear on auscultation and is a febrile, and well-hydrated
- Parents verbalize knowledge of the above listed aspects of patient and family teaching as well as knowledge of follow-up care.

Parents with a Preterm or Sick Baby

- Parents may have strong guilty feelings and sense of failure
- They may find it difficult to accept and understand the situation
- Keep the baby and mother together as much as possible
- Allow free visiting for the parents
- Discuss and explain child's condition, investigation and treatment
- Explain what the different equipment is for and why it is or may be used on their baby
- Keep the parent informed of the daily progress of the baby
- Encourage the mother to breastfeed, cuddle, change the nappy and bath her baby
- Continue to support the family, when the baby is in hospital
- Explain the parents, what is the management plan for the baby
- Advise against harmful local treatments at home, but understand that the parents can only do the best for their child.

Parents with Dying Child

1. Parents faced with a dying child have usually not expected any problem and often they have had little or no time to prepare for the death of the baby.
2. The death of a child makes a major impact on their lives and expectations for the future.

3. Parents may be angry with the medical and nursing staff, and blame them for what has happened. This is just a way of expressing their grief and if the staff understands this, it is easier for everyone to deal with the situation.
4. Have an area or a room that can be used by the parents of a dying baby.
5. If possible, an experienced neonatal nurse to care for the baby and the parents.
6. The same nurses for continuing of care and support for the baby and parents.
7. Common errors of all medical staff, doctors and nurses are (which should not occur):
   - Separation of parents from the child
   - Hiding deformities
   - Cheering with irrelevance; cheer up, you will soon get over it
   - Advise for another pregnancy, have another baby soon
   - Giving sedatives to parents
   - Little respect for the parent's feelings by joking and behaving as if all is normal in spite of hearing to the parents
   - Gossiping about the baby's problems with other parents on the ward or other staff
   - Ignoring the need for privacy of these parents
   - Ignoring the parents because of fear as how to behave when they need sympathy and support.
8. Need of the parents are as follows:
   - Respect, understanding empathy and permission to grieve
   - Opportunity to get to know the child they have lost
   - Professional conduct of the staff
   - Confidentiality, respecting their privacy
   - Time to observe religious practice
   - Directness and honesty with humane feelings
   - A support system for follow-up care.

ASSIST IN EXCHANGE TRANSFUSION

Hemolytic Disease

Hemolytic disease of the newborn, also known as hemolytic disease of the fetus and newborn or erythroblastosis fetalis, is an alloimmune condition that develops in a fetus, when the IgG molecules (one of the five main types of antibodies) produced by the mother, which pass through the placenta. Among these antibodies are some, which attack the red blood cells (RBCs) in the fetal circulation, the RBCs are broken down and the fetus can develop reticulocytosis and anemia. This fetal disease ranges from mild to very severe and fetal death from heart failure (hydrops fetalis) can occur. When the disease is moderate or severe, many erythroblasts are present in the fetal blood and so these forms of the disease can be called erythroblastosis fetalis.

Hemolytic leads to elevated bilirubin levels. After delivery bilirubin is no longer cleared (via the placenta) from the neonate's blood and symptoms of jaundice (yellowish skin and yellow discoloration of the whites of the eyes) increase within 24 hours after birth such as any other severe neonatal jaundice, there is the possibility of acute or chronic kernicterus, profound anemia can cause high output heart failure with pallor, enlarged liver and/or spleen, generalized swelling and respiratory distress. The prenatal manifestations are known as hydrops fetalis; in severe forms this can include petechiae and purpura. The infant may be stillborn or die shortly after birth.

Causes

Antibodies are produced when the body is exposed to a foreign antigen to the makeup of the body, if a mother is exposed to a foreign antigen and produces IgG (as opposed to IgM, which does not cross the placenta), the IgG will target the antigen, if present in the fetus, and may affect it in utero and persist after delivery. The three most common models in which a woman becomes sensitized toward (i.e. produces IgG antibodies against) the particular antigens are:

1. Fetal maternal hemorrhage can occur due to trauma, abortion, child birth, ruptures in the placenta during pregnancy or medical procedures carried out during pregnancy that breach the uterine wall in subsequent pregnancy, if there is a similar incomparability in the fetus, these antibodies are then able to cross the placenta into the fetal bloodstream to attach to the RBCs and cause hemolysis in other words, if a mother has anti-RhD (D being the major rhesus antigen) IgG antibodies as a result of previously carrying a RhD-positive fetus, this antibody will only affect a fetus with RhD-positive blood.
2. The women may receive a therapeutic blood transfusion. The ABO blood group system and the D antigen of the rhesus blood group system typing are routine prior to transfusion. Suggestions have been made that women of child bearing age or young girl should not be given a transfusion with RhC-positive blood or Kell-positive blood to avoid transfusion services.
3. The third sensitization model can occur in women of blood type O, the immune response to A and B antigens that are widespread in the environment, usually leads to the production of IgM anti-A and IgM anti-B antibodies early in life on rare occasions, IgG antibodies are produced in contrast, rhesus antibodies are generally not produced from exposure to environmental antigens.

ABO system

The ABO hemolytic disease of the newborn can range from mild to severe, but generally it is a mild disease it includes:

- Anti-A antibodies
- Anti-B antibodies.

Rhesus system

1. Rhesus (Rh) D hemolytic disease of the newborn (often called Rh disease) is the most common form of severe hemolytic disease of the newborn (HDN) the disease varies from mild to severe.
2. Rhesus E hemolytic disease of the newborn is a mild condition.
3. Rhesus hemolytic disease of the newborn can range from a mild to severe disease. This is the third most common form of severe HDN.
4. Rhesus C and hemolytic disease of the newborn are rare.

Kell system

- Anti-Kell hemolytic disease is the second most common cause of severe HDN
- Anti-K1 antibodies disease ranges from mild to severe, over half of the cases are caused by multiple blood transfusions.

Diagnosis

The diagnosis of HDN is based on history and laboratory findings:

1. Blood tests done on the newborn baby:
   - Biochemistry tests for jaundice
   - Peripheral blood morphology shows increased reticulocytes erythroblasts re (also known as nucleated RBCs may be pronormoblast, basophilic normoblast, orthochromatic normoblast) occur in moderate and severe disease
   - Positive direct Coombs' test (might be negative after fetal intrauterine blood transfusion).
2. **Blood tests done on the mother:** Positive in direct Coombs' test.

Note: Erythroblastosis fetalis is the hemolytic diseases of the newborn usually due to Rh incompatibility or ABO mismatching.

Treatment

Before birth, options for treatment includes intrauterine transfusions or early induction of labor when pulmonary maturity has been attained, fetal distress is present or 35–37 weeks of gestation have passed. The mother may also undergo plasma exchange to reduce the circulating levels of antibody by as much as 75%.

After birth, treatment depends on the severity of the condition, but could include temperature stabilization and monitoring; phototherapy transfusion with compatible packed RBCs, exchange transfusion with a blood type compatible with both the infant and the mother, sodium bicarbonate for correction of acidosis and/or assisted ventilation.

Rhesus-negative mothers, who have had a pregnancy with/or pregnant with a Rh-positive infant are given Rh immune globulin (RhIG) at 28 weeks during pregnancy, at 34 weeks and within 72 hours after delivery to prevent sensitization to the D antigen. It works by binding any fetal RBCs with the D antigen before the mother is able to produce an immune response and form anti-D IgG. A drawback to prepartum administration of RhIG is that it causes a positive antibody screen when the mother is tested, which can be difficult to distinguish from natural immunological responses that result in antibody production.

Exchange Transfusion

Indications

1. The most important indication for exchange transfusion is an indirect bilirubin concentration of 20 mg/dL in stable term infants. In sick premature infants, however, kernicterus may occur when bilirubin concentrations are below 10–15 mg/dL.
2. The purpose of exchange transfusion are to prevent the bilirubin from rising to a level that could lead to kernicterus and to correct the anemia caused by the hemolytic process. More specifically, an exchange transfusion removes circulating antibodies and replaces sensitized erythrocytes and lowers the bilirubin level in the blood.
3. Fresh donor blood that is compatible with the blood of both mother and infant should be used for exchange transfusion. If the blood is prepared before delivery, packed O Rh-negative cells mixed with AB plasma may be used.
4. Rapidly developing jaundice with unconjugated bilirubin above 5 mg%.

Start Exchange Transfusion

1. Blood should be freshly collected.
2. Check the blood type and group against the neonate's blood before administering it to prevent a hemolytic reaction caused by mismatched donor blood.
3. Blood for exchange should be Rh-negative whole blood from unsensitized donors with system ABO grouping to that of the baby or group 'O'.
4. The blood should be crossmatched with the mother's serum.
5. The blood is kept refrigerated prior to its use; it is gradually warmed to a temperature between 22 and 37°C, which is maintained throughout the transfusion.
6. The neonate's temperature is maintained under a radiant warmer and blankets should be used.
7. Maintain aseptic technique.

Complications

- Hypoglycemia
- Cardiac failure
- Coagulopathies
- Clotting.

After the procedure, the infant must be observed for bleeding from the transfusion site. The infant blood glucose levels should be checked hourly.

GUIDE TO SOME OF THE CONDITIONS, WHICH MAY BE RECOGNIZED

1. It is essential that all pediatrician, obstetricians, gynecologists, nurses, midwives and health visitors or anyone, who has contact with newborn children, to have a sound working knowledge of the possible surgical conditions, which may be encountered.
2. Any deviation from the normal range of pulse, respiratory rate, color or temperature, or any of the abnormal physical signs and symptoms in the newborn should result in a high index of suspicion, and possible early diagnosis.
3. A detailed history noting maternal hydramnios, meconium-stained liquor, difficulty in delivery, etc. are important.
4. Note and record, when the baby first passes urine or meconium.
5. All the orifices must be inspected, especially the perineum and anus, in girls make sure three orifices are present. If there is any doubt about the presence of an anal orifice, try to pass just the tip of a thermometer into the anal canal, for not more than 2 cm to establish patency. If it does not enter easily, consult pediatrician.

Genitourinary

1. It is worth remembering that gastrointestinal signs such as vomiting, abdominal pain and distension and diarrhea may be indicative of an underlying urinary anomaly.
2. Two third of all neonatal abdominal masses are due to renal enlargement. 90% of the renal masses are either hydronephrosis or multicystic kidneys. Polycystic kidneys and renal tumors are rarer conditions. All these, however need early assessment though not necessarily early intervention.
3. Posterior urethral valves must be considered in a male child with a poor urine stream, palpable bladder with or without palpable kidneys. They may also present as urinary ascites. Emergency management consists of catheter drainage of the bladder. If interventional radiology is considered, the child must first be stabilized and given antibiotics.

Intestinal Obstruction

Four cardinal signs of intestinal obstruction:

- Pain
- Vomiting
- Distension
- Absolute constipation.

Intestinal obstruction may be suspected because of the four above cardinal signs.

Note the Exceptions

- Abdominal pain (this may not be noticed in the newborn)
- Vomiting, especially if the vomit is not bile stained
- Abdominal distention (which may not be present in high lesions of the duodenum or jejunum)
- No passage of meconium or delayed passage of meconium, more than 24 hours in a full-term baby
- Passage of meconium one or two times, does not exclude intestinal atresia
- Any baby having these cardinal signs of obstruction should have an NG tube passed to empty the stomach and examine the contents, and see if any bile is present
- In any suspected case of intestinal obstruction, a plain X-ray of the abdomen in the erect and supine position is usually required for a diagnosis
- An X-ray will confirm the presence and the level of obstruction, and give a possible clue to etiology
- If there are dilated bowel loops and fluid levels, the baby should be referred to a consultant.

Diaphragmatic Hernia

Diaphragmatic hernia may have been suspected on prenatal ultrasound. It should certainly be suspected in any baby having tachypnea, cyanosis or dextrocardia after delivery. An X-ray chest is essential as soon as any of these signs are detected as clinical auscultation may be misleading.

An NG tube size 8 or 10 should be passed to decompress the stomach and should be left open (not spigotted) at all times so that any air, which may reach the stomach by crying or pushed in by bagging with a face mask, could be expelled. Using a mask with a 100% oxygen, if an NG tube is in place and left open to the atmosphere, is probably safe. Bagging with a mask in diaphragmatic hernia may actually aggravate the situation by distending the stomach further and compressing the thoracic content further.

If the baby's condition remains desperate with severe cyanosis, poor general condition, and there are no means of locally intubation or resuscitation, then the baby is perhaps best left without any further attempts at vigorous resuscitation. If the baby survives 6 hours or so, then he/she should be referred for further treatment.

Myelomeningocele and Spina Bifida

1. A baby with a large myelomeningocele together with lower limb, bladder and anal paralysis, should be treated actively.
2. It is decided that treatment should be offered if the baby has a large meningocele with a ruptured sac, either a wet swab with saline should be placed over it or a piece of cling film placed over the lesion, to prevent contamination and fluid loss is essential first aid treatment.
3. The baby should be sent for assessment, as to whether operation or no operation is deemed desirable and the parents should not be misinformed that surgery is going to cure the baby.
4. Always look for presence or absence of severe hydrocephalic, severe cardiac anomaly and any other congenital abnormalities.

Esophageal Atresia and Tracheoesophageal Atresia

1. The passage of the NG tube is essential in any baby who is frothing or salivating excessively, to determine patency of the esophagus and exclude esophagus atresia.
2. These babies do not vomit; the suspicion of a baby having esophageal atresia is suspected, when a mother gives a history of hydramnios or the baby is noted to have a constant amount of frothy saliva in the mouth after delivery, which needs frequent suctioning.
3. If this is noted then an NG tube has to be passed and a X-ray with radiopaque tube in the esophagus is taken. If the diagnosis is confirmed, an NG tube (FG 8 or 10) on continuous suction or certainly half hourly aspiration should be performed. Change of position with the upper pouch full of saliva, causes cyanotic attacks, as the saliva spills into the lungs. The most dangerous event however is abdominal distention with vomiting of gastric contents into the lungs. This distention cannot be prevented by the NG tube in the upper pouch.
4. If the baby is crying a lot and closes the glottis, air reaches into stomach and distends it via the tracheoesophageal fistula and vomiting may ensure urgent operation is needed in this situation.
5. The ideal position in which to nurse, the baby is debatable. Head up, head down or flat is thought by some, to be the best position. Probably nursed flat with a replogle double lumen tube (if available) or a suction tube of the upper pouch is ideal for transportation.

Scrotal Swellings

1. Remember that hydroceles are common, easily confirmed by transillumination. Over 90% disappears spontaneously by the age of 2 years. Therefore the majority do not require treatment or referral before the age of 2 years.

2. A hernia does require early operation because of the risk of strangulation.
3. Undescended testes should be reviewed at 3 months and if the testis is not in the scrotum, operation is necessary. The best time is between 1 and 2 years of age.
4. Remember that testicular torsion can occur antenatally and it may be seen in the neonatal period; pain is not a feature.

RELIEF OF CHOKING IN INFANTS

Early Recognition

Early recognition of airway obstruction is the key to successful outcome. It is important to distinguish this emergency from fainting, stroke, seizure, drug overdose or other conditions that cause sudden respiratory failure, but require different treatment. The trained observer can often detect signs of choking.

Types of Airway Obstruction

Foreign bodies may cause either mild or severe airway obstruction

Mild Airway Obstruction

Signs
- Good air exchange
- Responsive and can cough forcefully
- May wheeze between cough.

Rescuer action
- As long as good air exchange continues, encourage the victim to continue spontaneous coughing and breathing efforts
- Do not interfere with the victim's own attempts to expel the foreign body, but stay with the victim and monitor his/her condition
- If mild airway obstruction persists, activate the emergency response system.

Severe Airway Obstruction

Signs
- Poor or no air exchange
- Weak, ineffective cough or no cough at all
- High-pitched noise, while inhaling or no noise at all
- Increased respiratory diffculty
- Possible cyanosis (turning blue)
- Unable to speak

- Clutching the neck with the thumb and fingers, making the universal choking sign
- Unable to move air.

Rescuer action

Ask the victim if he/she is choking. if the victim nods yes and cannot talk severe airway obstruction is present and you must activate the emergency response system.

Management/Treatment

On a Responsive Child Victim

Follow these steps to perform abdominal thrusts on a responsive child who is standing or sitting:

1. Stand or kneel behind the victim and wrap your arms around the victims waist.
2. Make a fist with one hand:
   - Place the thumb side of your fist against the victim's abdomen, in the midline, slightly above the navel and well below the breastbone
   - Grasp the fist with your other hand and press your fist into the victim's abdomen with quick upward thrust
   - Repeat thrusts until the object is expelled from the airway or the victim becomes unresponsive
   - Give each new thrust with a separate, distinct movement to relieve the obstruction.

On Unresponsive Victim

Action to relieve choking in the unresponsive victim

1. Choking victims initially may be responsive and then may become unresponsive. In this circumstance, know that choking one must caused the victim's symptoms and has need to look for a foreign object in the pharynx.
2. If one is alone with a child choking victim, who becomes unresponsive, then open the airway remove an object if you see it and begin cardiopulmonary resuscitation (CPR). After about 5 cycles or 2 minutes of CPR, activate the emergency response system (ERS) if you have not already done so.
3. For child victim, every time you open the airway to give breaths, open the victim's mouth wide and look for the object, if you see an object, remove it with your fingers. If you do not see an object, keep doing CPR.
4. At other times, the choking victim may be unresponsive when you first encounter him/her. In this circumstance, you probably will not know that an airway obstruction exists. Activate the ERS and start CPR.

Action after relief of choking

You can tell you have successfully removed an airway obstruction in the unresponsive victim if you:

- Feels air movement and see the chest rise when you give breaths
- See and remove a foreign body from the victim's pharynx.

Follow these steps after you relieve choking in the unresponsive victim:

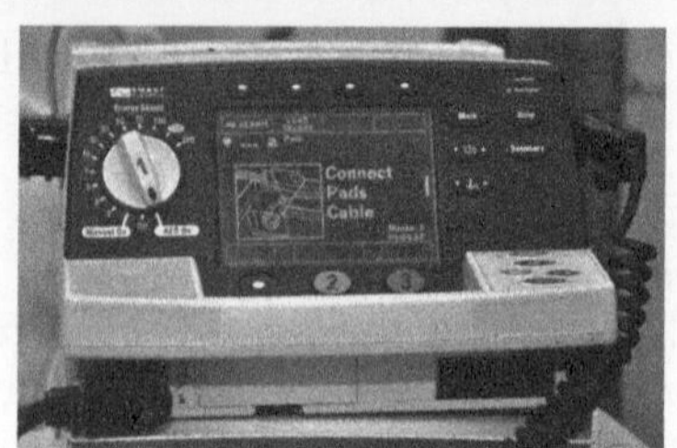

Fig. 24.3: Automatic external defibrillator (*Courtesy:* Anil Baghi, Multispecialty Hospital, Ferozepur, Punjab).

1. Provide two breaths.
2. Check for pulse (Table 24.3).

Table 24.3: Pulse checking in an unresponsive victim after chok relief

Pulse	Breathing	Action
No	No	Perform chest compression and attach the automatic external defibrillator (AED) (Fig. 24.3)
Yes	No	Continue rescue breathing and check for pulse every 2 min
Yes	Yes	Later place the victim in the recovery position

3. If you successfully relieve choking with abdominal thrusts, encourage the victim to seek immediate medical attention to ensure that the victim does not have a complication from abdominal thrusts.

Chapter 25 Genetics Influences in Child Health

GENETICS

Genetics is the branch of biology concerned with heredity and individual characteristics.

GENES AND CHROMOSOMES

The human body is made up of billions of cells. At the center of each cell is a special compartment called the nucleus, which stores threads of deoxyribonucleic acid (DNA) arranged in chromosomes.

A chromosome is rod-like structure present in the nucleus of the body cells, with the exception of the red blood cells (RBCs), which stores genetic information in the form of genes. The chromosomes are in their turn composed of 50,000–100,000 genes located on 46 chromosomes, which contain the genetic blue print determining individuals' characteristics. These 46 chromosomes occur as 23 pairs. We got one of each pair from mother in the egg or ovum and one of each pair from father in the sperm.

Simply, chromosomes are the structures that hold our genes. Genes are the individual instructions that tell our bodies how to develop and keep our body intact and healthy. The ovum and sperm each carry 23 chromosomes and on fertilization the chromosomes combines to give a total of 23 pairs, 46 chromosomes in total. One pair of chromosomes determines the sex of individual, males have X and Y chromosomes, while females have two X chromosomes.

KARYOTYPE

The chromosomes of an individual can be examined with a chart called karyotype. A karyotype is prepared form a photograph of the chromosomes of a single cell. The chromosomes are cut out of the photograph and are arranged in matched pairs according to length. These matched chromosomes are then numbered. The first 22 pairs, called autosomes, contain genes that determine a variety of physical and mental traits. The last 23rd pair contains the sex chromosomes; there are two X chromosomes in a normal. Female contains two X chromosome and in male one X and one Y chromosome. These sex chromosomes contain genes that control the development of the primary and secondary sex characteristics and the various other sex-linked traits.

CELL DIVISION AND REPRODUCTION

In the process of mitosis or ordinary cell division, cells divide and duplicate themselves exactly. There are number of steps in the process. First DNA of each gene unzips and replicates itself. Then each chromosome splits and reproduces the former chromosomes arrangement of the first cell. Thus, two new cells are formed. Each containing 23 pairs of chromosomes exactly similar to those in the original cell.

The process of cell division that creates reproductive cells (ova or sperm) is called meiosis. The reproductive cells formed during meiosis have only one half of the genetic materials of the parent cell 23 chromosomes. The rearrangement of genes and chromosomes resulting from meiosis is similar to the shuffling and dealing of cards. The chance that any two siblings may receive the same assortment of chromosomes is about 1 in 281 trillion. This figure does not even allow for the fact that the individual genes on a chromosome often make a crossover to the opposite chromosomes during cell division. It is therefore virtually impossible for the same combination of genes to occur twice.

BEHAVIORAL GENETICS

Behavioral genetics is one thing to consider the impact of genetics on the shape of one's nose or the color of the one's eyes, but it is quite another to wonder, if our short-tempered aggressiveness is in part, genetically determined. Human behavior seems nowhere near as prescribed or preprogrammed, as animal behaviors seem no terms do exist, highly modifiable, depending on the culture and circumstance. Nevertheless, the study of the genetic components of behavior has been a highly controversial field for decades. Researchers first look at genetic influences on the development of behaviors for the whole human species. These influences include the typical patterns of growth and also patterns of perceptual and motor skills. The genetic influence is evident beyond the prenatal period, in fact, genetic programming is involved throughout the development pubescence, e.g. occurs in adolescence as the organism become capable of sexual reproduction. There are physical aspects of this change that are genetically programmed, as well as some behavioral tendencies that are part of this sequence. While certain tendencies can be altered slightly with health care and nutrition, the underlying pattern remains (Scar and Kidd, 1983).

Interaction of Genetics and Culture

The ancient argument of heredity versus environment is still raging and is likely to continue. The important issue is not which influence on the personality is more powerful. But now heredity and environment interact in the development of human behavior studies, identical twins show that to some extent our genes control social traits introversion or extraversion, also some serious mental disorders, such as schizophrenia and manic depression, appear to have their roots in genetic makeup.

Our physical appearance whether we are tall or short, dark or light, plain or beautiful is genetically determined, but the way in which our culture views, these physical attributes can have a profound effect on personality development.

GENETIC ABNORMALITIES

Genetic Disease or Disorder

Traditionally, a genetic disease or disorder has been defined as a disease directly caused by a mutation or defect in a person genetic makeup (DNA). Today the definition of genetic disease may also include disease that are influenced by a particular genetic makeup or are found more commonly in persons with a particular genetic makeup.

Genetic Influence on Development

Genetic disorder account for about 20% of pediatric hospital admissions, with even higher percentage for children who require long-term hospital stays for this reason. It is important for nurses involved in the care of children to understand genetic factors that influence growth development and health.

Chromosomal Abnormalities

A numerical chromosome error occurs when an abnormal number of chromosomes during conception results in a major physical and mental defect. For example, if an extra chromosome develops in each cell, the defect is called trisomy. When there is a missing chromosome in each cell, the defect is called monosomy. A variety of numerical chromosome errors can take place at conception or after fertilization of the ovum. During germ cell formation in the mother, nondisjunction, the separation and migration of chromosome during cell division, may occur. Following fertilization nondisjunction can also occur and results in mixed mosaics. Variations in chromosomal counts may be discreetly identified and are called trisomies, e.g. trisomy 21 (Down syndrome) and XXY (Klinefelter's syndrome).

A structural chromosome error occurs when chromosomes break and reunite. As a result of this action, some chromosome part is exchanged between chromosomes in a process known as translocation. As a result of the translocation, chromosomes may:

- Contain a normal makeup
- Be balanced or rearranged chromosome
- Combine with missing or duplicated chromosome segments.

The child may have an appropriate number of chromosomes (46), but with a different structure. Infants born with missing or extra chromosomal segments are likely to have severe mental and physical handicaps. The presence of 45 chromosomes is not compatible with life and the embryo or fetus is usually spontaneously aborted. A child who has an extra chromosome (for a total of 47) can live, but will have a trisomy such as trisomy 21.

Monogenic Disorders (Single Gene)

Monogenic disorder result from a defect in a single gene located on specific chromosomes or from a defective gene on gene the X chromosome. Defective genes may be either recessive or dominant; they are inherited according to Mendelian principles. A disorder caused by a recessive gene is expressed only in the presence of two recessive genes, one from each parent. In a person who inherits just one recessive gene, the normal gene on the paired chromosome overcomes the effect of the recessive gene. Thus, this person is a carrier for the attributed disorder, but does not manifest the disorder. In contrast, a dominant gene produces its effect even in someone with one normal gene for a given trait.

Disorder caused by X-linked inheritance patterns are transmitted through a defect in gene on X chromosome, because males have only one X chromosome, a defective gene on that chromosome always leads to expression of the disease. X-linked disorders may follow either a dominant or recessive inheritance pattern. Disorders of X-linked dominant inheritances may occur in both males and females, disorders of X-linked recessive inheritance occurs only in males, they are transmitted through carrier females who pass on the disorder to their sons. X-linked dominant disorder is rare.

Multifactorial Disorders

Multifactorial disorders have no clear inheritance pattern, but are believed to be genetic, because certain families show an increased susceptibility. Presumably, these disorders result from interaction among many genes and environmental influences.

Teratogenic Disorders

A teratogenic disorder is a genetic disorder caused by exposure to external factors that have harmful effect on an embryo otherwise would have developed normally. It is also important to recognize the role of the environment. Teratogens are agent, such as drugs and pollution that affect the developing fetus and can results in abnormalities and increase the incidence of infant morbidity and mortality. Knowledge of environmental factors can help nurses to assesses the health of patients through early identification of exposure, anticipatory care planning, health teaching that includes measures to avoid or reduce exposure and coping strategies used to deal with the consequences of negative-environmental exposure. Environmental causes of developmental defects in humans have been attributed to four major sources:

- Drugs and environmental chemicals (including pollution)
- Infections
- Maternal metabolic imbalances
- Ionizing radiation, such as X-rays.

PRENATAL DIAGNOSIS

Prenatal diagnosis of genetic disorders involves ultrasonography, amniocentesis, chorionic villi sampling and fetal blood sampling. Ultrasonography may reveal physical manifestations of neural tube defects and hydrocephalus. Amniocentesis and chorionic villi sampling may detect abnormalities in chromosome number, include sickle cell anemia, etc. Fetal blood sampling may reveal a deficiency in coagulation factors.

POSTNATAL DIAGNOSIS

Postnatal diagnosis is accomplished through a comprehensive history and physical examination for typical manifestations of certain disorders such as chromosome analysis, enzymes and serologic studies.

THERAPEUTIC MANAGEMENT OF GENETIC DISEASE

There is no cure for genetic disease at present, although preventive and corrective therapy is helping number of conditions. At present, the major goal of the therapy is modification of the internal or external environment to correct or minimize the effects of the genetic defect.

Therapeutic Modalities

The therapeutic modalities available for genetic disorders are few when compared with the infinite variety of conditions affecting the population.

Surgical Repair

Surgical repair of structural defects has made it possible to prolong life in number of multifactor disorders, such as congenital heart disease, pyloric stenosis, etc.

Diet Modification

For disorders in which an enzymes deficiency causes a toxic accumulation of a substances often prevents irreversible damage from the improper metabolism of these compounds. For example, in heredity lactase deficiency elimination of dairy products containing lactose for these infants and children.

Product Replacement

In some deficiency diseases, supplying the missing product that cannot be synthesized prevents undesirable effects. For example, thyroid extract is given to prevent the damaging effects of hypothyroidism, also in the following condition such as hemophilia, diabetes and adrenogenital syndrome.

Avoidance of Drugs

In drug-induced disease such as glucose-6-phosphate dehydrogenase (G6PD) deficiency, avoidance of the drugs that precipitate reaction provides a simple preventive measure.

Removal of Toxic Substances

Removal of toxic substances that accumulate in vital tissues as a result of a heredity disease, e.g. β-thalassemia, serious complications can prevent. Excess accumulation of iron in the liver and pancreas can be reduced by administer chelating agents, e.g. deferoxamine.

Transplantation

Replacement of non-functioning organs with normal organs in increasing the survival of children, e.g. hereditary polycystic kidneys.

Cofactor Administration

Diet supplements can be given when the body is unable to synthesize or effectively use some substances needed as cofactor in metabolism, such as vitamin B_{12} in pernicious anemia in which absorption of vitamin is absent.

Recombinant DNA

The transfer of modified genetic material from one organism (a virus) to another causes the viral DNA, to become integrated into the cellular DNA of a recipient cell, often a bacteria cell. This recombinant DNA multiplies, producing the missing substances in the host cell. This technology has been applied in growth hormone therapy and factor VIII synthesis.

Gene Transfer

Fragment of DNA from a normal gene can be introduced directly into a recipient cell lacking such a gene. These approaches has been attempted in human with the transfer of normal gene copies of β-hemoglobin into bone marrow cells in an effort to treat a form of β-thalassemia and has been used in sickle cell diseases. Gene therapy research is the hope of the future for more effective treatment of cure of genetic disorder. But, thus for many patients have had inconsistent result.

Environmental Manipulation

Inherited diseases or defect for which there is no therapeutic modality can be modified to enhance the quality of life for the affected individual. Some examples of environmental manipulation include hearing aids for deaf children, glasses or vision enhancer such as enlarged print and books in Braille for the visually impairment, prosthetic devices for limb deficiencies and infant stimulation program to maximize the potential of children who are mentally retarded.

Advances in Genetic Research

Human Genome Project

An organism's genome is its full set of genes. It is not known for certain how many genes the human has, but it could be as many as 10,000 consisting of a total of 3,000 million base pairs. Techniques are now available, which make it possible to find out not only how many genes we have but also whereabouts they occurs on the individual chromosomes and which features they control. We already know about some of our genes and the scientists world over are working had to discover the rest. It will take years to complete the human genome project, but when it is complete it will pave the way to finding remedies for some of the disease caused by faulty genes. At present these disease afflict about 60 million people worldwide.

Genetic Counseling

Genetic counseling aims to provide the family with complete and accurate information about genetic disorders. The goals of genetic counseling include:

- Promoting informed decisions by involved family members
- Clarifying the family's option, available treatments and prognosis
- Examining alternatives to reduce the risk of genetic disorders
- Decreasing the incidence of the genetic disorders
- Reducing the impact of the disorders.

To achieve these goals, genetic counseling must include an accurate diagnosis and non-directive counseling, which provides information in a non-threatening, unbiased manner and reserve related decisions for the family, such counseling also must be confidential and completely truthful. Upholding the family's right to know what to expect including the prognosis of the child.

A team approach that involves the physician, nurse and social worker is essential. The nurse plays important role in follow-up clarifying information, providing continuous support to the family and assisting the family with the grieving process as appropriate. Medical geneticists and genetic counselors are healthcare professionals with specialized training and experience in human and medical genetics and counseling who can give information and supportive counseling, concerning numerous disorders or abnormalities.

Chapter 26 Principles of Preoperative Care of Infants and Children

PREOPERATIVE NURSING MANAGEMENT

Surgery imposes a stress on all body systems. It imposes psychological stress both on the client and their significant with others. The nurse responsibilities include recognition of on stress. Accurate assessment of their anticipation to the extent and prevention of consequences. By keeping the client informed of these stress, accurate assessment of what to expect, reinforcing the physician's explanations in understandable terms and frankly addressing spoken and unspoken concern about pain and disability, the nurse can make a major contribution to the client's effort to recovery.

It is important for the nurse to emphasize the parents that the child need for their presence during this potentially stressful experience. During preoperative period, the nurse parents and child have an opportunity to become acquainted and to establish a trusting relationship. When the nurse has assessed the level of knowledge and anxiety of the child and parents and their coping resources, preoperative teaching can be tailored to their general and specific needs. Teaching becomes more meaningful and the results are more productive. Successful preoperative teaching generally reduces anxiety, resulting in a decrease in the need for pain, medication, their occurrence of vomiting, the number of psychological problems and complications, and length of the hospital stay. Preparation for surgery begins with preparation for admission to the hospital; children can be prepared for their admission for surgery. Children need their parents when they are facing the unknown. They need their parent's strength to help them cope with potentially threatening situations.

Preoperative Preparation

- Physiological preparation
- Psychological preparation
- Legal preparation
- Physical preparation.

Physiological Preparation

Physiological preparation includes information about the following.

Age: Infants, young children have the lowest tolerance to the stressful effects of surgery. Their needs differ from those of older children, adolescents and adults.

Fluid and electrolyte balance: Dehydration and hypovolemia predisposes a child client to complications during and after surgery. Control prolonged vomiting, diarrhea and bleeding if any, and correct electrolyte imbalance before surgery through diet and intravenous (IV) infusion.

Infection: Any infection adversely affects surgical outcome during assessment of document symptoms such as sneezing, coughing, sore throat, elevated temperature and the skin condition.

Nutritional status: The client, who is well-nourished preoperatively, is better prepared to handle surgical stress and return to optimal health after surgery.

Cardiovascular function: Rule out cardiac conditions, which increase the operative risk. Assess blood pressure, pulse, cold, weakness, shortness of breath. Conduct diagnostic studies such as electrocardiogram (ECG) and hemoglobin test.

Pulmonary function: Assess child client for shortness of breath, wheezing, coughing, respiratory allergies and infection (get a chest X-ray).

Renal function: The surgical child client needs adequate renal functions to eliminate protein wastes, preserve fluid and electrolyte balance, and clear anesthetic agents. Condition that increases operative risk is acute nephritis; observe and report for such condition.

Gastrointestinal function: Impaired nutrition may be related to an altered gastrointestinal (GI) function; ask for any problem related to GI function.

Liver function: An impaired liver is unable to detoxify medications and anesthetic agents or to metabolize carbohydrates (CHO), fats and amino acids. Inadequate liver function is associated with poor wound healing and higher rate of infection.

Endocrine function: Monitor endocrine carefully.

Neurological function: Neurological assessment is done to determine the child's baseline function.

Hematological function: Child's blood coagulation disorders are at risk of hemorrhage and hypovolemic shock. Obtain history of bleeding tendencies, get bleeding and clotting time, and platelet counts done before surgical procedures.

Psychological Preparation

Discuss surgical procedures with parents and child, and evaluate their understanding, discuss limitation on diet if appropriate. Depending on order of the surgeon, describe what 'nil per os' (NPO) is discuss premeditation, anesthesia and demonstrate preoperative exercise. Explain the use of equipment postoperatively. Assure child that parents will be nearby, waiting for him/her after the operation is over.

Legal Preparation

Anyone undergoing an invasive procedure, must sign a permit. This legal document signifies that the client is giving informed consent. The permit guards the client against unwanted invasive procedures. It also protects the healthcare facility and healthcare professional. The child/parent must receive full explanation of the operation before signing the permit and understand complete surgical procedure. He/She/Parent should be told about potential risks, complications and disfigurement, anesthesia, etc. ensure that the client receives an honest, accurate and fair statement of what to expect during and after surgery, and understand the consent form before signing.

Physical Preparation

Record vital signs such as pulse, respiration, temperature and blood pressure. Any abnormal vital signs, report to the surgeon. Prior to surgery prescribed NPO for the period and follow the checklist (Box 26.1) as per institutional policy:

- Bathe the child and record in the chart
- Dress the child in clean hospital gown or other attire according to the institutional policy
- Observe for loosened teeth, remove any dental appliances
- Remove nail polish, if present
- Administer premedication as per instruction
- Ensure consent form is signed by the parent or legal guardian
- Ensure that all laboratory reports are enclosed with child chart
- Fasten side rails of crib or bed securely after preoperative medication has been given
- Document child hand bracelet (name, ID attached)
- When transporting, side rails of the bed should be raised always.

Box 26.1: Preoperative checklist

- Health agency name: ....
- Address: ....
- Hospital number: ....
- Name of the child: .... Age: ....
- Ward: .... Bed number: .... Date: ....
- Proposed operation: ....
- Name of the surgeon: ....
- Consent signed: Yes/No
- Premedication given: Yes/No, by .... at .... other drug given ....
- Height: .... Weight: .... Pulse..........
  Respiration: .... Blood pressure: ....
- Urine result: .... Glucose: ....
  Ketone: .... Protein: ....
  Fasting blood sugar ....
- Identification band: Yes/No
- Crowns: Yes/No

Contd...

Contd...

- Denture removed: Yes/No
- Hairpins removed: Yes/No
- Nail polish removed: Yes/No
- Nasogastric tube in place: Yes/No
- Bladder emptied: Yes/No
- Catheter present: Yes/No
- Theater gown: Yes/No
- Skin preparation: Yes/No
- Nurse (checking ward): ....
- Date: .... Time: ....
- Nurse (while receiving in theater): ....
- Date and time: ....

DIFFERENCES BETWEEN CHILDREN AND ADULTS

Anatomical, Physiological and Psychological Differences

1. Children have higher respiratory rates than adults. Higher respiratory rates lead to proportionately higher minute volumes.
2. Children have thinner skin than adults. Their epidermis is thinner and under-keratinized, compared with adults. As a result, children are at risk for increased absorption of agents that can be absorbed through the skin.
3. Children have a proportionately larger body surface area (BSA) than adults. The smaller the patient, the greater the ratio of surface area (skin) to size. BSA also parallels certain body functions including basal metabolic rate (BMR) and minute volume. As a result, children may be more susceptible to agents that affect the integrity of the skin or are absorbed through the skin pulmonary route than adults with the same exposure. Children may also respond more rapidly to such agents. Signs and symptoms in children may be an 'early warning' of a chemical, biological or radiological incident.
4. Since children are generally shorter than adults, their breathing zone is lower to the ground. At the same time, many agents that are aerosolized are heavier than air. As a result, children may be more susceptible to agents absorbed through the pulmonary route than adults with the same exposure.
5. Children have immature blood-brain barriers and enhanced central nervous system (CNS) receptivity. As a result, children may exhibit a prevalence of neurological symptoms. Nerve agents may produce more symptoms in pediatric patients, requiring levels of treatment for children that are not indicated for adults with the same level of exposure.
6. Children have a higher proportion of rapidly growing tissues than adults and some agents including ionizing radiation and mustard gas, significantly affect rapidly growing tissues. As a result, children are more prone to ionizing radiations and other agents that affect rapidly growing

tissue than adults. Children may be more symptomatic and show symptoms earlier than adults. Exposure can have a significant impact on children's bone marrow and developing CNS, especially in children under 2 years of age.

7. Children have relatively small airways compared to adults. The smaller the caliber of the airway, the greater the reduction in airflow, which is a result of increased pulmonary secretions that occur following exposure to chemicals or edema from inhalation of hot gases. As a result, children suffer more pulmonary pathology than adults at the same level of exposure.
8. While IV medications may be the recommended prescription, vascular access in children can be difficult. The smaller the child, the more difficult vascular access becomes. Managing many size-related issues that arise in acute emergencies presents problems; the variation in children's sizes further complicates the issues a result, errors and delays in treatment, and discomfort in drug dosing, may occur. The use of intramuscular (IM) and intraosseous (IO) medications may be of practical value in a mass casualty situation.

Psychological and Developmental Considerations

Children's psychological immaturity has many implications for emergency preparedness. Take a moment to think about some of the ways one can imagine children's psychological or developmental needs playing out in an emergency situation. In an emergency or disaster, it will be important to recognize the various psychological vulnerabilities and developmental issues that may affect children's risk factors and needs. Some examples are as follows:

1. Children's developmental ability and cognitive levels may impede their ability to escape danger. Indeed, their natural curiosity may actually attract them to an emergency or disaster site.
2. Depending on age and developmental maturity, children may not comprehend the situation.
3. Children cannot be expected to follow complex directions or instructions given to a group. Simple, individualized guidance will be required to help children through the process of obtaining care or escaping danger.
4. Children require more intensive and continuous psychological support during an emergency or disaster situation.

Children who are separated from families and other familiar persons can experience substantial fear, anxiety and agitation, all of which can complicate treatment. All of these issues will require a significantly higher level of individualized attention and staffing resources than would be typical when dealing with an adult population.

Chapter 27 Congenital Heart Disease

ACYANOTIC HEART DEFECTS

Description

1. Acyanotic heart defects are the condition, in which deoxygenated or poorly oxygenated venous blood enters systemic arterial circulation.
2. Types of cyanotic heart defects includes:
   - Left-to-right shunting through an abnormal opening, e.g. patent ductus arteriosus (PDA), atrial septal defect (ASD) and ventricular septal defect (VSD)
   - Obstructive lesions that restrict ventricular outflow (e.g. aortic valve stenosis, pulmonic stenosis and coarctation of the aorta).

Etiology and Incidence

1. In over 90% of congenital heart defects, the exact etiology is unknown.
2. Factors associated with increased incidence of congenital heart defects include:
   - Fetal and material infection during the 1st trimester (especially rubella)
   - Maternal use of other drugs with teratogenic effects
   - Maternal age over 40 years
   - Maternal dietary deficiencies
   - Maternal insulin-dependent diabetes
   - Other congenital defects.

Incident for acyanotic heart defects is as follows:

1. **Patent ductus arteriosus:** Occurs in 1 of every 2,000 live births and accounts for 10% of congenital heart defects.
2. **Atrial septal defect:** Accounts for about 10% of congenital heart defects; occurs almost twice as often in females as in males.
3. **Ventricular septal defect:** The most common congenital heart disorder, accounting for up to 30% of all congenital heart defects.
4. **Pulmonic stenosis:** Accounts for 5–8% of all congenital heart defects.
5. **Coarctation of the aorta:** Accounts for about 7% of all congenital heart defects; twice as common in males as in females.

Pathophysiology

Patent Ductus Arteriosus

1. The PDA results from persistence of the fetal ductus arteriosus between the pulmonary artery and aorta.
2. Oxygenated blood flows form the aorta to the pulmonary artery through the patent ductusarteriosus; eventually, this places a greater volume burden on the left heart.
3. A large PDA may result in left atrial and left ventricular enlargement, pulmonary edema due to increased pulmonary pressure; and congestive heart failure (CHF); in a small defect, these effects are minimal.

Atrial Septal Defect

1. Atrial septal defect refers to an abnormal opening in the septum between the left and right atria.
2. This opening may be located at the center of the atrial septum (ostium secundum) or at the base of the atrial septum (ostiumprimum).
3. Oxygenated blood flows through the defect from the left atrium to the right atrium and mixes with systemic venous blood returning to the lungs.
4. This increases the total blood flow to the lungs and leads to volume overload of the right ventricle, producing right-sided heart enlargement.
5. Increased volume of blood pumped through pulmonary circulation can lead to pulmonary edema and eventually CHF.
6. Excessive pulmonary resistance and right atrial pressure increase may cause reversal of the left-right shunt, producing cyanosis.

Ventricular Septal Defect

1. The VSD involves an abnormal opening in the septum between the right and left ventricles.
2. Oxygenated blood flows through this opening from the left ventricle to the right ventricle.
3. Thus, an increased amount of blood enters the pulmonary circulation; this may result in increased pulmonary vascular resistance and right-sided heart enlargement.
4. Right ventricular and pulmonary arterial pressures increase, leading eventually to obstructive pulmonary vascular disease.
5. High pulmonary resistance and excessive right ventricular pressure increase may cause reversal of the left-right shunt, producing cyanosis.

Assessment Findings

1. In PDA, clinical manifestations and diagnostic findings may include:
   - A continuous machinery-like murmur heard at the left infraclavicular area in older children
   - Widened pulse pressure
   - Slow weight gain and feeding difficulties
   - Recurrent respiratory infections
   - Signs and symptoms of CHF
   - Cardiomegaly
   - Increased pulmonary vasculature
   - Possible left ventricular hypertrophy.
2. In ASD, clinical manifestations and diagnostic findings may include:
   - Absence of symptoms in a small ASD
   - Slow weight gain
   - Easy fatigability
   - Dyspnea on exertion
   - Frequent respiratory infections.
3. Clinical and diagnostic findings in VSD may include:
   - Absence of symptoms in a small VSD
   - Slow weight gain, failure to thrive, feeding difficulties
   - Pallor and diaphoresis
   - Frequent respiratory infections
   - Tachypnea
   - Signs and symptoms of CHF
   - Characteristic loud murmur, usually developing a few weeks after birth and best heard at the lower left sternal border
   - Biventricular hypertrophy, pulmonary artery enlargement and left atrial enlargement.

Signs and Symptoms of Congenital Heart Failure

- Systolic injection, murmur heard most prominently at the second left intercostals space
- Abnormal S2 heart sound
- Prominent main pulmonary artery
- Right-sided hypertrophy
- Cardiomegaly
- Electrocardiogram changes.

Nursing Diagnoses

Nursing diagnoses depend on specific manifestations of the defect. Refer also to nursing diagnoses for CHF:

- Activity intolerance
- Anxiety
- Altered family processes
- Anticipatory grieving
- Altered growth and development
- High risk for infection
- High risk for injury
- Knowledge deficit
- Altered nutrition: Less than body requirements
- Self-esteem disturbance.

Planning and Implementation

1. Help to maintain optimal nutritional status by:
   - Promoting a well-balanced diet, which is rich in iron and potassium, and low in sodium
   - Providing small, frequent meals, if the child tires easily
   - Providing nipples that make it easier for an infant to suck and limiting feeding to 45 minutes or less, if the in front is not able to suck
   - Evaluating weight gain regularly.
2. Help to decrease cardiac workload by organizing nursing care to provide for periods of uninterrupted rest, preventing excessive crying in infants, and providing diversional activities that involve only limited energy expenditure for older children.
3. Observe for and assist in managing CHF.
4. Observe for and assist in managing respiratory distress (marked by manifestations such as tachypnea, cyanosis, bradycardia, retractions, grunting, nasal flaring, cough and cyanosis) by:
   - Administering oxygen therapy as ordered
   - Positioning the child to ease breathing.
5. Observe for and assist in managing hypoxia (marked by manifestations such as tachypnea, cyanosis, bradycardia, tachycardia, restlessness, progressive limpness and syncope) by:
   - Positioning the child to knee chest position
   - Administering oxygen, as ordered
   - Administering medication, as ordered
   - Documenting hypoxic spells.

6. Observe for and assist in managing infective carditis (characterized by fever, pallor, petechiae, anorexia and fatigue) by:
   - Ensuring prophylactic administration of antibiotics before dental work, surgery or laceration repair
   - Preventing the child's exposure to ill persons.
7. Monitor for signs and symptoms of thrombosis such as irritability, restlessness, seizure activity, coma, paralysis, edema, hematuria, oliguria and anuria. To reduce the risk of thrombosis, prevent dehydration, especially during acute illness.
8. Help to prevent infection through careful hand washing, avoiding contact between the child and with infected persons, ensuring that the child's immunizations are up to date, and providing for adequate rest.
9. Help to prevent hypokalemia secondary to diuretic therapy by maintaining a high-potassium diet and administering supplemental potassium, as ordered.
10. Help prevent animal by administering iron preparations as ordered.
11. Enhance the child's self-concept by encouraging the child to express feelings about the defect, clarifying any misconceptions he/she expresses concerning the defect and its treatment, and supporting positive coping mechanisms.
12. Help to decrease the child's and family members anxiety, and increase their understanding by providing needed information on medical and surgical treatment for the specific defect.
13. Provide the following information for PDA:
    - Surgery may be performed electively by age 1–2 years, earlier if CHF develops. Ligation of PDA is not open-heart surgery and does not require cardiopulmonary bypass
    - In premature infants, PDA sometimes can be closed using prostaglandin synthease inhibitors such as indomethancin, which stimulate closure of the ductus
    - Some children experience transient unexplained hypertension following repair.
14. Provide the following information for ASD:
    - Surgical closure by suture or patch requires cardiopulmonary bypass and usually is performed between age of 4 and 6 years
    - Some children develop dysrhythmias despite surgery.
15. Provide the following information on VSD:
    - Most VSDs close spontaneously
    - Early surgery, involving closure with a Dacron patch and requiring cardiopulmonary bypass, is recommended for children with pulmonary arterial hypertension, CHF, recurrent respiratory infections, and failure to thrive

- Surgery is complex, pulmonary artery banding may be done as a palliative procedure for infants who are poor surgical candidates.

16. Provide the following information for aortic valve stenosis:
    - If symptomatic, surgical aortic valvotomy or prosthetic valve replacement is necessary
    - Children with this defect may be restricted from sports and physical exertion.
17. Provide patient and family teaching, covering:
    - Nature of the defect, diagnosis, treatment and potential complications
    - Infection prevention and control measures
    - Administration, dosage and side effects of prescribed medications
    - The child's nutritional requirements and any special diet information
    - The child's need for adequate rest periods and any physical or activity limitations
    - The significance of normal developmental tasks and the importance, of avoiding overprotecting the child through overstrict activity limitations.

Evaluation

1. Parents verbalize knowledge of their child's defect, treatments and potential complications.
2. The child verbalizes and age-appropriate understanding of the disease and its treatment.
3. The child maintains adequate oxygenation, as evidenced by normal color and improved blood gas values.
4. The child remains free from infection.
5. The child's breathing is nonlabored.
6. The child gains or maintains adequate weight.
7. Parents verbalize the date and time of next scheduled follow-up appointment.

CONGESTIVE HEART FAILURE

Description

Severe circulatory congestion due to decreased myocardial contractility resulting in the heart's inability to pump sufficient blood to meet the body's needs.

Etiology and Incidence

1. The primary cause of CHF in the first 3 years of life is congenital heart disease.

2. Other causes in children include:
   - Other myocardial disorder such as cardiomyopathies, dysrhythmias and hypertension
   - Pulmonary embolism or chronic lung disease
   - Severe hemorrhage or anemia
   - Adverse effects of anesthesia or surgery
   - Adverse effects of transfusions or infusions
   - Increased body demands resulting from such conditions as fever, infection and arteriovenous fistula
   - Adverse effects of drugs such as doxorubicin
   - Severe physical or emotional stress
   - Excessive sodium intake.

Pathophysiology

1. In CHF, the heart is unable to meet the body's oxygenation and nutrition needs, most commonly due to excessive volume or pressure load on the heart, or to diminished myocardial function.
2. The body attempts to compensate through the following mechanisms:
   - Increased heart rate and increase stroke volume, resulting in cardiomegaly
   - Release of catecholamines, which increases systemic vascular resistance and leads to decreased renal blood flow
   - Decreased glomerular filtration rate (GFR) and increased tubular reabsorption, leading to diminished urinary output and sodium retention.
3. Further myocardial stretching results in progressively ineffective contractions, leading to diminished cardiac output and pulmonary, and systemic circulation congestion.

Assessment Findings

1. Signs and symptoms of CHF vary somewhat depending of the child's age and on whether failure occurs on the right or left side of the heart; manifestations of combined right-and left-sided CHF (the usual condition) may include:
   - Respiratory distress, marked by tachypnea, dyspnea, orthopnea, retractions, nasal flaring and grunting
   - Cough
   - Tachycardia, S3 ventricular gallop
   - Pallor, mottling or cyanosis
   - Feeding difficulties and failure to thrive

- Restlessness and irritability
- Weakness, easy fatigability
- Unexplained weight gain
- Diaphoresis
- Abdominal distention
- Neck vein distention
- Hepatomegaly.

2. Chest radiograph reveals cardiomegaly and pulmonary congestion.
3. Laboratory study results commonly reveal dilutional hyponatremia, hypochloremia and hyperkalemia.

Nursing Diagnoses

- Activity intolerance
- Anxiety
- Ineffective breathing pattern
- Decreased cardiac output
- Altered family processes
- Excess fluid volume
- High risk for injury
- High risk for infection
- Altered nutrition: Less than body requirements.

Planning and Implementation

1. Monitor for signs of respiratory distress. Provide pulmonary hygiene as needed, administer oxygen as ordered keep the head of the bed deviated, and monitor arterial blood gas values.
2. Monitor for signs of altered cardiac output such as signs and symptoms of pulmonary edema, dysrhythmias including extreme tachycardia or bradycardia and characteristic ECG and heart sound changes.
3. Evaluate fluid status by keeping strict intake and output records, monitoring daily weights, assessing for edema and severe diaphoresis, and monitoring electrolytes values and hematocrit level. Maintain fluid restrictions, as ordered.
4. Help prevent infection through scrupulous hand washing and limiting the child's exposure to persons with infections.
5. Reduce cardiac demands by keeping the child warm and clustering nursing care activities to allow for periods of uninterrupted rest. Do not allow an infant to feed for more than 45 minutes at a time and gavage feed if the infant becomes fatigued before eating an adequate amount.
6. Help to ensure adequate nutrition. As necessary, provide small frequent meals. Maintain a high-calorie and low-sodium diet, as ordered.

7. Help to decrease the child's and parents' anxiety by providing developmentally appropriate explanations, encouraging expression of feelings and concerns, and encouraging parental involvement in the child's care, as appropriate.
8. Administer medications as ordered, which may include:
   - Digoxin, given to increase cardiac performance
   - Diuretics such as furosemide, hydrochlorothiazide and spironolactone, given to reduce venous and systemic congestion
   - Iron and folic acid supplements, given to improve nutritional status.
9. Monitor for medication side effects, including:
   - Digitalis toxicity: Extreme bradycardia is a cardinal symptom of toxicity; hold the drug if the child's heart rate falls below the normal range for age, unless the physician specifies a different guideline
   - Hypokalemia, due to diuretic therapy: Monitor potassium level closely and administer supplemental potassium, if necessary.
10. Provide patient and family teaching, covering:
    - Signs and symptoms of CHF to watch for which and report
    - Diet and fluid restrictions
    - Dosage, administration and side effects of prescribed medications.

Evaluation

1. The child exhibits improved cardiac output as evidenced by clinical condition and laboratory values.
2. The child has normal fluid and electrolyte values, and decreased edema.
3. The child exhibits improved oxygenation as evidenced by normal color and blood gas values within the normal range.
4. The child maintains adequate nutrition for optimal weight gain.
5. Parent verbalize an understanding of signs and symptoms of CHF, and possible complications, correct dosage and administration of medications, and necessary follow-up care.

RHEUMATIC FEVER

Description

An inflammatory disease that affects the connective tissue of the heart, joints, central nerves system (CNS) and subcutaneous tissue.

Etiology and Incidence

1. Rheumatic fever (RF) follows by untreated, group A beta-hemolytic *Streptococcus* of pharyngitis tonsillitis.
2. Rheumatic fever usually occurs in children between 6 and 15 years of age with peak incidence at 8 years of age.
3. Incidence peaks in the winter months.

Pathophysiology

1. The pathophysiology of RF is uncertain.
2. It is generally thought to an immune reaction to antigens of group A *Streptococcus.*
3. Changes in the connective tissue.
4. The structures most often affected are the mitral and aortic valves, which may become swollen and edematous.

Assessment Findings

The findings typically involve the following clinical manifestations.

General

- Low-grade fever usually spiking in late afternoon
- Abdominal pain
- Arthralgia without arthritic changes
- Weakness, fatigue, pallor, loss of appetite and weight loss.

Major Manifestations

1. **Carditis:**
    - Tachycardia
    - Cardiomegaly
    - Precardial pain
    - Changes in ECG.
2. **Migratory polyarthrities:**
    - Swollen, hot, red and painful joint(s)
    - After 1–2 days affects different joint(s)
    - Favors large joints-knees elbow, hips, shoulders and wrists.
3. **Erythema marginatum:**
    - Erythematous macules with clear center and well-demarcated border
    - Non-pruritic primary affects trunk and extremities.
4. **Chores (Saint Vitus Dance or Sydenham's chorea):**
    - Subcutaneous nodes
    - Non-tender swelling
    - Located over body prominences
    - May persist for some time, then gradually resolve.

Laboratory Study and Diagnostic Test Results

- Complete blood count with differential indicates leukocytosis and anemia
- Erythrocyte sedimentation rate (ESR) elevated
- Creative proteins are elevated
- An increased or rising antistreptolysin O (ASO) titer is the most commonly used serologic test to detect previous group a streptococcal infection
- Electrocardiography may indicate a prolonged PR interval and non-specific PR interval, and non-specific ST or T wave changes
- Chest X-ray may reveal cardiomegaly or pulmonary edema.

Chapter

28

Child with Special Needs

OVERVIEW

1. A child with serious chronic illness or developmental disability often has complex needs that differ from those of unimpaired agemates.
2. A chronic illness is any disorder that disrupts daily functioning for more than 1 month in any given year.
3. Development disability refers to a severe physical or mental disability that occurs before age of 22 years and usually results in substantial limitation of function. Chronic illness affects an estimated 10–15% of all children under age of 18 years. Asthma and congenital heart defects account for almost 67% of these chronic illnesses leukemia, congenital heart defects and spina bifida carry the highest mortality of all childhood illness.
4. Adding speech, learning, sensory, cognitive and emotional problem is estimated 40% of children between kinder garden and sixth grade have significant long-term disabilities.
5. In contrast to care of unimpaired children, health care for the child with special needs is related more to developmental age than to chronologic age. Accurate assessment of the child's level of development and adaptation is crucial to planning appropriate interventions.
6. Nursing interventions should be aimed at promoting optimal adjustment of each family member.

TRENDS IN HEALTH CARE

1. The Education for All Handicapped Children Act of 1975 (Public Law 94-142), probably the most significant recent federal legislation affecting children, provides for the following:
   - Free appropriate public education for all handicapped children
   - Identification and evaluation of all handicapped children
   - Preparation of an individualized education program for each handicapped child
   - Provision of education in the least restrictive environment possible
   - Procedural safeguards for parental grievances (due process)
   - Protection of the rights of children placed by the state in private schools
   - In-service training for educators.
2. National organizations and local support groups geared to the needs of children with specific disabilities (and their families).

Provide opportunities for children and parents to improve their understanding of the disability and its management to develop networks for self-help.

3. In hospitals, parent care units and rooming-in arrangements provide parents of a disabled child with the opportunity to learn the specialized care measures that their child requires and free the child from the stress associated with separation from family, allowing the child to mobilize all of his/her emotional resources to cope effectively with the threat posed by the disability.
4. The advent of pediatric home care agencies has enabled shorter hospital stays by providing a variety of continuous or episode services for disabled children in their home environment.

MENTAL RETARDATION

1. As defined by the American Association on Mental Retardation (AAMR), mental retardation is "significantly subaverage intellectual function coexisting with deficits in adaptive behavior and manifested during the developmental period (before age 18)."
2. Mental retardation is classified by the AAMR based on the intelligence quotient (IQ) level as follows:
   - Mild (educable mentally retarded)—IQ of 50–55 to about 70
   - Moderate (trainable mentally retarded)—IQ of 35–40 to 50–55
   - Severe—IQ of 20–25 to 35–40
   - Profound—IQ below 20–25.

Etiology and Incidence

1. The most common developmental disability, mental retardation affects up to 3% of the population.
2. Causes are classified as idiopathic, acquired, inherited or genetic and endocrine as follows:
   a. Idiopathic, all cases of unknown cause (the most common classification).
   b. Acquired—perinatal infections (e.g. maternal infections such as rubella, toxoplasmosis, syphilis, cytomegalovirus), other maternal illnesses, are teratogenic effects of prescription or non-prescription drugs used by the mother during pregnancy; birth injury; prenatal, perinatal, or postnatal hypoxia, kernicterus, trauma in infancy or childhood, lead poisoning, malnutrition, brain tumor, severe psychosocial or psychological deprivation.
   c. Inherited or genetic, chromosomal abnormalities such as Down syndrome, Turner's syndrome and Klinefelter's syndrome; autosomal dominant disorders such as Huntington's chorea, spinocerebellar degeneration, tuberous sclerosis and neurofibromatosis; autosomal recessive disorders such as galactosemia, glycogen storage disease,

phenylketonuria (PKU), Tay-Sachs disease, Niemann-Pick disease and Hurler's disease.

d. Endocrine—coal hypothyroidism.

Pathophysiology

1. Clinical manifestations vary according to the child's age and degree of impairment general signs include developmental delays in motor, social, language or cognitive skills.
2. Diagnostic evaluation typically includes some or all of the following:
   - Neurological examination including computed tomography (CT), to rule out nervous system pathology
   - Radiological studies to detect lesions
   - Endocrine studies including urine screening for abnormal metabolic activity
   - Developmental screening tests such as the Denver Developmental Screening Test (DDST), to identify apparent developmental delays
   - Intelligence evaluation with standardized tests such as the Stanford-Binet intelligence scale, the Wechsler intelligence scale for children, and Gesell developmental schedules
   - Adaptive behavior evaluation is to be done using tools such as the American Association on Mental Deficiency (AAMD) adaptive behavior scale
   - Chromosomal analysis and genetic screening, in cases of a family history of mental retardation or chromosomal abnormalities.

Nursing Diagnoses

- Impaired verbal communication
- Altered family processes
- Altered growth and development
- Altered health maintenance
- High risk for infection
- Altered role performance
- Self-care deficit
- High risk for impaired skin integrity
- Impaired social interaction
- Social isolation.

Planning and Implementation

1. Support the family at time of initial diagnosis by actively listening to their feelings and concerns and assessing their composite strengths.

2. Perform a task analysis before attempting to teach the child any new task. Break tasks into specific steps with each step building on the last.
3. Facilitate the child's self-care abilities by encouraging parents to enroll the child in an early stimulation program establishing a self-feeding program, initiating independent toileting and establishing an independent grooming program (all developmental level appropriate).
4. Promote optimal development by encouraging self-care goals and emphasizing the universal needs of children such as play, social interaction and parental limit setting.
5. Promote anticipatory guidance and problem solving by encouraging discussion regarding physical maturation.
6. Assist the family in planning for their child's future needs; refer them to available community agencies.
7. Provide patient and family teaching covering:
   - Normal developmental milestones and appropriate stimulating activities, including play and socialization activities
   - The need for patience with the child's slow attainment of developmental milestones
   - Information regarding stimulation, safety and motivation
   - Measures to help prevent skin breakdown keeping the child's skin clean and well-lubricated applying lip balm during dry weather and using soap sparingly
   - The need for discipline that is simple, consistent and appropriate to the child's developmental level
   - Demonstration as a better way of fostering learning than verbal explanation, since the child is better able to deal with concrete objects than abstract concepts
   - The benefits of motivating the child to learn through positive reinforcement and shaping and fading principles
   - The role of positive self-esteem built by accomplishing small success in motivating the child to accomplish other tasks.

Evaluation

- The child exhibits no evidence of infection or respiratory distress
- The child's skin remains clean and intact with no evidence of breakdown
- The child participates in self-care activities appropriate for his/her mental capabilities
- The child and family are actively involved in early intervention programs and appropriate special education programs
- Parents verbalize understanding of appropriate discipline and recreational and social activities
- Family members express feelings and concerns regarding the child's limited mental abilities

- Family members verbalize realistic goals for care of the child
- The family demonstrates acceptance of the child into the family structure.

PARENTS OF A CHILD WITH SPECIAL NEEDS

Essential Concepts

1. Parenting a child who must master the same developmental achievements as all children in accordance with individual potentials and limitations, leaves the family unit vulnerable to psychological and physical problems.
2. Response of family members to the child's disability is influenced by many factors including perception of the situation, previous coping skills and support systems.
3. Depending on such variables, a stressful situation may or may not become a crisis for the family.
4. Parents of a disabled child need information, guidance and support to help them:
    - Understand and manage their child's illness or problem
    - Assist their child in understanding and coping with the disability
    - Meet the needs of the child
    - Meet the needs of all other family members.

Parental Coping Strategies

1. Once parents accept the reality of their child's disability, the task of making adjustments in family life begins. The emerging coping parents may be adaptive or maladaptive.
2. Adaptive patterns may include:
    - Assigning special meaning to the disability that provides hope and places the hardship in the context of a meaningful future (e.g. "God selected us to care for this child for his/her purpose")
    - Focusing on the child's positive attributes rather than on the negative aspects of the disability
    - Sharing hardships with others outside the family such as friends, church members and formal support groups
    - Adapting daily family life to the child's special needs without major disruptions in family functioning
    - Becoming involved in support groups to help parents of other children with similar disabilities.
3. Maladaptive strategies can include:
    - Overprotecting the child and not providing proper discipline and limit setting

- Rejecting or becoming emotionally detached from the child or other family members
- Directing anger or blame toward the child, spouse or self.

Assessing the Family

1. Successful parenting of a child hinges on numerous factors including the parents' reaction to the disability, perception of the disability parenting style coping behaviors, composite family strengths, available support systems concurrent stressors and the child's developmental level.
2. Common reactions to chronic illness or disability include:
   a. Shock and denial: Initial intense emotions usually adaptive to cushion or soften grief reaction to any type of loss; healthy enabling reaction until it becomes protracted or maladaptive with no or limited recognition of diagnosis; denial allows individual to maintain sense of hope.
   b. Adjustment beginning acknowledgement that disability or disorder exists; initially manifested by intense feelings of guilt, self-accusation, anger, bitterness with the most common result being 'benevolent overreaction', consequence of unresolved guilt. It is cycle of guilt, over permissiveness and anger.
   c. Reintegration and acceptance: Realistic expectation of child's abilities and reintegration of child into family life; acceptance is interspersed with 'chronic sorrow' (periods of intensifies sorrow or sadness of loss), especially at times child would have normally been achieving particular developmental milestone.
   d. Freezing-out phase behavior not experienced by many; not always maladjusted; decision based on need to permanently place child in residential setting, usually institutionalization.
3. The parents' perception of their child's disability involves the meaning or significance that they attach to the situation. This is influenced by such factor as previous knowledge, religious or cultural influence, imagined cause, child's gender and birth order, child's previous health status and child's prognosis.
4. Common parenting style includes:
   a. Authorization: Parental control of child's behavior by series of rigid, inflexible rules that dictate standards of conduct.
   b. Permissive: Laissez-faire style of control over the child's actions with few or no rules determining standards of conduct.
   c. Authoritative: Parental direction and guidance of the child's behavior by discussion of reasons for rules with standards of conduct regulated by exchange of ideas between parent and child, but with the parent retaining ultimate control.
5. Coping behaviors include actions aimed at reducing tension by crisis and disruption reflect reactions to previous crisis:

a. Approach behaviors: It is used to move a person toward adjustment and resolution (e.g. asking for information, seeking support, anticipating future, expressing feelings, planning realistic goals for the future).
b. Avoidance behaviors: They are usually maladaptive aimed at protecting a person by moving him/her away from adjustment and resolution (e.g. failing to recognize the seriousness of the child's condition refusing to agree to treatment avoiding staff members or the child using magical thinking).

6. The family's composite strengths encompass individual family members' strengths, coping behaviors and reactions to the child's disability; these can help achieve or impede the goal of optimal development for the family or individual members.
7. Available support systems include:
   a. Marital relationship: Prime source of potential support, best predictor of coping behaviors, single parent family structure or poorly adjusted family unit contribute to already stressful circumstance of disabled child leaving family unit vulnerable to psychological trauma.
   b. Alternate support systems: Those available outside marital relationship.
   c. Economic support system: Financial sources are available for health and rehabilitative care.
   d. Emotional support system: System that sustains individual family members during period of vulnerability.
   e. Communication support system; verbal and non-verbal symbols that convey meaning to event; open communication system is one in which verbal and non-verbal cues are congruent with intended message.
8. Concurrent stress within family involves any other difficulties with which family is attempting to deal (e.g. financial, marital, social isolation).
9. The child's development level: Chronically ill child have the same needs and concerns their well-counterparts. However, age of onset influences reaction to diagnosis and psychological adjustment. Early age of onset predisposes child to additional psychological problems, since critical development stages are interrupted; these stages include:
   a. Infancy: Sensorimotor experiences are critical, as well as establishment of sense of trust and attachment to significant other.
   b. Childhood: Mastery of locomotion and language skills; separation anxiety is at its height; illness interferes with critical foundation of sense of autonomy.
   c. Preschool: Social development, sexual identity and body image are developing; interruption in development can interfere with development of sense of initiative and influence development of sense of guilt.

d. School age: Striving for sense of achievement and accomplishment, while overcoming sense of doubt; relationships with peers is taking on more importance.

e. Adolescence: Self-esteem, self-image, striving for independence and identity are hallmarks and illness interferes with incorporate disability into self-image; illness or disability is greatest thereat during middle adolescence (age 14–16 year) when energy is devoted to meet normal development demands.

Nursing Diagnoses

- Ineffective family coping
- Altered family progress
- Altered growth and development
- Parental role conflict
- Altered parenting
- Self-esteem disturbance.

Planning and Implementation

1. Promote parental functioning by offering support at times of diagnosis, providing follow-up information and coordinating services with healthcare agencies.
2. Promote parental understanding by giving clear and simple explanation of illness or disability and opportunity to ask questions; always remain active and empathetic listener.
3. Promote the child's development by focusing on his/her strengths and asset and by sharing his/her expected developmental achievements.
4. Promote parenting skills by sharing universal developmental milestones, discipline guidelines and methods of effective communication.
5. Prevent ineffective coping and dysfunctional parenting by guiding parents to support groups of parents who have children with similar special needs.
6. Promote optimal family functioning by including all significant others and siblings in understanding child's condition; allow family members to vent feelings and concerns; guide family members to identify composite strengths.

Evaluation

- Parents verbalize appropriate use of resources
- Parents cope adaptively to stress
- Parents demonstrate positive parent-child interaction and use effective discipline without anger, violence or belligerence
- Parents express realistic perception of the child's abilities and disabilities

- Parents express realistic expectations of the child's skills and behaviors
- Parents express feelings and concerns regarding the child's future
- The child's behavior is developmentally appropriate
- Parents verbalize support and affirmation of the child's abilities
- Parents verbalize understanding that chronic illness or disability will require continuing therapeutic management.

BEHAVIORAL DISORDERS IN CHILDREN

The changing trends towards younger members of our society influence the society and parents and children, all members have responsibility in the nurturing of children, the development of future behavior and character of the children. Children learn to understand culture, tradition, religion, social obligation as they grow from infancy through adolescence to adulthood, they must be aware of the meaning of wellness behavior as it is practiced by other members of the community. Children need to be motivated to participate actively in making the kind of behavioral choices that will lead to wellness and to have such behavior reinforced.

The ancient argument of heredity verso environment is still raging and is likely to continue. The important issue is not which influence on the personality is more powerful, but how heredity and environment interact in the development of human behavior, studies identical twins shows that to some extent, the genes control social traits introversion or extraversion, also some serious mental disorders, such as schizophrenia and manic depression, appear to have their roots in genetic make up. The physical appearance whether we are tall or short, dark or light, plain or beautiful is genetically determined, but the way in which the culture views these physical attributes can have a profound effect on personality development.

SOCIALIZATION OF CHILDREN

The school age years a period of dynamic change and maturation as the child becomes increasingly involved in more complex activities, decision-making and goal-directed activities. As a school age child becomes more knowledgeable about his/her body, social development centers on the body and its capabilities.

Social Adjustment

1. School serves as a formal agent for transmitting societal values to each generation, it is second in importance only to the family as a socializing agent and has a lasting influence on a child social development.
2. Most children adjust to this new structure with little difficulty.
3. The readiness of the child and parents for separation is an important factor in the adaptation process.

4. In many families both parents work outside the home, and the child is at home alone after school these latchkey children need guidance for safety precautions, productive activities.
5. Children begin to internalize their own controls and need less outside direction.
6. The child does however need a parent or other caretaker to answer questions and provide guidance for decisions and responsibilities.
7. When disciplining a child parents and other care takers should set reasonable concrete limits and provide plausible explanations and keep rules to minimum.
8. Children will have bouts of bad behaviors; they may have temper tantrums or talk back to their parents or teachers. When things start to get out of hand, however it may be a clue that something in the child life needs attention.
9. Good parenting practice can help the child and benefit the family as a whole. Behavior disorders can be identified in house, school and in social gathering. It is important to understand that children can start acting out when there are other stresses in their lives. It may be that there has been a death in the family or their parents are having argument or dysfunctional family or they are bullied at school, reassuring the child and providing extra care may help to get them through these stressful times. But if the child does not feel better and their behaviors does not improve, it is important to seek professionals help particularly if the problems last many months and are severe

DESTRUCTIVE BEHAVIORS DISORDERS

The most common destructive behavior disorders include oppositional defiant disorders (ODD), conduct disorders (CD) and attention deficit hyperactivity disorders (ADHD) these three behavioral disorders share some common symptoms, so diagnosis can be difficult.

Oppositional Defiant Disorders

Typical behavior of a child with ODD occurs below 12 years of age include:

- Easily angered
- Temper tantrum
- Argues with parents
- Low self-esteem
- Blaming other
- Occurs below 12 years of age.

Conduct Disorders

Delinquent behavior, not accepting rules. Typical behavior are:

- Not obey the parents
- Prone to use drugs, use of cigarette smoking and alcohol
- Lack of empathy for others
- Sadistic behavior, cruel to animal
- Indulge in physical fight, using dangers weapon or instruments
- Lying, staling, breaking into house
- Tendency to run away from home
- Suicidal tendency.

Attention Deficit Hyperactivity Disorders

1. **Inattention:** Difficulty in concentrating, forgetting instruction, skipping from one task to other before completing one.
2. **Impulsivity:** Not tolerating others and accident prone.

Risk Factors

- The causes of ODD and ADHD
- Gender—boys suffer more than girls from behaviors disorders
- Genes—parents or in the family had the similar problems
- Gestation and birth—difficult pregnancies and difficult labor.
- Family—dysfunctional families, such as domestic violence, poverty, poor parents skills
- Learning difficulties, intellectual disabilities, brain-retarded growth.

Diagnosis

Depth interview by pediatrician, psychiatrist and psychologist with parents and child:

1. **Parental education:** Teach parents what to expect from children and problem-solving skills (normal and abnormal behavior expected).
2. **Family therapy:** This will be decided by professionals depending on type of behavior disorders and therapy required.
3. **Cognitive behavior therapy:** Therapy help child to control their thought and behavior.
4. **Social behavior:** How to behave in society, teach important social skills to parents and child.
5. **Anger management:** Child is taught how to control anger.
6. Relaxation therapy and stress management.
7. Extend professional help to doctors, nurses, social workers.
8. Encourage the parents and child to build self-esteem, help to recognize their (child) talent.

ANXIETY DISORDERS

Anxiety disorders is normal for a child to feel anxious about his/her 1st day of school or for adolescents to feel anxious about a major examination and also it is normal for parents to feel anxious for their children. Normal anxiety is a good thing, because it prepares the body to handle a situation that may be more stressful or may require more concentration than usual.

Definition

An anxiety disorders is characterized by having feelings of anxiety that are so severe they interfere significantly with daily living, when there is no reasons to worry.

Etiology

- Genetic disorders
- Environmental factors
- Social demand
- Starting school
- Not recognized early anxiety and not treated
- Learning disability.

Identifying Anxiety Disorders

- Difficulty to identify
- Behavioral clue such as nail bitting, finger picking or hair twirling
- Socially isolating
- Adolescents turn to drug abuse and alcohol
- Anxiety can appear different from indifferent time.

Behavior disorders leads to poor academic achievement, socializing difficulties in getting along with others.

Types

- General anxiety disorders (GAD)
- Obsessive compulsive disorders (OCD)
- Panic disorders
- Post-traumatic stress disorders
- Separation anxiety disorders
- Social anxiety disorders.

Management

- Careful diagnosis and assessment
- Medication
- Psychotherapy
- Evaluate coexisting condition
- Parent teaching
- Teach parents to observe child's anxiety how often does the child become anxious, when does anxiety occurs intensity and duration
- If you notice that there is an increase in frequency seek help of professionals.

BED WETTING

Bed wetting can be symptoms of an underlying disease; majority children who wet the bed have no underlying disease. Child who wets the bed can control it or is doing it on purpose. Bed wetting is most often a developmental illness.

Types

There are two types of bed wetting primary and secondary. Primary means bed wetting that has been ongoing since early childhood. Secondary bed wetting that starts up after the child has been dry at night for a significant period of time at least 6 months.

Etiology

1. Lack of toilet training, too early or severe training.
2. Child cannot hold urine for entire night.
3. Child does not waken when his/her bladder is full.
4. Large amount of urine produced during the evening and night hours.
5. Problems, which they cannot solve.
6. Child has poor daytime toilet habit.
7. Secondary bed wetting can be a sign of an underlying medical or emotional problems, such as urinary tract infection, structural or anatomical abnormalities, neurological problems, emotional problems such as stressful home life as parents are in conflict, starting school, new baby arrival in the house, moving to new house, children physically or sexually abused sometimes begin bed wetting.
8. Heredity, parents also had the same problems as they grow it stopped.

Management

- Parental training, should be examined by physician and by psychologist
- Physical examination of urinary tract

- Verify condition of toilet place like distance and light
- Child may reluctant to get out from warm bed, counsel the child
- Giving less fluid during night
- Examine parents and child relation
- Help the child to achieve dry night and develop confidence in ability to control elimination
- Keep alarm on 4th hour duration.

ANOREXIA NERVOSA

Often referred to simple as anorexia. Eating disorders characterized by a low weight. Fear of gaining weight; a strong desire to be thin and food restriction.

Causes

- Genetic factors
- Cultural factors that value thinner body having high recognition
- Professional concern such as dancer, actress, modeling have more percentage than general population.

Signs and Symptoms

- Individual see them self as over weight even though are under weight
- Desire to be thin personality
- Eat only small amount of food and eat certain food only
- Some individual will exercise excessively
- Use laxative.

Complications

- Osteoporosis
- Infernality
- Heart damage.

Treatment

- Restoring healthy weight
- Treating underlying psychological problems
- Treating behavior problems
- Family therapy—teaching parent
- Cognitive therapy and behavioral therapy
- Sometimes hospitalization may require
- Educate the parents to manage the behavior.

PHYSICALLY CHALLENGED CHILDREN

Some children are physically handicapped from birth and others develop infirmities after accidents, there are many physical disabilities such as blindness, deafness, dumbness, etc. There are other children who may not have any physical abnormality, but they must be abnormally short fat with julting teeth, small and sunken eyes and several such features.

Physically handicapped person defined as a person who has a disability of locomotors and neurological origin, which constitute a disadvantage or restriction in one or more aspects of daily living activities, including work.

Disability

Disability is the consequence of an impairment that may be physical, cognitive, mental, sensory, emotional development or some combination of these disability may be present from birth or occur during lifetime.

Types

- Sensory disability
- Vision impairment
- Hearing
- Olfactory and gustatory impairment
- Somotosensory impairment
- Balance disorders
- Intellectual disability
- Mental health and emotional disability
- Pervasive developmental disorders.

Government Policies and Support

On December 13, 2006, the United Nation formally agreed on the convention on the rights of person with disabilities. The first human rights treaty of the 21st century to protect and enhance the right and opportunities of the world estimated 650 million disabled people.

Countries that sign the convention are required to adopt national laws and remove old one, so that person with disabilities will, e.g. equal right to education and employment and cultural life. The right to own and inherit property, to not be discriminated against in marriage, etc. in 1976, the United Nation launched its international year of disabled person (1981). Later renamed international year of disabled person.

Effect of Physical Problems on Educating Physically Challenged Children

1. Mobility and physical fitness: Physical handicapped may cause various degrees of weakness and incoordination of the limbs, which may affect

mobility, posture and manual dexterity. Other physical problems such as heart problems may cause poor exercise tolerance and low level of physical fitness, all these may directly result in pupil's difficulty to cope with ordinary school routine and limit their ability in exploring and understanding the environment.

2. Neurological impairment may also cause sensory deficiencies or over stimulation, which may disturb perception and concentration inducing specific learning difficulties for the pupils.
3. The disadvantage which physically handicapped pupils are placed may cause them some of the emotional problems including low self esteem. Lack of self confidence.
4. Fear of changes in environment, apathy; over dependence on others low level of aspiration anxiety and frustration. Some brain damaged children may also be hyperactive, aggressive or lack of emotional control

Aims in Educating Physically Handicapped Children

The aim of education for physically handicapped pupils focused on the total development of pupils is similar to that for special education on the whole.

Following Specific Aims in Education

- Offer general education in ordinary, special day or special residential school setting according to their needs
- To prepare them for integration into ordinary school or society, and to meet their psychological needs for security love and affection acceptance and success
- Teach them the basic daily living skills for independent living
- To help them to realize their limitation and their potential, and hence develop a realistic and positive outlook towards life
- Enhance their social development
- Provide medical services.

Teacher, parents and experts all have the same goal to enable the child to become a creative, assertive, warm and friendly person.

FRACTURES (ORTHOPEDICS DISORDERS)

Trauma in a child is a common occurrence, children depending on their age, accidents and injury depends. Fracture means a break in continuity of bone. Injury to musculoskeletal system may be caused by the following:

- Falling
- Climbing, running into a solid object
- Play in the school
- Risk taking behavior
- On bicycles/motor cycle.

Classification of Fracture

1. Complete fracture, in this bone is completely broken across, may be transverse or a fracture at right angles to the bone. Oblique, a fracture in which the break extends in an oblique direction.
2. Spiral fracture in which the bone has been twisted apart.
3. Incomplete fracture is one where fracture not completely destroy the continuity of the bone.
4. Closed fracture is one where fracture not produce an open injury in the skin.
5. Open fracture is one where there is an external wound leading to the break in the bone or it is called compound fracture.

Assessment of Fracture

- History collection
- Physical examination
- Assess the pain
- Identify deformities
- Observe color and temperature of the injuries parts
- Observe for cyanosed area, examine carefully to elicit the sensation
- Check the pulse in the area and radial pulse.

Laboratory Examination

- Complete history
- X-ray examination
- Blood test, Hb%, complete blood count (CBC).

Management

- Management depends on child's age and type of fracture
- Immobilization
- Reduction by traction.

Types of Fracture Reduction

Traction

Traction is force applied in a longitudinal direction to reduce a fracture closed reduction, by manipulation and manual traction open reduction. Some fracture require surgery or open reduction under direct visualization, internal fixation devices in the form of metallic screws, plates or rods may be used to hold the fragments of bone in position until solid bone healing takes place. After the wound is closed, external immobilization of the fracture is achieved by applying an external fixation device such as a splint or cast.

Fracture Immobilization

Immobilization can be achieved with external fixation devices including plates, screws and rods.

Casts Application

A process of applying plaster of Paris to a body parts for aligning malpositioned tissues such as clubfoot, congenital hip dislocation or for the purpose of immobilization.

Purpose

- To immobilize a reduced fracture
- To immobilize a body part in a specific position
- To correct deformity
- To Provide support and stability for weakened joints.

Equipment

- Rolls of cast materials
- Stockinet
- Padding
- Scissors
- Lubricant
- Bucket with fresh water at the right temperature
- Disposable gloves
- Adhesive tape
- Plastic splints.

Procedure (Table 28.1)

Table 28.1: Procedure for assisting, applying plaster of Paris (POP)

Sl No.	Actions	Rationales
1.	Explain the procedure to the patient	Get parents and child cooperation
2.	Place water proof padding under affected body parts	Protects bed wetting
3.	Keep ready stockinet as per measurement	Enough to cover the cast
4.	Roll the stockinet	Ensure application facilities
5.	Hold the affected limb in a neutral position	

Contd...

Contd...

Sl No.	Actions	Rationales
6.	Hold the affected limb, while the physician applies one to three layers of padding	Provide soft protection between stockinet and surface cast
7.	Immerse the cast roll in water for required period	Moistens the hardening agents, activating the hardening agents
8.	Support the body parts, while physician unrolls the cast material and forms the cast dressing	Facilitates easier application of the casting materials
9.	Adjust the edges and create smooth finishing trim with scissors as necessary	Creates a rounded smooth and soft edge for the cast
10.	Remove excess materials and clean the area as needed	
11.	Observe the client response to the cast, discomfort, pain, chilling, movement and sensation of distal parts of castled extremities	
12.	Elevate the casted limb above the level of the client heart by using pillows, blankets under the cast	Facilitates venous return to the heart
13.	Reassess the neuromuscular and circulatory status of the distal part every 2 hours	
14.	Neuromuscular status is assessed, such as unusual coldness, paleness and cynasis of the toes or fingers of a casted extremity	
15.	If noticed weak or absent peripheral pulses, inform concerned doctor	Prevent further complications
16.	Reported abnormal findings obtained from client; record all findings	

Note:

- The child with hip spica is turned routinely
- Ambulation is encouraged as soon as possible
- A sling is used to support a casted arm
- A child with a casted leg is encouraged to use crutches
- Food and fluids are offered in frequent intervals.

CANCER IN CHILDREN (ESSENTIAL CONCEPTS)

Cancer is a group of diseases with different causes that begins when an abnormal cell is transformed by genes, abnormal cell begins to proliferate abnormally ignoring, ignoring growth regulating signals in the surrounding cell the cells infiltrate these tissues and gain access to lymph and blood vessels, which carry the cells to other areas of the body.

General Characteristics

- Cancerous cells are described as malignant neoplasms, as uncontrolled cell growth that follow no physiologic demand
- The cell membranes are altered in cancer cells, which affect fluid movement in and out of the cell
- Mitosis occurs more frequently in malignant cell than in normal cells
- Cancer is a group of disease processes characterized by uncontrolled proliferation of abnormal cell
- In adults, cancers most commonly involve epithelial cells (carcinoma), which are largely environmental in origin
- Cancers involving connective tissue (sarcomas) occur in both children and adults
- Embryonal tumors, which probably originate in intrauterine life generally are manifested during childhood
- Lymphoreticular cancers (leukemia and lymphomas) occur more frequently in children but also occur in adults
- Although relatively rare, childhood cancers remain the leading cause of death by disease and the second leading cause of death overall (exceeded only by accidents) in children of age 1–14 years
- Leukemia is the most common form of childhood cancer
- In recent years, cancer survival rates have increased so significantly that the term cancer is now being used cautiously.

Invasion and Metastasis (Table 28.2)

- Malignant cell have ability to transfer cancerous cells from one organ to another by invasion and metastasis
- Spread of malignant cells from origin to distant sites, cavities through lymphatic and blood circulation
- Lymph and blood are main circulation, breast tumor are best example of metastasis.

Classification (by Tissue of Origin)

1. Blood and related cell cancers include:
   a. Leukemia originating in hematopoietic cells.
   b. Lymphomas originating in lymphoid tissue; Hodgkin's disease and non-Hodgkin's lymphoma.

Table 28.2: Difference between Malignant neoplasms and benign tumor

Malignant neoplasms	Benign tumor
Destruction of tissue, and ability to cause death	Benign tumor grows by expansion and does not infiltrate the surrounding tissues, usually encapsulated
Rate of growth is variable, the faster its growth	Does not spread to other areas
Gain access to blood and lymphatic system and spread to other areas of body	Does not cause death
Ability to spread cancerous cells to other organs	Does not infiltrate to surrounding areas

2. Connective tissue tumors include:
   a. Fibrosarcoma originating in fibrous tissue.
   b. Osteosarcoma originating in the bone-producing (mesenchymal) cells.
   c. Ewing's sarcoma, originating in the midshaft of long bones and flat bones.
3. Muscle tissue tumors include rhabdomyosarcoma originating in striated muscle.
4. Nerve tissue tumors include:
   a. Neuroblastomas originating from the neural crest during embryonic development from ganglion.
   b. Glioblastomas originating from glial cells.
   c. Retinoblastoma originating in the retinal tissue.
5. Renal tissue tumors include Wilms' tumor (nephroblastoma) originating in the kidneys.

Staging

1. Cancer staging is a system for describing and classifying the extent of malignant neoplasm and its metastases, used to guide therapy and predict prognosis.
2. Various staging criteria and terminology are used depending on the specific tumor or treatment center, examples include:
   a. The tumor node metastasis (TNM) staging classification: Primary tumor size (T) and involvement of regional lymph nodes (N).
   b. The national Wilms' tumor: A guide to staging Wilms' tumor or to guide treatment (total or partial nephrectomy radiation, chemotherapy or transplantation) groups one and two completely respectable disease, most curable (90% chance for cure); group two partially respectable with no evidence of metastasis, group four evidence of metastasis group five and bilateral kidney involvement.

Diagnostic Studies

Based on clinical assessment and functional changes. As given below:

- Tumor marker identification
- Genetic profiling
- Magnetic resonance imaging
- Computed tomography
- Ultrasonography
- Endoscopy
- Nuclear medicine imaging.

Management of Cancer

Based on type of cancer treatment option available grading of cancer, age of the patient or relief of symptoms.

Surgery

Surgery is most often preferred choice of treatment, however, depends on diagnostic surgery, curative or it may be reconstructive or palliative.

Biopsy

Tissue excision depends on size and location of tumor. Types of surgery used as follow:

- Electrosurgery
- Cryosurgery
- Laser surgery.

Radiation Therapy

- Radiation may be used to cure the cancer
- To control the spread of primary cancer
- Radiation therapy depends on size of the tumor and surrounding tissue condition
- Radiation will be given in several weeks and daily doses basis
- Repeated radiation dose treatment to increasing tumor cell death.

Types

- Internal radiation
- External radiation.

Chemotherapy

Antineoplastic agents used to destroy or kill the tumor cells, chemotherapy maybe combined with surgery or radiation, or both. The goal of chemotherapy, cure, control and palliation.

Nursing Care

- Obtain thorough history from client and family
- Assess complication of chemotherapy and radiation therapy
- Observe for bleeding tendencies
- Avoid visitors with any infection such as respiratory infection
- Monitor laboratory values
- Monitor bleeding disorders
- Do not give any intramuscular injection
- Do not give medication containing aspirin
- Avoid mucosal injury
- Administer antiemetics as ordered
- Discuss dietary requirements
- Assess pain and manage pain medications
- Nursing reprovided by or undersupervision of a doctor concerned
- Providing counseling service to family
- Educating the care takers
- Follow-up of care
- Care giver when the patient is no longer able to care themselves with them continuously
- After treatment initiation, client will returns to home and frequent visit to hospital, educate who to contact, what the family has to follow.

Overview of Cancer in Children

Assessment

1. Specific clinical findings X-ray depending on particular body system involvement.
2. Cardinal signs and symptoms of cancer in children include:
   - Fever
   - Pain
   - Palpable masses
   - Purpura and petechiae
   - Changes in behavior, gait and balance
   - Unexplained weight loss
   - Fatigue.

Laboratory Studies and Diagnostic Tests

Laboratory studies commonly used to detect, stage and track cancer include:

- Complete blood count (CBC)
- Blood chemistry analysis, especially creatinine
- Peripheral blood smears: Cell types and level of cell maturity
- About 24 hours urine for homovanillic and vanillylmandelic acid (VMA) and catecholamine
- Bone marrow aspiration or biopsy for definitive diagnosis of leukemia
- Lumbar puncture to analyze cerebrospinal fluid for leukemia cells.
- Radiological and other imaging studies include:
  - Intravenous pyelography
  - Computed tomography
  - Radiographs.

Psychosocial Implications

1. A child his/her family adjusts to the process of living with a life-threatening illness in phases.
2. The first stage, 'crisis of discovery' begins with announcement of the diagnoses. In most cases, the child and family initially do not realize the seriousness of the situation.
3. Parents typically respond with shock and disbelief, followed by guilt and self-blame.
4. The child's reaction largely depends on his/her age, the information of the child is given and the physical impact of the disease process on his/her energy level and coping strategies; common responses include:
   a. Under 3 years of age: Views death as a reversible event.
   b. Ages 3–6 years: Understands death as something that happens to others, may view cancer as a retribution for his/her 'bad' thoughts or actions.
   c. Ages 6–11 years: Begins to view death as a personal event.
   d. Preadolescent: Vulnerable to intense feelings of guilt in association with death.
   e. Early adolescent: Intellectually understands the universality and permanence of death; the prospect of 'death before fulfillment' is extremely difficult for a youth who is experiencing illness during a period when physical beauty and activities are important standards of self-worth and self-esteem.
5. After the discovery stage, the child gradually becomes aware of the change in his/her condition and comes to terms with his/her illness and possible impending death; phases of this process include:
   a. Expressions of anger and guilt.
   b. Reorganization of relationship with others.

c. Resolution of the loss through active grieving.
d. Reorganization of identity, incorporating the changes that have taken place.

6. These phases do not necessarily occur in a linear path, but rather can occur in any order and can recur with each disease exacerbation.
7. School is the child's 'work,' a school-age child should engage in school activities to the greatest extent possible throughout the course of illness.
8. Regardless of which family member has cancer, each person in the family is affected by the disease and in turn affects the adjustment of other family members.

LEUKEMIA

Leukemia is an increased level of leukocytes in the circulation; leukemia is a neoplastic proliferation of one particular cell type. The defect originates in the hematopoietic stem cell, the myeloid or the lymphoid stem cell. Leukemia is an unregulated proliferation of leukocytes in the bone marrow.

Description

Leukemia is a malignant neoplastic disorder of the blood-forming tissues. It can be classified according to its predominant cell type and level of maturity, as follows:

- Lymphoma: Involving the lymphoid or lymphatic system
- Myeloma of bone marrow origin
- Blastic and acute involving immature cells
- Cystic and chronic involving mature cells.

Causes

- Genetic factors (children with down syndrome develop leukemia)
- Exposure to ionizing radiation
- Exposure to chemicals
- Congenital abnormalities
- Siblings of a child with leukemia have higher risk
- Radiation during pregnancy may develop leukemia.

Classification

- Acute lymphocyte leukemia
- Acute myeloblastic leukemia
- Chronic leukemia
- Monocytic leukemia.

Acute Lymphocyte Leukemia

- Common childhood leukemia
- Caused by a block in the differentiation of cells in the hematopoietic cells
- Massive accumulation of immature non functional cells
- Acute lymphoblastic leukemia (ALL) is most common in children (median age,10 years).

Acute Myeloid Leukemia

- Defect in hematopoietic stem cell line, the result is a massive accumulation of immature, non-functional cells or in the bone marrow
- All age group are affected
- Prognosis highly variable
- Patient age is significant.

Clinical manifestation

- Result from insufficient production of normal blood cells
- Fever
- Weakness and fatigue from anemia and bleeding tendencies from thrombocytopenia
- Pain from enlarged liver
- Severe infections
- Anemia, pallor, fatigue
- Weight loss
- Enlarged organs (splenomegaly, hepatomegaly)
- Headache and disorientation.

Diagnosis

- Complete blood count (CBC)
- Platelets counts
- Bone marrow aspiration/analysis
- Lumbar puncture (very rarely done to find the abnormality presence of blasé cells.

Complications

- Bleeding and infection
- Low platelets counts
- Increased risk of infection, bleeding
- Fungal infection.

Management

- Children with lymphocytic leukemia, number of treatment option are used
- Vincristine, prednisone and cyclophosphamide included
- After remission of therapy the maintenance therapy will follow

- Chemotherapy
- Bone marrow transplantation therapy
- Supportive care
- Antimicrobial therapy
- Blood transfusion
- Pain management
- There is no clear criteria for duration of therapy.

Chronic Myeloid Leukemia

- Starts with a mutation in the myeloid stem cell
- Uncontrolled proliferation of cells
- The marrow expands into cavities of the long bones result in enlargement of organs
- Chronic myeloid leukemia (CML) is uncommon in people younger than 20 years.

Clinical manifestation

- Clinical manifestation varies and many patients are asymptomatic
- Leukocytes increased
- Shortness of breath.

Management

- An oral formulation of a tyrosine kinase inhibitor
- Imatinib mesylate.

PSYCHOSOCIAL CARE

- Nursing responsibility during this stage involve detailed assessment, planning and implementation
- Nursing history contribute to voluble information
- Psychosocial assessment helpful to gain understanding of family members, child and parents
- Discuss with parents and client
- Provide activities, which child enjoy
- Nurses should take cue from family members and child
- Educate the family and child about care and treatment
- It is important to parents to recognize the consistent with child adherence to treatment. Allow parents to feel that they are able to manage their child.

Nursing Management

- Assessment of child, physical and psychological status
- Prepare the child for investigation

- Clear the misconception
- Provide information as per child and parents understanding
- Explain the parents about preparation for diagnosis, therapy and complications
- Avoid exposing child with person having respiratory infection
- Prepare the child and family for all type of therapy
- Promote optimum nutrition to maintain and rebuild healthy tissue
- Serve frequent small feeds
- Provide careful personal hygiene, mouth care and skin care
- Monitor vital signs
- Providing care for postchemotherapy and radiation therapy side effect
- Help to prevent constipation
- Encourage high fiber diet.

LYMPHOMAS

Tumors originating from the lymphatic system:

- Lymphoma will be non Hodgkin's lymphoma
- Hodgkin's lymphoma.

Hodgkin's Disease

Hodgkin's disease is a cancer of the lymph, appear as enlarged lymph nodes.

Etiology

- Epstein-Barr virus
- Individual with immunodeficiency diseases
- Genetic causes.

Clinical Manifestation

- Lymph nodes becomes necrosis
- Spread to surrounding structure
- Painless lymphadenopathy
- Usually occurs in supraclavicular, cervical and mediastinal region
- Non-productive cough
- Lymphadenopathy
- Weight loss
- Night sweats skin irritation
- Alteration in body temperature
- Jaundice, increased bilirubin
- Anemia

- Edema face and neck
- Increased erythrocyte sedimentation rate (ESR).

Management

Medical and nursing management

- Chemotherapy, with or without radiation therapy
- Radiation therapy:
  - Vincristine is the first standard of drugs
  - Doxorubicin
  - Follow-up treatment is required
  - Bone marrow transplant
  - Symptoms management
  - Managing complication
  - Follow-up care
  - Informing client and family about the therapy, health education
  - Dosage management.

Etiology and Incidence

1. Genetic influences: Children with Down syndrome develop leukemia at a rate 15 times higher than the general population.
2. Familial predisposition: Siblings of a child with leukemia have higher risk of developing leukemia themselves.
3. Immunologic influences: Immune deficiencies increase the risk of developing many cancers.
4. Viral infection: Research suggests the possibility of an oncogenic virus that facilitates the development of cancer (although no direct link has been proved).
5. Environment influences: Evidences suggests that radiation during pregnancy contributes to the development of leukemia in childhood.

Pathophysiology

1. Malignant leukemia cells arise from the precursor cells in blood- forming organs.
2. These cells accumulate and crowd out normal bone marrow elements, spill into peripheral blood and eventually can invade all body organs and tissues.
3. Replacement of normal hematopoietic elements by leukemia cells results in bone marrow suppression, marked by decreased production of red blood cells (RBCs), normal white blood cells (WBCs) and platelets.
4. Bone marrow suppression results in anemia from decreased RBC production, predisposition to infection due to neutropenia and bleeding tendencies from decreased platelet production. This puts the patient at increased risk of death from infection or hemorrhage.

5. Infiltration of reticuloendothelial organ—the spleen, liver and lymph glands causes marked enlargement and eventually, fibrosis.
6. Leukemic infiltration of the central nervous system (CNS) results in increased intracranial pressure (ICP) and other effects depending on the specific areas of involvement.
7. Other possible sites of long-term infiltration include the kidneys, tests, prostate, ovaries, gastrointestinal (GI) tract and lungs.
8. The hypermetabolic leukemic cells eventually deprive all body cells of nutrients necessary for survival. Uncontrolled growth of leukemic cells can actually result in metabolic starvation.
9. Leukemia treatment commonly involves a combination of chemotherapy and radiation therapy, provided at four levels:
   a. Number of leukemia cells drugs used commonly include a combination of oral prednisone [intravenous (IV)] vincristine and L-asparaginase (IV).
   b. Sanctuary therapy: The goal is to attack leukemic cells in the CNS, which are protected by the blood-brain barrier (BBB) or in the testes which are protected by their peripheral location. Therapy consists of intrathecal chemotherapy typically a combination of methotrexate, cytosine arabinoside and steroids or irradiation, usually beginning during the first 6–8 weeks after diagnosis and lasting for 2 weeks (*Note:* Irradiation of the testes remains controversial).
   c. Continuation (maintenance) therapy: The goal is to preserve remission and continue to reduce the number of leukemic cells. Therapy begins when CBC values approach normal levels and commonly lasts for 1½–3 years.
   d. Reinduction therapy: The goal is to reduce the number of leukemic cells in a child who has relapsed; chemotherapy commonly involves prednisone and vincristine combined with other drugs not used previously in therapy.
10. Bone marrow transplantation may be performed in children facing almost certain death without the procedure. If successful, it destroy the leukemic cells and replenishes bone marrow with healthy cells. Prognosis for long-term survival after transplantation is 25–50%.

Assessment Findings

Common clinical manifestations include:

1. Signs and symptoms of anemia: Pallor, fatigue, lethargy, cardiac.
2. Poor wound healing, fever, anorexia, lymphadenopathy related to neutropenia.
3. Petechiae, ecchymosis, purpura, epistaxis, easy bruising blood in urine or emesis related to decreased platelet production.
4. Bone and joint pain related to leukemic cell invasion into the periosteum.

5. Headache, vomiting, papilledema and other signs and symptom of increased ICP related to leukemia cell invasion of the CNS. Laboratory and diagnostic study results typically reveal:
   - Anemia: Normochromic and normocytic with a low reticulocyte
   - Thrombocytopenia
   - Neutropenia
   - Blast cells on peripheral blood smear
   - Extensive replacement of normal bone marrow elements by leukemic cells seen on bone marrow examination, which confirms diagnosis.

Nursing Diagnoses

- Activity intolerance
- Fatigue
- High risk for infection
- Altered nutrition: less than body requirements
- Pain
- Impaired skin integrity.

Planning and Implementation

1. Set realistic patient goals depending on the type of therapy prescribed:
   a. Curative goal is complete disease eradication.
   b. Adjuvant: Goal is eradication of disease and subclinical micrometastases with systemic adjunctive modulates.
   c. Palliative: Goal is not to cure, but to provide quality survival with symptom control.
2. Prepare the child for diagnostic tests and treatments by:
   a. Assessing the child's level of understanding.
   b. Addressing specific fears and misconceptions.
   c. Providing information appropriate to the child's age and development level.
   d. Explaining what he/she will see, smell, hear and feel rather than merely specifying what will happen.
3. Helps to prevent complications related to bone marrow suppression such as infection and sepsis through scrupulous hand washing, limiting the child's exposure to persons with infection (particularly with potentially lethal organisms such as varicella virus) and if ordered, maintaining reverse isolation (Note: Reverse isolation a controversial measure).
4. Prepare the child and family for bone marrow transplantation, if this procedure is scheduled.
5. Promote optimum nutrition to maintain and rebuild healthy tissue. Serve small, frequent meals in a pleasant, relaxed environment and involve the child in food selection as appropriate.

6. Take measures to prevent hemorrhage including:
   a. Turning the patient frequently to relieve pressure on bony prominences.
   b. Providing meticulous mouth care and good skin care.
   c. Measuring temperature via the oral or axillary routes only by avoiding rectal temperature measurement.
7. For a child receiving blood transfusion, assess for blood transfusion reaction.
8. Promote adequate rest by providing a calm, quiet environment and by clustering nursing care activities and other procedures to ensure long periods of uninterrupted rest.
9. Take steps to prevent nausea and vomiting resulting from chemotherapy, such as:
   a. Administering an antiemetic agent 30 minutes to 1 hour before a chemotherapy session.
   b. Continuing the antiemetic every 2–6 hours for 24 hours after chemotherapy.
10. Help to prevent constipation resulting from neuropathic side effects of chemotherapy by:
    a. Encourage a high-fiber diet.
    b. Promoting physical activity according to the child's tolerance.
    c. Administering a stool softener.
11. Help to minimize hemorrhagic cystitis resulting from chemotherapy by:
    a. Encouraging increased fluid intake and frequent voiding.
    b. Administering chemotherapy early in the day to allow adequate time significant fluid intake.
12. Helps to prevent renal damage resulting form chemotherapy by:
    a. Administering allopurinol as ordered.
    b. Alkalinizing the urine with an acid-ash diet.
    c. Providing adequate hydration.
13. Help to minimize alopecia resulting from chemotherapy by applying a scalp tourniquet before therapy as ordered (Note: This measure is controversial).
14. Provide for appropriate play activities based on the child's age developmental level and health status.
15. Provide patient and family teaching, covering:
    a. Diagnosis and nature of the disorder.
    b. All treatments and other procedures.
    c. Side effects of chemotherapy and radiation therapy.

Evaluation

1. The child or parents verbalize an understanding of the signs and symptoms of infection. The importance of monitoring for these signs and symptoms promptly and notifying the physician, if they occur.

2. The child exhibits no evidence of abnormal bleeding.
3. The child engages in usual activities and routines as appropriate for his/her age and developmental level.
4. The child consumes adequate calories balanced among the basic four food groups.
5. The child verbalizes decreased discomfort or absence of pain and appears to rest comfortably.
6. The child or parents verbalize an understanding of treatment protocols and prescribed drugs including the side effects of medications and treatments to watch for and report.
7. Family members know the dates and times of scheduled follow-up appointments.

Chapter 29

Pediatric Emergencies

Congenital heart disease appendicitis, diarrhea, croup, dental problems asthma, dehydration, diabetes, fever, fracture, head injury, poisioning, seizure, burns, bites, foreign bodies, pneumonia and some emergencies in children.

CONGENITAL HEART DISEASE

Congenital heart disease (CHD) can describe a number of different problems affecting the heart, it is the most common type of birth defect and CHD causes more death in the 1st year of life than any other birth defect. Congenital heart disease is often divided into two types, i.e. cyanotic (blue skin color caused by a lack of oxygen) and noncyanotic.

Common Congenital Heart Disease

- Metrology of fallot
- Aortic stenosis
- Atrial septal defect (ASD)
- Patent ductus arterious (PDA)
- Pulmonic stenosis.

Most congenital heart defect are found during a pregnancy when defect is found a pediatrician, surgeon other specialists can be there the baby is delivered to deal life and death. Some CHD can be treated with medication alone. Others need to be treated with one or more heart surgeries.

Prevention

Women with pregnancy avoid:

- Using drugs, and alcohol
- Visit hospital for screening
- If during pregnancy diabetes appear, control blood sugar level, follow the correctly follow the doctor instruction.

PEDIATRIC ASTHMA

Childhood asthma is the most common chronic disease in infants and children.

Clinical Manifestation

- Wheezing, labored breathing, dyspnea
- Cough
- Chest pain
- Nasal congestion.

Etiology

- Hereditary
- Allergen
- Malnutrition.

Diagnosis

- Physical examination, clinical evaluation
- Blood complete blood count (CBC), hemoglobin (HB), platelets counts
- Routine urine analysis
- Chest X-ray
- Pulmonary function test.

Management

- Bronchodilator such as theophyline, salbutamal
- Steroids
- In severe condition intravenously (IV), aminophyline
- Oxygen administration
- Cough syrup
- Antibiotics to treat infection
- Maintain electrolytes balance
- Maintain semi-fowler's position
- Meter dose inhaler, nurses should teach child and parent (children above 5 years)
- Nebulization.

CROUP

Croup is a common pediatric viral respiratory tract illness, generally affect trachea, its also called laryngotrachobronchitis, and result in audible harsh high-pitched sound on inspiration.

Signs and Symptoms

- Hoarseness of voice
- Respiratory distress

- Airway obstruction may result in respiratory distress and even death
- Barky cough, noisy breathing, condition worse in night, morning lessened.

Etiology

- Contact with fomites, allergen
- Contact with parainfluenza virus
- Rhinovirus
- Influenza a and b.

Influenza A is associated with severe respiratory disease and it has been detected in children with marked respiratory compromise.

Management

- Routine management of respiratory distress
- Removing mucus secretion
- Bronchoscope, helps in diagnosis
- Humidification.

INTESTINAL OBSTRUCTION

Four cardinal signs of intestinal obstructions:

- Pain
- Vomiting
- Distension
- Absolute constipation

Intestinal obstruction may be suspected because of the above four cardinal signs, note the exception:

1. Abdominal pain (this may not be noticed in the newborn).
2. Vomiting, especially if the vomitus is not bile stained.
3. Abdominal distention (which may not be present in high lesions of the duodenum or jejunum).
4. No passage of meconium or delayed passage of meconium more than 24 hours in a full-term baby.
5. Passage of meconium one or two times does not exclude intestinal artesia.
6. Any baby having these cardinal signs of obstruction should have an nasogastric (NG) tube passed to empty the stomach and to examine the contents and see if any bile is present.
7. In any suspected case of intestinal obstruction a plain X-ray of the abdomen in the erect and supine position is usually all that required for a diagnosis.

8. An X-ray will confirm the presence of an obstruction, the level of obstruction and give a possible clue as to etiology.

If there are dilated loops and fluid levels, the baby should be transferred for further management.

POISONING

Any substance that impairs health or destroys life when ingested, inhaled or absorbed by body. All substances are poisons. Many experts says that it is impossible to categorize any chemical as either safe or toxic and that the real concern is the risk or hazards associated with the use of any substance such as the high-risk that may be associated with a life-saving drug that would not be acceptable as a food additive.

Substances when swallowed intentionally or by accident, which can cause damage to the body or body structure and function by its chemical action called poison.

Poison or toxic substances accessible to the children, the parents and care giver able to identify as the child consumed poison that immediate treatment can be started, if they notice child consumed poison immediately bring the child to the hospital for first aid or for treatment.

Common Types of Poison

- Food poisoning
- Heavy metal poison
- Petroleum distillate poisioning
- Carbon monoxide poison
- Pesticide poisioning
- Antihistamines and cold medication
- Kerosene poison
- Lead poison
- Mercury poison
- Acids
- Barbiturates
- Camphor
- Mercury poison
- Boric acid
- Alkali
- Cathartics (mineral oil, e.g. phenolphthalein).

Common Signs and Symptoms of Different Kinds of Poison

1. Some poison cause immediate effect and other type of poison cause slow action.

2. Gastrointestinal disturbances, nausea, vomiting, abdominal pain and diarrhea.
3. Respiratory and circulatory symptoms, unexplained cyanosis, shock and collapse.
4. Central nervous system, lethargy, and loss of consciousness and convulsions.
5. Effect of poison depends on types of poison, overdosage of sedatives or rate poison have slow effect.
6. Lead, paint poison depends on type of poison.

Immediate Action

Immediate action, if found child consumed poison are:

1. The symptomatic and supportive care given a patient who has been exposed to or who has ingested a toxic drug, commercial chemical, or other dangerous substance.
2. In case of oral poisioning, a primary effort should be directed toward recovery of the toxic substance before it can be absorbed in the body tissues. If vomiting doesnot occur spontaneously, it should be induced.
3. If the poison is a petroleum distillate such as kerosene, or a caustic or coressive substances vomiting should not be induced.
4. The decision on whether to induce vomiting is dependent on the substances ingested.
5. Try to remove by inducing vomiting, while child still at home.
6. Vomiting is induced by use of large quantity of water drinks or by syrup ipecac 5–15 mL repeated after 10 minutes.
7. Gastric lavage for removing poison through gastrointestinal tract.
8. If poison is coressive or acid inducing vomiting is contraindicated.
9. Shift the child to hospital as early as possible.
10. Preserve content of poison.
11. Emotional support to child and parents.
12. Intake of water depends on child age and type of poison.
13. Nurse should observe child condition, respiration and pulse.
14. Gastriclavage to reduce amount of poison absorption, excretion of poison.
15. To increase excretion of some poison diuresis as per doctor's instruction.
16. If required cardiopulmonary resuscitation (CPR) may be initiated.
17. Observe for restlessness, convulsions or stupor or coma.
18. Follow antidotes available for poison taken and administer antidote as per instruction.

Prevention of Accident Poison in Home

1. Effective storage and handling of all poisonous substances.
2. Parents should label poison substances.

3. All poison substances including drugs, foods, should be kept away from reach of children domestic chemicals.
4. All medications and chemicals are kept out of reach of children.
5. Drugs are administered under the supervision.
6. Potential house hold substances such as toilet materials, kerosene, insecticide, pesticides kept under supervision.

BURNS

Injuries that result from direct contact with or exposure to any thermal, chemical, electrical or radiation source are termed burns. Burn injuries are classified according to the mechanism of injury.

Etiology

The most common cause of burn in children, which occur in less than 15 years of age group are:

1. Thermal burns are caused by exposure to or contact with flame, hot liquids, semiliquids, etc.
2. Scald injuries from moist heat (children from 3 to 5 years, because of their activities.
3. Flame injury occurs over the age of 5 years, children are reaching flame because flame creates curiosity.
4. Electrical injury: Contact with faulty electrical wiring.
5. Chemical injury: Contact with acids, alkalis or organic compounds, such as house hold cleaning materials.
6. Inhalation injury.

Assessment of the Burn Wound

The cause of the injury and the time that it occurred should be ascertained and recorded Even quite experienced staff can mistake the depth of a burn and at this stage it is sufficient to distinguish between erythema and actual skin damage, if the history is of a corrosive or chemical burn, irrigation with water should be continued. A thermal burn should not be interfered with at t his time. There is a need to make a quick estimate can be made mentally by using the rule of nines, which indicates in an easily remembered form. The percentage of total body surface area accounted for by various part of the body 9% each for arms and head; 18% each for legs, front of trunk and back of trunk for part of the body that have only small areas of burn it is useful to remember that the palmar surface of the patients hand constitutes about 1% of the body surface area.

Simple erythema is excluded from the estimate and if the total burn is more than 15–20% in an adult, or 10–15% in child intravenous infusion is indicated with extensive burns 30% and more it is both essential and urgent.

The nurse should obtain through incident report on where, when and how the injury occurred. The nurse should note, condition of the child parental attitude, coping skills and availability of support system.

Size of the Burn or Percentage of Burns

It calculated using rule of nines, which is adjusted for the age of the child. It should be noted that child who is younger than 2 years has 10% of burn injury is greater risk than compared with adult can tolerate 10% as minor burn injury.

Depth of Injury

- Superficial partial thickness injury
- A scald injury, which occurs in toddlers
- Partial thickness injury includes first degree burns
- Full thickness injury.

Management

At the Scene

First aid

The first priority is to remove the causalty from further damage, e.g. extinguish burning cloths. Flames travel upwards and continue to burn the face, neck and scalp, if the casualty is upright. With the casualty horizontal on the ground, smoother the flames with a coat rug or similar heavy materials, if the fire was in an enclosed space and there is smoke present. Remove the casualty to fresh air. If clothing is still smoldering, douse with water, clothes saturated with hot liquids act like a hot poultice. They should be removed quickly or cooled by drenching with cold water. With these exceptions, the active cooling of extensive thermal burns is of debatable value and should never be allowed to delay the removal of the casualty to hospital.

Corrosive burns

The removal of coressive chemicals from the skin is just as urgent as extinguishing the flames of blazing clothing copious quantities of water should be used and particular attention must be paid to the eyes. Contaminated clothing should be removed, irrigation of the affected parts should continue until the ambulance arrives and if possible be continued during the journey to the hospital. Any known information concerning nature of the chemical should accompany the casualty to hospital.

In the accident and casualty department

Airway and breathing

Fires kill more people by asphyxia than by burns and as with any other accident. The first medical priority is the management of the airway and breathing, if the fire is in an enclosed space, carbon monoxide poisoning may occur, sometimes to the extent of producing unconsciouness. In this case, control of the upper airway will be important, as well as providing 50% oxygen in air to breathe. The specific problems of smoke inhalation will be considered.

Upper airway obstruction

The main threat to the upper airway occurs when laryngeal edema develops following direct thermal injury caused by the inhalation of flame, hot gases or steam occasionally, aspiration of hot liquids during scalding of the face produces similar damage. Whenever there are burns or scalds of the face, consider the need for airway support. In general, the more severe the thermal injury the earlier will laryngeal obstruction become apparent in the most severe cases, obstruction is virtually inevitable within a few hours and may occur with little warning.

Pulmonary damage

The inhalation of hot gases can produce burns down to the terminal bronchi, but only steam can carry sufficient heat into the lungs to produce thermal damage in the alveoli, an unusual injury with a very bad prognosis. Much commoner is smoke damage essentially a corrosive burns of the lungs, resulting from products of combustion.

Protection burn area

Regardless of the cause of the burn injury, is covered with clean dry cloth or dressing

Setting up the intravenous drip

Fluid management

Major threat to life is fluid and electrolytes imbalance, shock due to loss of electrolytes

IV fluid should be started immediately in children with more than 15% of burns and less than 2 years with 10% of burns. A large bore catheter should be inserted IV or cut down methods.

Unless both arms are burned to the extent of deep charring it will be possible to find a vein in one or other forearm or anticubital fossa. If the vein can be seen,venipuncture is satisfactory, otherwise a cut down should be performed. In either case, the largest possible cannula should be inserted and secured firmly. A long narrow catheter is a bad choice.

Fluid and electrolytes imbalance

Evaporative water loss through the burn contributes to the client's diminished fluid volume and compromised hydration status. Evaporative loss are evidenced by a low blood pressure, decreased urine output, dry mucous membranes and poor skin turgor:

- Urine output diminishes to less than 30 mL/h
- Elevated blood, urea, nitrogen (BUN) until the client adequately hydrated
- Absence of bowel sounds

- Nausea and vomiting, and abdominal distention
- Approximately 18–36 hours after burn injury capillary membrane integrity begins to be restored.

Blood samples
If a blood sample can be obtained from the cannula before the drip set is connected it will save time and the need for a venipuncture a few minutes later.

Choice of infusion fluid
Fluid resuscitation is used to minimize the fluid shifts. The goal of fluid resuscitation is to maintain vital organ perfusion, while avoiding the complications related to either inadequate or excessive fluid administration. Seveeral formula recommended by the American Burn Life Support (ABLS), e.g. consensus formula for fluid resuscitation.

If burned client is delayed 2nd hour in reaching an emergency department those 2 hours must be considered in any calculation of needed fluid. However adjustment to the fluid infusion rate is based on client physiologic response, e.g. urine production, vital signs and lung sounds.

The infusion rate is adjusted, so that half of the estimated volume is administered in the first 8 hours post burn. The remaining half of the estimated resuscitation volume is administered over the 16 hours.

Analgesia

The requirement for analgesia during the shock phase of burns is often small. With full thickness skin burns there is seldom any complaint of pain because sensory end organs in the skin have also been destroyed. Even when the burns are partial thickness and the survival of sensory end organs can clearly be demonstrated by pinprick, it is unusual for the patient to complain of continuing pain.

However some children will complain of pain and most will be affected by fear and discomfort and the provision of analgesia at an early stage depends on child age, percentage and depth of injury will guide to advice drugs.

Cauterization of the Bladder

Because knowledge of the flow rate and composition of the urine provides vital information concerning both the effectiveness of resuscitation and the functional status of the kidneys themselves an indwelling catheter should be inserted. The bladder is emptied, the urine volume measured thereafter.

Reassessment
When the above priorities in treatment have been attended to the patients conditions should be reassessed. Use of rule of 9 of 10 results in an over estimate of the extent of the burn and at this stage, a more accurate assessment should be made.

Wound care

Stop the burning process, all burn wound care begins at the scene of the injury. Clothing that continue to smolder should be carefully removed, once the clothing is removed the client should be covered with a dry sheet and preserve the body heat. In chemical burns injuries, all clothing should be promptly removed and any chemical powder brushed off the skin irrigated for chemical eye injuries, irrigate the eyes with a gentle stream of normal saline.

Wound care should consist of covering the wound with sterile towels, and placing clean dry sheets and blankets over the client.

Prevent tetanus

Burns even minor ones are susceptible to tetanus, tetanus toxoid should be administered.

Clinical Observation

- Nausea
- Vomiting
- Diarrhea
- Septicemia
- Drug reaction.

Box 29.1: Diet approaches for pediatric burns patients (above 2 and 12 years of age and > 10% total body surface area (TBSA) burns)

Performa

Patients name: ....

Age/Sex: .... IP no: ....

Body weight: .... Date of burns: ....

Time of burns: .... Post burn day: ....

Diet approach (oral/nasogastric tube): ....

Parental nutrition if any: ....

Recommended/Required diet allowance: ....

Post burn	Calories		Protein (g)	
Week	Require intake	Deficit	Required intake	Deficit
1.				
2.				
3.				
4.				

Additional Intervention

- Fluids may be adjusted to achieve a urine output of 30–50 mL/h (0.5–1.0 mL/kg/h) in a adult 1 mL/kg/h in a child

- Indwelling urinary catheter is needed to monitor response to fluids therapy
- Elevate extremities
- Monitor peripheral pulses
- Administer humidified oxygen through a nasal cannula or ventilator support
- Nothing by mouth (NPO) status until bowel sounds returns 5/10 mL/h tube feeding are typically started with 24 hours to maintain function of gastrointestinal tract
- Nutritional management to combat acute nutritional deficiency (Box 29.1).

Appendices

APPENDIX I

EMERGENCY DRUGS REQUIRED DURING RESUSCITATION

- Required for correcting metabolic acidosis
- Correcting hypovolemia
- Correcting a systole
- Correcting hypoglycemia.

Table 1: Drugs for resuscitation of the newborn

Name of the drugs	Dose/Route	Indication/ Actions	Precautions
Sodium bicarbonate 8.4%	2 mL/kg/dose Intravenously or via umbilical vein	Correction of acidosis Severe asphyxia Poor response to resuscitation	Give only after adequate ventilation, dilute 1:1 Give slowly over 60 S
Adrenaline 1:10,00 (0.1 mg/mL)	10 µg/kg/dose (0.01 mg) Chart: 1.0 kg = 0.1 mL 2..0 kg = 0.2 mL 3..0 kg = 0.3 mL 4.0 kg = 0. 4 mL 5.0 kg = 0.5 mL Intravenously or endotracheal	Severe bradycardia Asystole Increase cardiac contractility and heart rate	Prime tube and tap Administer drug rapidly Remove catheter adverse reaction, ventricular tachycardia
Plasma protein fraction (PPF) 5% 5% albumin Normal saline	10–20 mL/kg/ dose Intravenously or via umbilical vein	Hypovolemic shock Poor capillary refill Hypotension increase blood pressure (BP)	Monitor BP Monitor heart rate Measure urine output
Dextrose 10%	2–3 mL/kg/dose intravenously or via umbilical vein	Correction of hypoglycemia Raises blood sugar	Rebound hypoglycemia Monitor blood glucose level
Narcon (0.2 mg/ mL) (naloxone)	0.02 mg/kg/dose Intravenously or via umbilical vein	Respiratory depression due to pethidine/ sedation given to mother 2–4 hour prior to delivery	Anticipation can repeat dose Baby usually has good heart rate But not respiratory effort

When to Stop Resuscitation

1. Irreversible brain damage will occur, if the infant remains profoundly asphyxiated and unresponsive.
2. Repeat the cycle of evaluation, ventilation, chest compressions and drugs three times.
3. If the baby remains unresponsive after full resuscitative measures, do not continue resuscitation.

Do not continue resuscitation after 10 minutes if:

1. There is no heart beat.
2. There is no spontaneous response.
3. The pupils are fixed and dilated.

Do not continue resuscitation after 30 minutes if:

1. There is severe bradycardia (heart rate < 40/min).
2. There is no spontaneous breathing.
3. It is important to tell the mother what is happening to her baby.
4. Whether resuscitation is successful, or not the baby should be wrapped in a towel and given to the mother, so that she can see and hold her baby.
5. She may want to see the whole body; and her wishes must be respected.

Care After Resuscitation

If the baby has required a prolonged period of resuscitation or if there was diffculty in establishing respiration, then arrange for a period of observation. Monitor the vital signs every 15 minutes for 1 hour and then every 30 minutes for 1 hour and then hourly for few hours. An explanation by the pediatrician/nurse, as the parents may feel anxious with regard to the need for resuscitation of her baby.

APPENDIX II

ADVANTAGES OF BREASTFEEDING VS FORMULA

1. Breastfeeding is the best and most natural way of feeding the newborn.
2. It is very satisfying and rewarding for a mother to feed her own baby. Breast milk and breastfeeding have many unique advantages for the mother and baby.
3. Breastfeeding develops a loving relationship between the mother and baby.
4. Breast milk has easily digested proteins, lactose or milk sugar and fats.
5. It gives the baby all the required nourishment.
6. It contains antibodies to protect the baby against infections.
7. It protects the baby from allergic reactions.
8. Breast milk is the most hygienic and cleanest milk, which does not require any preparation.
9. Immunoglobulin supply antiviral and antibacterial to protect baby from certain diseases.
11. It is cheep and does not cost money.
12. Breastfeeding helps the woman to regain her figure and health more quickly in the following ways:
    - It causes the uterus to contract, which prevents prolonged blood loss
    - The pelvic muscles regain their tone quicker
    - The extra weight gained during pregnancy is used up in breastfeeding.

Preparation for Breastfeeding During Pregnancy

1. Mentally prepare the mother from early pregnancy.
2. Advise her to eat a well-balanced diet.
3. Check that her nipples are prominent enough to breast feed. she can be given advice if they are flat or inverted.

At the Time of Delivery

1. Anesthesia, strong sedation, prolonged labor and other sources of stress, discomfort and fatigue for mothers and infants are a deterrent for breastfeeding, but with persistence it is possible.
2. A woman's experience during labor and delivery can affect her motivation toward breastfeeding.
3. After delivery.
4. A baby's rooting and sucking reflexes are particularly strong immediately after normal delivery and a mother is usually keen to touch and cuddle her baby.

APPENDIX III

COMPOSITION OF BREAST MILK

Breast milk is always in perfect condition for a baby even if the woman is ill, pregnant, menstruating or malnourished. Breast milk contains all the nutrients that a baby requires for the first 4-6 months of life.

Colostrum

Colostrum is secreted by the breasts from about the 16th week of pregnancy. It is yellow and thicker than later milk. It is rich in protein, low in fat and contains antibodies for many common infections, which protects the baby against infection, until he/she can make his/her own antibodies. Colostrum is secreted in a small amount, but it is adequate for a newborn baby.

How a Baby Sucks?

A healthy full-term baby has three reflexes, which help him/her to feed. They are:

1. Rooting reflex: This reflex helps him/her to find the nipple. If something touches the side of his/her mouth and he/she is hungry, he/she opens the mouth and turns toward the touch.
2. Sucking reflex: When something goes into his/her mouth far enough, he/she sucks it. The sucking reflex is very strong immediately after birth.
3. Swallowing reflex: If the baby's mouth is filled with milk, he/she swallows it. There is a reflex to help the baby to find the nipple and a reflex to make him/her suck, but there is no reflex to help the baby to take the nipple into his/her mouth. This is some thing that the baby has to learn for himself/herself and for which he/she needs the mothers help. To suck effectively the baby must take enough of the nipple and areola into his/her mouth. Breastfeeding is the natural way to feed a baby. Most women need some help at the beginning, especially with their first baby or if they are very young.

How to Put a Baby to the Breast Correctly?

1. Let the mother sit or lie somewhere comfortably, so that she is relaxed. A low seat or lying on a bed, so that she is not in pain.
2. Show the mother how to hold the baby in her arms, so that he/she faces the breast and his/her stomach is against the mother if the mother wants, she can support him/her on a cushion. Make sure the whole baby faces the breast. Do not just turn his head.
3. Hold the baby at the back of his/her shoulders, not at the back of his/her head.

4. The mother should hold and offer the whole of her breast, not just the nipple.
5. The mother touches the baby's cheek or the side of his/her mouth with the nipple to stimulate his/her rooting reflex.
6. She waits until the baby's mouth is open and he/she wants start feeding. Then the mother should aim his/her lower lip toward the base of the areola. Quickly move the baby well into the breast.
7. A bad sucking position may be the cause of many common problems.
8. Sore nipple, not enough milk, refusal to feed.

APPENDIX IV

PROCESS OF BREASTFEEDING

1. Stimulate the baby by tickling the side of his/her mouth with the nipple.
2. When baby's mouth is wide open, move him/her firmly on to the breast holding the back of his/her head.
3. To be in the correct position most of the areola should be in the baby's mouth and he/she should be able to suck deeply and this should feel comfortable for the mother.
4. If the baby does not take the areola into his/her mouth, the mother will have sore nipple.
5. If the position is wrong, release the nipple by pushing a finger against the baby's chin to release the suction and start again.

Signs of Breastfeeding

Signs certain that the baby has fixed on to the breast in a good position

- The baby's whole body is close to the mother
- His mouth and chin are close to the breast
- The baby's mouth is wide open
- You cannot see much areola
- You can see the baby taking slow deep sucks
- He/She is relaxed and happy
- The mother does not feel the nipple pain.

Establishing Breastfeeding

It is important to establish breastfeeding early and to emphasize the mother, the importance of giving the baby the colostrum. Ideally, the baby should be put to the breast within the first hour of delivery. However, this may not always be possible if the condition of the mother or the baby is not satisfactory. Explain the mother that it is natural for there to be little milk in the breasts for the first few days after delivery. The colostrum is all that the baby requires and feeding should be on demand.

Rooming In

1. There is normally no need for the mother and baby to be separated after delivery. The baby should be in a cot at the mother's bedside. She can then respond to his/her needs and feed him/her as necessary.
2. Babies feed very irregularly at first and it may take a week or two to settle down into some sort of rhythm.
3. Frequent sucking stimulates the production of prolactin, which is necessary for the secretion of milk.

4. Babies should feed from both breasts. Larger babies may suck from both breasts at each feed, where as a smaller baby may be satisfied after feeding from only one breast. It should be explained to the mother that she should start feeding from alternate sides, so that both breasts get equal sucking time.
5. A breast fed baby does not require any other milk feeds or water.

APPENDIX V

COMMON PROBLEMS ENCOUNTERED DURING BREASTFEEDING AND ITS SOLUTIONS

Sore Nipples

The nipples should not become sore, if the mother is shown how to breast feed correctly. And it is common in the first 4 weeks if they do become sore

Solutions

1. Check that the baby has the nipple and the areola well into his/her mouth, failure to ensure than this is the commonest cause of cracked nipple.
2. Advise the mother to breast feed more often and to limit sucking time.
3. Encourage the mother to relax and get into a comfortable position before starting to feed, so that the milk flows more easily.
4. Suggest that starts the flow by hand by expressing some milk before the feed.
5. Advise the mother to start feeding on the side, which is less sore as sucking is strongest at the beginning of a feed.
6. Teach the mother how to take the baby off the breast, i.e. by putting a finger in the baby's mouth or by pressing down on his/her chin and never pull the baby off the breast.
7. Advice the mother to breast feed in different position to see which is most comfortable.
8. Advise the mother not to wash her nipples with soap, as this will dry the skin.

Short or Flat Nipples

1. For short nipples, press the areola on either side of the nipple. This makes most nipples stand out and look longer. Gently try to roll the nipple and areola with the thumb and forefinger to form a teat.
2. Daily pull and stretch the nipples in all directions. This should be done even before delivery.
3. Place thumbs on either side of the nipple. Press in firmly against the breast tissue and at the same time push the thumbs away from each other. This stretches the nipple out. Do these exercise 5 times a day.

Engorgement

When the milk first comes in the breast they feel full and heavy. They may be swollen, hard, painful and engorged—engorgement is partly due to the milk that fills the breast and partly due to the increase in the blood and tissue fluid. This will resolve after a few days, but in the mean time, the mother needs help:

1. The breast will be so full that the nipple becomes flattened and the baby cannot fix and suck.
2. It is painful for the mother.
3. The milk supply decreases, because the baby does not suckle often enough.
4. The breast may become infected, because the milk is not removed.

Prevention: Allow the baby to feed on demand immediately after birth.

Treatment: Help the mother to express her breasts manually or by using an electric pump, so that they will become softer and more comfortable. The baby will then be able to fix and suck. Continue to express the breasts as often as necessary to empty the breasts and until engorgement stops.

Blocked Milk Duct

Sometimes, a milk duct becomes blocked; preventing milk flow and that develops a painful limp.

Treatment: Are as follows:

1. Start the baby on the affected side and empty it at each feed.
2. Gently massage inwards toward the nipple, while the baby is sucking.
3. Wipe dried secretions with a warm cloth; apply warm compresses between feeds.
4. Try alternative positions.

Leaking Breasts

1. Likely in the first few weeks or when it is time for a feed.
2. It usually stops by itself after a few weeks, when the breast becomes softer.

Treatment: Are as follows:

1. Put clean piece of cloth inside the bra to soak up the milk. Change the cloth frequently and wash them thoroughly.
2. Working women may express the milk periodically to relieve the breasts and discard it if it is not possible to give it to the child immediately.

How to Ensure Good Nutrition for Breastfeeding?

Weight gain during pregnancy is normal and essential. The extra body reserves are converted into breast milk. A good amount of fluid intake is necessary; about 6–9 glasses per day. Also continue taking the prescribed iron and folic acid tablets for 3 months after delivery. After delivery, continue eating a well-balanced diet of fresh fruits, vegetables, legumes, meat, fish, cheese, eggs, milk and bread. Prevent anemia by eating leafy green vegetables, lean meat, kidney, heart, whole wheat bread, dried peas, beans and fruits.

APPENDIX VI

BREASTFEEDING POLICY

Breastfeeding is the most nutritious and beneficial food for newborn and babies. Breast milk provides an infant's total nutrient requirement. It is an invaluable source of nourishment until 2 years of age. It is the policy adopted in all health institutions, government or private, through implementation of the following steps by all health personnel:

1. Ensure that the mother starts breastfeeding immediately within the first half an hour after birth.
2. Do not separate newborn babies from mothers; allow mother and newborn to remain together for 24 hours a day.
3. Orient and train all staff on benefits and management of breastfeeding.
4. Inform every mother about the benefits and management of breastfeeding.
5. Show mothers how to breast feed and how to maintain lactation even if newborn baby and mother are separated for medical reasons. In such cases, mothers should be taught to express breast milk in order to maintain lactation and to feed using cup and spoon. Babies should be given only their mother's breast milk and not from another mother.
6. Encourage mothers to breast feed on demand and not on schedule.
7. Do not give milk substitute or water for newborn unless medically indicated.
8. Do not give artificial teats or pacifiers to newborn babies.
9. Do not supply bottle or milk substitute to newborns except when medically indicated. No free breastfeeding substitutes should be provided to any health facility. Such supplies are neither to be offered, nor accepted by health services or health workers at any level, whether private or government. Any such products, which are required by health institutions must be obtained through the normal procurement procedures.
10. Foster establishment of breastfeeding support groups in the hospital and in the community.

APPENDIX VII

IMPORTANT MILESTONES

Important Milestones from 3 to 60 Months

Babies develop at their own pace, so it is impossible to tell exactly when the child will learn a given skill.

Developmental Milestones by the End of 3 Months

Social and emotional

- The child begins to develop a social smile
- Enjoys playing with other people and may cry when playing stops
- Becomes more expressive and communicates more with face and body
- Imitates some movements and facial expression.

Movement

- The child raises head and chest when lying on stomach
- Supports upper body with arms when lying on stomach
- Stretches legs out and kicks when lying on stomach or back
- Open and shuts hands
- Pushes down on legs, when feet are placed on a firm surface
- Brings hand to mouth
- Takes swipes at dangling objects with hands
- Grasps and shakes hand toys.

Vision

- Watches the face intently
- Follows moving objects
- Recognizes familiar objects and people at a distance
- Starts using hands and eyes in coordination.

Hearing and speech

- Smiles at the sound of voice
- Begins to babble
- Begins to imitate some sounds
- Turns the head toward direction of sound.

Important Milestones by the End of 7 Months

Social and emotional

- Enjoys social play
- Interested in mirror images
- Responds to other people's expressions of emotion and appears joyful often.

Cognitive
- Finds partially hidden object
- Explores with hands and mouth
- Struggles to get the objects that are out of reach.

Language
- Responds to own name
- Begins to respond to no
- Can tell emotion by tone of voice
- Responds to sound by making sounds
- Uses voice to express joy and displeasure
- Babbles chains of sounds.

Movement
- Rolls both ways (front to back, back to front)
- Sits with and then without support on hands
- Supports whole weight on legs
- Reaches with one hand
- Transfers object from hand to hand
- Uses hands to rake objects.

Vision
- Develops full color vision
- Distance vision matures
- Ability to track moving objects improves.

Important Milestones by the End of 1 Year (12 Month)

Social and emotional
- Shy or anxious with strangers
- Cries when mother or father leaves
- Enjoys imitating people in his/her play
- Shows specific preferences for certain people and toys
- Tests parental responses to his/her action during feeding
- Tests parental responses to his/her behaviors
- May be fearful in some situations
- Prefer mother or regular caregiver over all others
- Fingerfeeds himself
- Extends arm or leg to help when being dressed.

Cognitive
- Explore objects in many different ways (shaking, banging, throwing, droping)
- Finds hidden objects easily

- Looks at correct picture when image is named
- Imitates gestures
- Begins to use objects correctly, drinking from cup, brushing hair, dialing phone and listening to receiver.

Language

- Pays increasing attention to speech
- Responds to simple verbal requests
- Responds to 'no'
- Uses simple gestures, such as shaking head for 'no'
- Babbles with inflection (changes in tone)
- Says 'dada' and 'mama'
- Tries to imitate words.

Movement

- Reaches sitting position without assistance
- Crawls forward on belly
- Assumes hands and knees position
- Creeps on hands and knees
- Gets from sitting to crawling or prone (lying on stomach) position
- Pulls self up to stand
- Walks holding on to furniture
- Walks two or three steps without support
- Hands and fingers
- Bangs two objects together
- Puts object into container
- Takes objects out of container
- Pokes with index finger.

Important Milestones by the End of 2 Years (24 Month)

Social

- Imitates behavior of others
- Aware of themself as separate from others
- More excited about company of other children.

Emotional

- Begins to show defiant behavior
- Separation anxiety increases toward midyear then fades
- Cognitive
- Finds objects even when hidden under two or three covers
- Begins to sort by shapes and colors
- Begins make-believe play.

Language
- Points to object or picture when it is named for him/her
- Recognizes names of familiar people, objects and body parts
- Says several single words
- Uses simple phrases
- Follows simple instructions.

Movement
- Walks alone
- Pulls toys behind his/her, while walking
- Carries large toy or several toys, while walking
- Kicks a ball
- Walks up and down stairs on to support.

Hand and finger skills
- Scribbles on his/her own
- Turns over container to pour out contents
- Builds tower of four blocks or more
- Might use one hand more often than the other.

Important Milestones by the End of 3 Years (36 Month)

Social and emotional
- Imitates adults and playmates
- Spontaneously shows affection for familiar playmates
- Can take turns in games
- Understands concept of mine and his/her.

Emotional
- Expresses affection openly
- Expresses a wide range of emotion
- Separates easily from parents
- Objects to major changes in routine.

Cognitive
- Makes mechanical toys work
- Plays make-believe with dolls, animals and people
- Sorts objects by shape and color
- Completes puzzles with three or four pieces
- Understands the concept of two.

Language
- Follows a two or three part command
- Recognizes and identifies almost all common objects and pictures
- Uses four to five words sentences
- Can say name, age, etc.

- Uses pronouns (i, you, me, we, they) and some plurals (cars, dogs, cats)
- Strangers can understand the language.

Movement
- Climbs wall
- Walks up and down stairs, alternating feet
- Kicks ball
- Runs easily
- Pedals tricycle.

Hands and finger skill
- Makes up and down, side to side
- Turns book pages one at a time
- Holds a pencil in writing position
- Screws and unscrews jar lids, nuts and bolts.

Important Milestones by the End of 4 Year (48 Month)

Social
- Interested in new experiences
- Cooperates with other children
- Inventive in fantasy play
- Dresses and undresses.

Emotional

- Imagines that many unfamiliar images may be monsters
- Views self as a whole person involving body, mind and feelings
- Often cannot tell the differences between fantasy and reality.

Cognitive
- Correctly names some colors
- Understands the concept of counting and may know a few numbers
- Try to solve problems from a single point of view
- Begins to have a clearer sense of time.

Language
- Has mastered some basic rules of grammar
- Speaks in sentence of five to six words
- Speaks clearly enough for stranger to understand
- Tells stories.

Movement
- Goes upstairs and downstairs without support
- Kicks ball forward
- Moves forward and backward with agility.

Hand and finger skills
- Copies square shapes
- Uses scissors
- Draws circles, squares and begins to copy some capital letters.

Important milestones by the end of 5 years (60 month)

Social
- Wants to please friends
- More likely to agree to rules
- Likes to sing, dance and act.

Emotional
- Aware of gender
- Able to distinguish fantasy from reality
- Sometimes demanding, sometimes eagerly cooperative.

Cognitive
- Can count 10 or more objects
- Correctly names at least four colors
- Understands better the concept of time
- Knows about things that are used everyday in the home
- Language
- Recalls part of a story
- Uses future tense
- Tells longer stories
- Says name and address.

Movement
- Stands on one foot for 10 seconds or longer
- Swings and climbs
- May be able to skip.

Hand and finger skills
- Copies triangle and other shapes
- Draws person with body
- Dresses and undresses without help
- Uses fork and spoon
- Usually cares for own toilet needs.

APPENDIX VIII

PROBLEMS OF IMMEDIATE NEWBORN

The newborn has serious conditions or problems such as the following:

- Gasping or not breathing
- Breathing with diffculty (less than 30 or more than 60 breaths per minute (bpm), indrawing of the chest or grunting)
- Central cyanosis (blueness)
- Preterm or very low birth weight (less than 32 weeks gestation or less than 1,500 g)
- Lethargy
- Hypothermia (auxillary temperature less than 36.5°C)
- Convulsions.

Immediate Management

1. Suction the mouth and nose to ensure that the airways are clear.
2. Give oxygen at 0.5 L/min by nasal catheter or nasal prong.
3. Transfer baby to the appropriate service for the care of sick newborns.
4. Ensure that the baby is kept warm. Wrap the baby in a soft, dry cloth, cover with a blanket and ensure the head is covered to prevent heat loss.
5. When using oxygen remember only, to use supplement oxygen for diffculty in breathing or cyanosis.
6. If the baby is having severe indrawing of the chest or is gasping for breath or is persistently cyanotic, the increase then concentration of oxygen by nasal catheter, nasal prongs or oxygen hood.

Note: Indiscriminating use of supplemental oxygen for premature infants has been associated with the risk of blindness.

APPENDIX IX

SIGNS AND SYMPTOMS IN ABNORMAL NEWBORN

- Prematurely
- Inactive 'sick looking' infant with decreased feeding
- Central cyanosis
- Respiratory distress
- Tachypnea at rest or during feeding (respiratory rate over 60/m)
- Subcostal and intercostal recessions
- Grunting, apnea and stridor
- Bleeding from any site—cord, mouth, rectum
- Petechiae
- Pallor and mottled skin coloration, dusky green appearance
- Temperature instability—hypothermia and hyperthermia
- Jaundice in the first 24 hours or prolonged more than 2 weeks
- Irritability, twitching and convulsion
- Persistent vomiting—especially bile-stained vomits
- Abdominal distension
- Failure to pass urine in the first 24 hours
- Failure to pass meconium in the first 48 hours
- In all cases, the nurse should notify the pediatrician to review the baby immediately since prompt investigation and special care is required.

APPENDIX X

DEVELOPMENTAL EXAMINATION

Table 1: Developmental examination

Completion of	Motor development		Language		Cognitive		Social psychological	
6 week	Fixes sight on mother's face	Yes No	Normal Crying	Yes No	Sucking Grasping Reflexes	Yes No	Smile	Yes No
3 month	Holding head Raises chin above table	Yes No	Coos and squeals	Yes No	Putting finger in mouth	Yes No	Smiles to mother more	Yes No
6 month	Sitting with or without support	Yes No	Produces vowel sound babbling	Yes No	Forgets rattle if hidden	Yes No	Recognizes the mother	Yes No
15 month	Walks alone	Yes No	Says 'mama' 'Papa' Vocabulary of 3–20 words	Yes No	Hidden objects are traced by child	Yes No	Assists and cooperate in dressing	Yes No
3 year	Runs rides, tricycle, up and down, stairs tip-toe	Yes No	3 words sentences 3 give name and sex	Yes No	Can identify name objects (symbolic play copies	Yes No	Feeds self well Puts on sandals	Yes No
6 year	Hops one foot Throws a ball	Yes No	Can name all colors Value of coin	Yes No	Identifies long- and short- copies	Yes No	Plays co operatively with peers Sex role behavior	Yes No
8–10 year	Can balance on board	Yes No	Can name 10 animals in 1 minute	Yes No	Abstract Reasoning	Yes No	Can use knife Combs hair	Yes No

Index

Page numbers followed by *f* refer to figure and *t* refer to table

A

Abdomen 23, 332
ABGs See Arterial blood gases
ABLS See American burn life support
Accident and casualty department 127
ACE See Angiotensin-converting enzyme
Acid, source of 97
Acid-base
  balance 97, 278
  control of 97
    disorder of 99
  disturbances 281, 282*t*
  imbalance, types of 98
Acquired immunodeficiency syndrome 307, 349
  pathophysiology 349
Acyanotic heart defects 397
ADH See Antidiuretic hormone
ADHD See Attention deficit hyperactivity disorders
Adolescents 163
Adrenaline 69
  infusion 70, 70*t*
Adult respiratory distress syndrome 80
Advanced cardiac life support 45, 143
Advanced critical care nursing 3
Advanced life support 8
Aed child system 43
Aed pads 43
AEG See Atrial electrocardiogram
AIDS See Acquired immunodeficiency syndrome
Air embolism 53, 210, 229*t*
Air embolism
  management of 227, 229*t*
  prevention of 227
Air in heart, entry of 228
Airway 8, 128, 328
  breathing 17, 64
  circulation 17, 64
  mask breathing unit 115
    bag 113*f*
  obstruction
    mild 380
    severe 380
    types of 380
    upper 128
  patency 17, 145
  pressure 132
    continuous positive 135
  ventilation 145
Albuminuria 166
Alcoholics 277
Allergic reaction, acute 13
Allergies 21
Alpha-receptor blockers 124
AMBU See Airway mask breathing unit
American Association on Mental Deficiency 410
American burn life support 128
Amiodarone infusion 71, 71*t*
Analgesia 129, 449
Anaphylactic shock 13
Anastomosing 196
Anger management 418
Angina
  pectoris 25
  types of 26
  unstable 26
  vasospastic 26
Angiotensin-converting enzyme 27
  inhibitors 124
Anions 279*t*
Anorexia nervosa 421
Anticoagulant 202
Antidiuretic hormone 181
Antimicrobial ointments 49
Antistreptolysin O 407
  positive 184
Anuria 166
Anxiety
  disorders 419
  minimizing 273
Aorta, coarctation of 398
Apgar score 343*t*

Arterial blood gas 30, 80, 92, 134
    analysis 15, 80, 97
    values 98t
    values by age 370*t*
Arterial catheters, peripheral 18
Arterial needle, insertion of 206
Arterial pressure monitoring 55, 99*t*
Arteriosclerosis 24
Arteriovenous fistula 196, 204, 205t, 208, 262
    postoperative care of 224
    preoperative care of 224
Arteriovenous graft 196
Artery venous 266
Artifacts 33
Artificial airway 145
Aseptic measures 140
ASO See Antistreptolysin O
Assess baby's color 326
Assisted mandatory ventilation 135
Atherosclerosis 24
Atracurium 70
Atria-atrial rhythm 37
Atrial
    dysrhythmias 38
    electrocardiogram 40
    fibrillation 38
    flutter 38
    pressure, left 152
    pressure, right 54, 58
    septal defect 397, 398, 441
Atrioventricular junction 37
Atropine 70
Attention deficit hyperactivity disorders 417, 418
Automated external defibrillator 43, 41, 382
    operation 41
Autonomic nervous system 124, 269
AVF See Arteriovenous fistula

B

Baby
    condition of 326
    in incubator, care of 358
Bacille calmette-guérin 330
Bacitracin 49
Back 333
    pain 164
Bactrim 171
Bag and mask 345
Bag mask ventilation 112, 113*f*
Basal metabolic rate 393
Basic life support 143
Bathroom
    cleaning 156
    disinfection of 156
BBB See Blood-brain barrier
BCG See Bacille calmette-guérin
Bed wetting 420
Beta blockers 27, 124
Biopsy 85
Birthmarks 334
Bladder
    cauterization of 449
    pain 164
Blocked milk duct 338, 461
Blood 262, 266, 276
    clot 230
    group 240
    leak 233*t*
        management of 231
        minor 232*t*
        severe 210
    matching 240
    pressure 13, 71, 114, 116, 123, 143, 213, 214, 228, 270
        apparatus 249
    samples 128
    test 96
    transfusion 237
        during hemodialysis 238t
    urea nitrogen 127, 284
        elevated 184
        level 61
Blood-brain barrier 437
BLS See Basic life support
BMR See Basal metabolic rate
Body fluid distribution 278
    composition 279
    proportions 278
Body surface area 393
Body weight, fluid percentage of 278*t*
Body's physical barriers 275
BP See Blood pressure
BPH See Benign prostate hyperplasia
Breast 334
    care 337
    hardness of 337
    leaking 461
Breast milk
    composition of 456
    expressed 358
Breastfeeding 304, 329, 335, 460
    during pregnancy 455
    establishing 458
    initiation of 329
    policy 462

process of 458
signs of 458
Breathing 8, 17, 128, 328
absent 44
circuit of ventilators 140
depth of 150
exercise 145
with difficulty 340
Bronchial asthma 368
Bronchiolitis 363
BUN See Blood urea nitrogen
Burn 12, 446, 450
etiology 446
management of 126
percentage of 447
size of 447
wound, assessment of 127, 446
Burning on urination 165

C

CABG See Coronary artery bypass grafting
CAD See Coronary artery disease
Calcium 285, 290
balance, disturbance in 288*t*
channel blockers 124
chloride 70
Cancer in children 426, 429, 430
biopsy 429
chemotherapy 430
diagnostic studies 429
diagnostic tests 431
laboratory studies 431
radiation therapy 429
staging 428
surgery 429
Cancer, management of 429
Capnography 97
Carbon dioxide 80
monitor, end-tidal 153
Cardiac arrhythmias 37
Cardiac massage, external 347
Cardiac monitor 17, 31, 32, 32*f*, 45*t*
basic components of 32
management of 31
operation of 34
Cardiac output 18
Cardiac surgical patient 151
Cardiac system 10, 20
Cardiogenic shock 12
Cardiopulmonary
bypass 153
resuscitation 10, 32, 42, 43, 134, 143
Cardiorespiratory pattern 326
Cardiovascular
assessment 24
disease 124
system 20, 395, 396
Casts application 425
Catheter 52, 53
inserting 48
maintenance 49
site 265
Catheterization of bladder 129
CBC See Complete blood count
CDC See Centers for disease control
Cell division 384
Central console 33
Central nerves system 13, 62, 80, 393, 405, 437
Central venous
catheter 229
line, care of 53
pressure 15, 45, 49, 84, 144, 191
lines 46
monitoring 52
Cerebrospinal fluid 61, 353
Cerebrovascular system 75
CHD See Coronary heart disease
Chemotherapy 272
Chest
drainage 101
system 102
drains, removal of 104
for placement of electrodes 35
tube
connected 103*t*
removing 104
CHF See Congestive heart failure
Child deaths, reduce 307
Child health 308
assessment 310
Child morbidity 306
cause of 307
Child mortality 306, 307
cause of 307
Child with special needs 408
Chloroxylenol solution 157
Chromosomal abnormalities 385
Chromosomes 383
Circulatory status 148
Clotting of bloodlines 210
CML See Chronic myeloid leukemia
Cognitive behavior therapy 418
Colostrum 456
Coma 60
Complete blood count 15, 424, 431, 433, 442
Condenser humidifier of ventilator 140
Conduct disorders 417

Conduction abnormalities 39
Congenital heart disease 395, 396, 441
  common 441
Congenital heart failure
  signs of 400
  symptoms of 400
Congestive heart failure 49, 226, 398, 402
  nursing diagnoses 404
Consciousness 60
  level of 17, 18, 22
Continuous ambulatory peritoneal dialysis 243, 250
COPD See Chronic obstructive pulmonary disease
Cord in hospital, care of 326
Core temperature 17
Coronary
  artery
    bypass grafting 29
    disease 24
  care units 33
  heart disease 25
  syndrome, acute 26, 27
Corrosive burns 126
Cradle cap 335
C-reactive protein 28
Creatine kinase 28
  muscle bone 26
Critical care area 5, 156
  admission criteria in 10
Critical care team 3
Croup 442
CRP See C-reactive protein
Cryptorchidism 185
CSF See Cerebrospinal fluid
Cuff deflation 116
CVS See Cerebrovascular system
Cyanosis 340
Cycling 135
Cystitis 168, 176
Cystoscopy 167
Cytomegalovirus 322

D

Daily fluid intake 280*t*
Daily living, activities of 31, 150
Decubitus 26
Deep vein thrombosis 81, 104, 150
Defiant disorders 417
Defibrillation 41
Dehydration 12, 282, 284, 285
Delivery, time of 455
Denver developmental screening test 410
Deoxyribonucleic acid 383
Destructive behaviors disorders 417
  diagnosis 418
  risk factors 418
Dettol 157
Diabetes
  hypertension in 123
  mellitus 105
    chronic complications of 122
Diabetic
  emergencies, managing 118
  foot 125
  ketoacidosis 119
  nephropathy 122
  neuropathy 124
  retinopathy 122
Dialysate bag exchange 254
Dialysis 191, 195, 204*f*
Diaphoresis 270
Diazepam 354
Diet
  approaches 450
  modification 387
Dietary habits 22
Dietitian 4
Discharge, advice on 266
Disease control, centers for 350
Disease prevention 308
Disinfection, chemical 236, 236*t*
Disorders in children, behavioral 416
Dispose of dead 276
DM See Diabetes mellitus
DNA See Deoxyribonucleic acid
Dobutamine infusion 74, 74*t*
Dopamine infusion 72, 72*t*
Drainage tubes 148
Dressing 129, 148
  at exit site 265
  changing 130
  material 49
  of incision site 265
Drug 341
  administration of 8
  avoidance of 388
  choice 15
  for resuscitation of newborn 453*t*
  infusion guidelines 70
  infusion, preparation of 69
  ingestion 11
  overdose 11
  therapy 27
  tray 69
Dysrhythmias 37
Dysuria 165

E

Eczema 335
Electrical hazards 34
Electrodes 34
Electrolyte
  balances, disturbances 281
  imbalance 127, 285
  sources of 279
Electronic calibration 226
ELISA See Enzyme-linked immunosorbent assay
Emergency care 15, 63
Emergency drugs 347, 453
Emergency medical
  service 7
  technician 7
Emphysema 85
End-expiratory pressure 132
  positive 135, 141
Endocrine 11
Endotracheal
  intubation 109, 346
  suctioning 110*t*, 115*t*, 117
  tube 109, 112*f*, 133, 145, 157
    management 116
    suctioning 114
Endourology 167
Enuresis 165
Environmental manipulation 389
Enzyme-linked immunosorbent assay 349
Epididymal pain 164
Erythrocyte sedimentation rate 29, 407, 436
Esophageal atresia 379
ESR See Erythrocyte sedimentation rate
Extracellular fluid 97, 278
Extrication casualties 8
Extubation, complications 117
Eye
  care of 328
  response 63

F

Face 331
Femoral vein catheter 215
Fever 277
First aid 126
Fistula 214, 241*t*
  care 240
Fluid 127
  and electrolyte
    balance 149, 290, 291, 294
    imbalance 294
  balance 146
    management of 191
  disturbance in 281
  imbalance 281, 282, 284, 285
  increasing 293
  replacement 16
  sources of 279
  volume
    deficit 281
    deficit, signs of 281
    excess 281
    excess, signs of 281
Flush solution 53
Foot care, rules of 125
Forearm 196
Fracture 423
  assessment of 424
  immobilization 425
  reduction, types of 424
FVC See Femoral vein catheter

G

Gambro machine 233
Gastrointestinal
  bleeding 16
  disorders 11
  status 153
  symptoms 164, 166
Gauze dressing pads 245
Gene 383
  single 386
  transfer 388
Genetic 383
  abnormalities 385
  behavioral 384
  counseling 389
  disease 385, 387
  influence
    in child health 383
    on development 385
  interaction of 384
Genitourinary 377
Genitourinary disorders 161
Gestational age 303, 323, 324, 356
Glomerular filtration rate 191, 403
Gloves, discard 223
Glutaraldehyde 140
Glyceryl trinitrate infusion 75, 75t
Gonorrhea 320
Graduated elastic compression stockings 105
Gross structure 161

H

Hand 332
  and finger skills 466-468
  exercise 224
HBSAG-positive mother 349
Head 331
Health
  care, trends in 408
  education 304
  promotion 308
Hearing 463
Heart 332
  block 39
  rate 116
Heat disinfection 236, 236*t*
Hematological investigation 154
Hematological status 153
Hematuria 166, 177
Hemodialysis 202, 227, 228*t*, 230, 231, 234, 234*t*
  hazards 230
  machine 203, 204, 205*t*, 208, 217, 219*t*
    maintenance of 235
  patient 197, 213
  shunt graft 240, 241*t*
  using anticoagulant 203*t*
Hemodynamic
  instability 11
  monitoring 17, 54
Hemofiltration 267
Hemoglobin 353, 442
Hemolytic disease 373
  of newborn 375
Hemorrhage 12
Hemothorax 107
Heparin 203
  free dialysis 203, 204*t*
  pump 203
  regime 267
Hepatitis B 349
Hernia, diaphragmatic 378
Herpesvirus type 11 323
Hips 332
HIV See Human immunodeficiency virus
Hodgkin's disease 435
Hospital
  admission to 126
  care, trends in 308
  cleaning 156
Human
  biological waste 156
  chorionic gonadotropin, administration of 186
  immunodeficiency virus 307, 349
Hyaline membrane disease 316
Hydrocephaly 321
Hyperbilirubinemia 318, 319
Hypertonic dehydration 283
Hypocalcemia 290
Hypoglycemia 118
  in newborn 351
  prevention of 119
Hypokalemia 289
Hypospadias 187
Hypotension, management of 227, 228*t*
Hypotonic dehydration 283
Hypovolemic shock 12

I

IABP See Intra-aortic balloon pump
IDDM See Insulin-dependent-diabetes mellitus
Ill patient 6
  critically 6
Immobilization 9
Immune
  response 276
  system 275
Immunization, expanded program on 330
Implantable cardioverter 44
  defibrillators 39
Implanted defibrillators 44
Impulse formation, disturbance in 37
Infants 163
  choking in 380
  preoperative care of 390
Infection 14, 176*t*
  control
    procedure 155
    provision of 305
  prevent 129
Inflammation 276
Infusion fluid 128
Injury
  defense against 275
  depth of 447
Inspiratory-expiratory ratio 132
Insulin-dependent-diabetes mellitus 120
Intelligence quotient 409
Intensive care unit 3, 49, 104, 154-156
Intensivists 4
International pneumatic compression 105
Intestinal obstruction 443
Intra-aortic balloon pump 152
Intra-arterial monitoring 57
Intracellular fluid 278
Intracranial pressure 437
Intramuscular 394
Intraosseous 394
Intrarenal 190

Intravenous
drip 127
fluid, administration of 9
pole 245
pyelogram 179
therapy 229
Intubation technique 113
Invasive cardiac test 23
Invasive techniques 17
IQ See Intelligence quotient
Ischemic heart disease 25, 105
Isoimmune hemolytic disease of neonate 319
Isoprenaline infusion 78, 78*t*
Isotonic dehydration 283

J

Jaundice 334
early 354
in newborn 354, 355
treatment 355
prolonged 354
Jugular vein
catheter 213, 215, 223
internal 46, 47
Junctional rhythms 37
JVC See Jugular vein catheter

K

Kernicterus, signs of 319
Kidney 189, 262
function 162
increase in 150
structure of 161

L

Labor room 305
Lactate dehydrogenase 28
Lactic acidosis 121
Laryngoscope blade 111*f*
Laryngotracheobronchitis, acute 361
Leg pain 164
Leukemia 432
Lifestyle considerations 40
Lignocaine 70
Live birth 303
Living with pacemaker 39
Local adaptation syndrome 269
Loop of Henle 161
Low birth weight 303, 356
Lower blood pressure in diabetes 124
Low-molecular-weight heparin 105
Lumen, avoid 254
spraying 257
Lungs 332
Lymphoblastic leukemia, acute 433
Lymphocyte leukemia, acute 433
Lymphomas 435
etiology 436
nursing diagnoses 438
pathophysiology 436

M

Maternal death 303
Mechanical ventilation, types of 134
Meconium 326
aspiration syndrome 317
etiology 317
Medical and nursing management 81, 106, 107, 189, 316, 317
Medical antishock trousers 16
Medical management 15, 82, 169, 171, 177, 179, 193
Medication history 21
Medications, administration of 215
Medullary loop 33, 161
Mental retardation 409
etiology 409
pathophysiology 410
Mental status 214
Metabolic acidosis 282
Metabolic alkalosis 282
Metabolism, increase in 150
Midazolam 70
Midclavicular line 45
Millennium development goal 307
Monocytes 276
Monogenic disorders 386
Moro reflex 315
Morphine 70
Motor response 63
Multifactorial disorders 386
Myeloid leukemia
acute 433
chronic 434
Myelomeningocele 379
Myocardial infarction 12, 13, 29, 105
acute 25, 27

N

Nail 23
Nalbuphine 70

Nasal
cannula 87, 88t
culture 97
Nasogastric 443
tube 134
Neck vein assessment 23
Needle biopsy of kidney 167
Neomycin 49
Neonatal
care unit, admission to 305
critical care 303
resuscitation 340
unit 303
drugs 304
equipment 304
Neonate
critical care for 301
high-risk 316
in warmer 358*f*
reflexes in 315
Neoplasms, malignant 428*t*
Neosporin 49
Nephrotic syndrome 172, 180
Neurogenic shock 13
Neurological disorders 10
Neurological status 148, 152
Neutrophils 276
Newborn
by pediatrician 331
conditions 340
convulsion in 352
infant from HIV, care of 349
problems of immediate 469
signs in abnormal 470
symptoms in abnormal 470
NIDDM See Non-insulin-dependent-diabetes mellitus
Nipples, flat 460
Nocturia 165
Nocturnal angina 26
Non-insulin-dependent-diabetes mellitus 120
Non-invasive techniques 17
Non-ketotic hyperosmolar hyperglycemic coma 121
Non-steroidal anti-inflammatory drugs 13
Noradrenaline infusion 76, 76t
NSAIDs See Non-steroidal anti-inflammatory drugs
Nurse
assisting 222, 244, 258, 259
critical care 3
registered 3
in-charge of intensive care unit 138
responsibility 53
role of 113
specialist's 308
Nursing
actions 216, 238
activity 239*t*
alert 233
care 93, 99, 103, 117
for clients 103*t*
for patient 45, 50*t*
of newborn 325
diagnoses 29, 130, 145, 169, 171, 179-181, 184, 186, 187, 189, 194, 272, 298
evaluation 300
implementation 299
planning 299
history 20, 93
implications 59
intervention 30, 58, 130, 141, 145, 169, 171, 177, 179, 180, 193, 194
management 18, 27, 60, 64, 65*t*, 83, 130, 136*t*, 169, 171, 173, 174, 176, 177, 179, 193
of stress 271
precaution 67, 67*t*
process 290
responsibilities 104, 108
Nutrition, maintain 149
Nutritional support 130, 139

O

Obsessive compulsive disorders 419
Obstetric death, indirect 303
Obstructive pulmonary disease, chronic 90
Occupational therapist 4
Octreotide infusion 77, 77*t*
Oliguria 165
Operation theater 55, 156
Organism causing cystitis, common 168, 176
Orogastric catheter procedure 345
Oropharyngeal airway 111*f*
Orthopedics disorders See Fractures
Oscilloscope 32
Osmosis 195
Oxygen 80
administration 85
in children 87
concentration, inspired 87*t*
fraction of inspired 87, 132
indications for administering 87
mask 87, 90
saturation 97
tent or canopy 88
therapy 87, 89*t*, 93*t*, 145

Oxygenation, improving 16
Oxyhood 87

P

Pacemaker 44
therapy 39
Pain 296
acute 295, 296*t*
assessment of 297
chronic 295, 296*t*
components of 295
in glans penis 164
management of 295, 299
referred 296
relieving 146
signs of acute 297*t*
types of 295
Pancuronium 70
Parasympathetic dominance 270
Parental education 418
Patent ductus arteriosus 397, 398, 441
Pediatric
burns patients 450
emergencies 441
nurse practitioner 308
ventilator 132*f*
Penile shaft pain 164
Pericardial tamponade 13
Peristalsis 275
increase in 151
Peritoneal dialysis 243, 245, 246*t*
machine 245, 257, 259
preparation of 243
Phenobarbitone 354
Phenylketonuria 321, 410
Phenytoin 354
Physical therapist 4
Physically challenged children 422
Plasma 261
exchange 262
separator 260
Plasmapheresis 260
Plaster of Paris 425*t*
Pleural aspiration 85
Pleural effusion 84
Pleurisy 84
Pneumococcal pneumonia 367
Pneumococci 365
Pneumonia 307, 365
Pneumothorax 105, 106
simple 105
types of 105
Poison, kinds of 444
Poisoning 444
signs of 444
symptoms of 444
Polymyxin 49
Polyuria 165
Postanesthesia care unit 143
admission to 143
Postanesthetic assessment t 144
Postdialysis assessment 214*t*
Postmaturity 324
etiology 324
problems 324
Postnatal diagnosis 387
Postnatal ward 306
Poststreptococcal glomerulonephritis, acute 173, 183
Potassium 79, 285, 289
balance, disturbances in 287*t*
levels, reduce 191
rich foods 286
Power failure during hemodialysis 230
Predialysis assessment 198*t*
Prehospital care 7, 8
protocols 8
treatment of 8
Prehospital transport 9
Premature
atrial complex 38
ventricular complex 38
Prenatal diagnosis 387
Preoperative nursing management 187, 390
Preoxygenation 112
Preparing for birth 325
Prerenal 190
Preschoolers 163
Pressure
inhalation, negative 138
support ventilation 135, 139
triggered 138
ventilation
negative 134
positive 134
Prinzmetal's angina 26
Prophylactic treatment 104
Prostate hyperplasia, benign 179
Proteinuria 166
Prothrombin time 28, 153
Psychogenic pain 296
Psychological
comfort 146
manifestation 270
Psychosocial
care 434
implications 163
Pulmonary artery 54, 56
catheter 56

occlusion pressure 56
pressure monitoring 55
values 57
wedge pressure 54
Pulmonary capillary wedge pressure 18, 56
Pulmonary damage 129
Pulmonary edema 184
Pulmonary embolism 13, 81
Pulmonary function
parameters 100*t*
test 100
Pulmonary system 10
Pulmonic stenosis 398
Pulse 44, 228
Pyelonephritis 170, 178
acute 171
chronic 171, 179

R

RBC See Red blood cell
Recovery room 145
discharge from 147
Red blood cells 166, 183, 373, 383, 436
Refrigerating breast milk 337
Renal calculus 161, 188
Renal endoscope 167
Renal failure 190
acute 190
chronic 192
Renal function test 166
Renal pain 164
Renal status 153
Renal system 162
Respiration status 152
Respiratory
acidosis 282
alkalosis 282
assessment 361*t*
distress syndrome, acute 80, 110
pattern 17
rate 132
status 148
syncytial virus 361
system 80, 93, 359
therapist 4
Resuscitation 341
care after 454
Rheumatic fever 405
etiology 405
pathophysiology 406
Rheumatoid arthritis 56
Rubella 322

S

Saline infusion 120
Saturation venous oxygen 56
School-age children 163
Scrotal pain 164
Scrotal swellings 379
Sensitivity 97
Sepsis 317
etiology 317
medical management 318
nursing management 318
Septic shock 14
Septran 171
Sex determination 187
Sexually transmitted disease 320
Shock 44
classification of 12
delivery 43
distributive 13
management of 1, 12
obstructive 13
stages of 14
Short-acting nitrates 27
Sinoatrial node 37
Sinus
arrhythmias 38
bradycardia 38
rhythm 37, 38
tachycardia 38
Skeletal system 332
Skin 23
care of 328
irritation 34
Sniffing position 112, 112*f*
Social behavior 418
Social worker 4
Sodium 285, 286
balance, disturbances in 286*t*
bicarbonate 70
low 227
sulfate 191
Sore nipples 338, 460
Special care baby unit 303, 330, 335
Speech 463
Spina bifida 379
Spinal cord injury 13
Spine 333
protection of 8
Spontaneous pneumothorax 106
Spots 334
Sputum culture 96
Stable angina, chronic 26, 27
Staphylococcal pneumonia 367

Staphylococci 365
Staphylococcus aureus 264
Stillbirth 303
Streptococcal pneumonia 367
Streptococci 365
Stress 268
  concept of 268
  incontinence 165
  manifestation of 269
Subclavian vein 47
  catheter 213, 215, 223
Sucking reflex 315
Swan-Ganz catheter 18
Sweat production 270
Synchronized intermittent mandatory ventilation 134, 135, 139
Syphilis 320
Syringe 203

T

Tactile stimulation 345
TB See Tuberculosis
Temperature monitoring 17
Temporary access 217
  to hemodialysis machine 216*t*
Temporary cardiac pacemaker support 40*t*
Tenckhoff catheter 263, 264
Tension pneumothorax 13, 105
Teratogenic disorders 386
Testicle, undescended 185
Tetanus, prevent 129
Therapeutic modalities 387
Thiazides 124
Three-chamber water seal system 102
Throat culture 97
Thromboembolism prophylaxis 104
Thrombolytic
  agents 51
  therapy 83
Thromboplastin time 153
Thrombus formation 83
Tidal volume 132
Tissue, damaged 276
TNM See Tumor node metastasis
Tonic neck 315
TORCH syndrome 322
Total parenteral nutrition 47, 266
Toxic substances, removal of 388
Toxoplasmosis 322
Tracheoesophageal atresia 379
Tracheostomy 108, 108*f*, 109*t*
  indication for 108
Transdermal medication patches 44
Transient tachypnea of newborn 316
  etiology 316
Transmembrane pressure 209, 211, 222, 227
Traumatic pneumothorax 105
Trunk incurvature 315
Tuberculosis 84
Tumor
  benign 428*t*
  node metastasis 428
Two-chamber water seal system 101

U

Ultrafiltration 195, 209
Ultrasonography 85
Unconscious patient 60
Unconsciousness 1, 60, 61
  causes of 60
Unfractionated heparin 105
UNICEF See United Nations International Children's Emergency Fund
United Nations International Children's Emergency Fund 307
Uremia 192
Ureter 189
Urethral
  brush biopsy 167
  meatus pain 164
  pain 164
Urethritis 170, 178
Urinalysis 166
Urinary
  acidity 166
  analgesics 179
  dysfunction 166
  frequency 165
  incontinence 165
  output 16, 18
  tract infection 168, 168*t*, 176
Urine 326
  clarity 166
  color 166
  odor 166
  retention 166
  values in children 163, 163*t*
Urodynamic measurements 167
Urofix 261
Urological disorders 176

V

Vagina 277
Vanillylmandelic acid 431

Vein open 29
Venous
  hemofiltration with hemodialysis 266
  line 201
  oxygen saturation monitoring, mixed 18
Ventilation
  adequate 145
  continuous mandatory 134, 135
  control 135
  intermittent mandatory 135
  mechanical 132, 133, 141
  modes of 135, 135*t*
  technique of artificial 345
Ventilator 138, 139
  alarms 137*t*
  asepsis of 140
  classification of 134
Ventilatory support 133
Ventricle physiology, single 152
Ventricles-ventricular rhythms 37
Ventricular dysrhythmias 38
Ventricular fibrillation 38
Ventricular septal defect 397, 398
Ventricular systole 38
Ventricular tachycardia 37, 38
Ventriculoatrial 40
Verbal response 63
Viral pneumonia 367
Viscera, eviscerated of 9
Vision 463, 464
Vital capacity pack, forced 260
Vital signs 22, 154, 198, 214
VMA See Vanillylmandelic acid
  Voiding, changes in 165

W

Waste
  categorization of 155
  chemical 155
  collection of 156
  disposal
    of collected 156
    policy 155
WBCs See White blood cells
WBCs in urine 168
Weaning 137
  from mechanical ventilator 137
  indications for 138
White blood cells 275, 436
  in urine 177
Wilms' tumor 174
Wound care 129

X

Xiphoid 264